A Clinician's Guide to Integrative Pediatrics

A Clinician's Guide to Integrative Pediatrics

Editor: Magan Gilbert

AMERICAN
MEDICAL PUBLISHERS
www.americanmedicalpublishers.com

AMERICAN
MEDICAL PUBLISHERS
www.americanmedicalpublishers.com

Cataloging-in-Publication Data

A clinician's guide to integrative pediatrics / edited by Magan Gilbert.
p. cm.
Includes bibliographical references and index.
ISBN 978-1-63927-845-9
1. Children--Diseases--Alternative treatment. 2. Integrative medicine. 3. Infants.
4. Children--Diseases. I. Gilbert, Magan.
RJ53.A48 C55 2023
618.92--dc23

American Medical Publishers,
41 Flatbush Avenue,
1st Floor, New York,
NY 11217, USA

ISBN 978-1-63927-845-9 (Hardback)

Contents

Preface

This book has been an outcome of determined endeavour from a group of educationists in the field. The primary objective was to involve a broad spectrum of professionals from diverse cultural background involved in the field for developing new researches. The book not only targets students but also scholars pursuing higher research for further enhancement of the theoretical and practical applications of the subject.

Pediatrics refers to the field of medicine concerned with the medical care of infants, children and adolescents. Integrative pediatric medicine is a branch of medicine that combines traditional medicine with complementary therapies supported by scientific research, primarily aimed at children and young adults. One of the most prominent clinical uses of integrative medicine in pediatrics includes the use of mind-body medicine treatments, such as biofeedback, guided imagery and hypnosis, for the management of pain. Another potential use for mind-body treatments is the reduction of toxic stress and its effects on children's health. The other areas include integrative approaches towards chronic illnesses, like bowel disease, cancer, arthritis, asthma and other conditions where conventional therapies are required but leave treatment gaps. These gaps can be filled with evidence-based integrative therapies that target lifestyle factors like sleep patterns, social support, dietary habits and physical activity levels that are frequently disregarded in the patients. This book includes some of the vital pieces of work being conducted across the world, on various topics related to integrative pediatrics. Its aim is to present researches that have transformed this discipline and aided its advancement. This book is appropriate for students seeking detailed information in this area as well as for experts.

It was an honour to edit such a profound book and also a challenging task to compile and examine all the relevant data for accuracy and originality. I wish to acknowledge the efforts of the contributors for submitting such brilliant and diverse chapters in the field and for endlessly working for the completion of the book. Last, but not the least; I thank my family for being a constant source of support in all my research endeavours.

Editor

1

Complementary Medicine: Risks to Infants and Children

Terry Polevoy

33-285 Sandowne Dr., Waterloo, ON N2K 2C1, Canada; drpolevoy@yahoo.com

Abstract: Complementary Alternative Medicine (CAM) that targets infants and children can place them at grave risk. Our plan is to review some of the major cases of CAM used by parents, and by unlicensed and even licensed health professionals. Complications from CAM are rarely the focus of regulatory bodies, or even the courts. Even regulated health professionals, who have profited by misrepresenting science-based evidence for treatment or prevention of disease, have been rarely sanctioned by their respective Boards or Colleges. This must change. In addition, there is a dire need for regulators, including the governments, who allow quack products and devices to be marketed in their respective countries, to prosecute them. Existing regulations must be coupled with more effective enforcement. Some of these cases have had a direct connection to me personally, while others are examples of just plain dangerous quackery.

Keywords: complementary alternative medicine; quackery; infants; children; regulation; anti-vaccine; autism; cancer; chiropractic; naturopathy; homeopathy; health fraud

---

1. Why Does Complementary Alternative Medicine (CAM) Seem to Thrive and Why Is It Almost Always Ignored by Regulators and the Government?

Misinformation about CAM for infants and children is just far too easy to find. Just search on Amazon for "pediatrics alternative medicine" and you can find hundreds of books that ignore science-based methods. The Internet is full of so-called "experts", including celebrities, hucksters, politicians who are in the pockets of the nutraceutical manufacturers, and yes, even licensed health professionals.

We will review some extreme CAM cases that have resulted in fatalities. This will include some deranged parental belief systems, which directly resulted in their child's death, with or without direct intervention by health professionals. Other cases directly involved licensed medical practitioners, who ignored everything they learned in medical school and residency training to flog their treatments, or lack of treatments (i.e., immunizations) on vulnerable families.

Some of the topics we will review include the CAM anti-vaccine movement, the quack treatment of children with cancer, cerebral palsy, and other chronic conditions. Extreme nutritional advice by parents has also killed children.

Here in Canada, where I trained in pediatrics, we have had our share of headline cases over the years. Some have left a deep impact on me personally, while others have stayed in the headlines for years. Others have been too often just forgotten. By writing this article, I hope that we will all be reminded of the risks when CAM endangers our children.

One of the major dangers to child health has been the regulators themselves. Medical, chiropractic, and naturopathic Boards and Colleges around the world have been lax in overseeing their members. Doctors of Medicine (MDs) have maintained their licenses, despite their opposition to immunizations. Some have promised parents that they can treat children with profound conditions, like mental retardation, cerebral palsy, and cancer. Even after numerous complaints, many practitioners have survived unscathed.

CAM professionals may or may not actually believe what they do. Some are just snake-oil salespeople, while others are gurus who spend their lives mesmerizing their flock of true believers.

2. Chiropractic Pediatrics

Chiropractors who treat infants, children, and even pregnant mothers have formed professional associations like the International Chiropractic Pediatrics Association (ICPA). In my opinion, they exist to sustain the unbelievable charade that infants and children should go to a chiropractor from birth [1]. This group claims to be experts. But, in fact all they do is to promote parental fear that their babies have been "damaged" when they go through the birth canal. They make bogus claims that this will result in serious health problems later on in life [2]. Marketing organizations are widespread, selling full-scripts, supportive flyers, magazines, web sites, and videos that target the vulnerable minds of parents [3].

A simple search of pediatric chiropractic web sites reveals most of their false claims. The trouble is that chiropractic regulatory bodies refuse to take any firm action against their members who violate their Standards or Policies. In 2013, a group of four chiropractic authors from Canada published a review of Vaccinations and Chiropractic [4].

In Ontario, the College of Chiropractors of Ontario (CCO) has a history of sitting on complaints for years, and then when complaints are appealed to our *Health Professions Appeal and Review Board (HPARB)*, and are sent back to the CCO, it again takes years for the CCO to respond.

One of the most egregious examples of the CCO's lack of firm action goes way back to the 1990s, when many of their members were known for anti-vaccine activities. It took years for them to pass any meaningful policies or standards to control it.

A prime example that I personally witnessed in 1997 here in Waterloo, Ontario, Canada, involved Jeffrey Winchester, DC. He placed himself in front of the *Bluevale Collegiate Institute*, our local high school, and told the students that they really did not have to get the meningitis vaccine. Two teenage girls had just died, but it did not stop his bizarre protest. I have many examples in my collection of anti-vaccine chiropractors here in Ontario, but very few of them were adjudicated.

Chiropractic promotions at health fairs, malls, and in the media, are sometimes more like a "Three Ring Circus". Over the years, I have attended a number of large and small presentations where chiropractors set up shop and try to sell various programs. Some of them targeted families with young children. One of the funniest was Dr. Roger Turner, a DC from Barrie, Ontario. He and his young son, who was not a chiropractor, claimed to be able to move the skull bones to improve kids with autistic spectrum disorder (ASD). I even volunteered to have my skull manipulated at a quack-filled alternative health convention in Toronto.

In May 2018, Sharon Kirkey, a reporter for Canada's National Post newspaper, authored one of the best articles on pediatric chiropractors [5]. It was met with applause from the usual science-based groups and authorities [6].

There is absolutely no debate that those who adhere to their title of "pediatric chiropractor" really love their stuff. In September 2018, one group organized the *Chiropractic Pediatric & Family Conference* in Newark, NJ, USA [7]. The usual anti-vax brigade will be there along with the usual sales people selling all sorts of goodies to help chiropractors build their practices. Among the speakers are Canadian and American chiropractors, along with a long history of anti-medical opinions. They have even invited Larry Palevsky, an anti-vaccine MD from NYC to round out the conference.

In Summary, the basic spin of pediatric chiropractors has never been confirmed in any major study. But, the case against them has not seemed to stop their marketing in any way. As more chiropractors graduate each year, they are having difficulty finding practice opportunities that would help them pay back their tuition. That is my belief! That is why there are so many of them who have swallowed the sales pitch of organizations who skillfully sell them expensive programs.

3. Dangers of Licensed and Unlicensed Quacks

There are thousands of unlicensed individuals who prey on children and their families around the world. In developing countries, they are called shamans, or "medicine men" or "medicine women". I will not be discussing this. But, I will attempt to identify an area of grave concern, especially when it comes to children in Canada.

Children are victimized because either their parents allow them to be treated by these quacks, instead of real medical professionals, or their health providers, who are licensed as regulated health professionals, treat them without regard for science-based medicine.

I will choose from a few of these tragic cases here in Canada, where even though we have "socialized medicine", the practice of quackery sadly exists. Little has changed over the last few decades. It is particularly troublesome here in Ontario, because we have authorized the regulation of naturopathy, homeopathy, and traditional Chinese medicine. Socialized medicine was supposed to provide oversight of these CAM professions, but we have found little has changed. Claims made by these "professionals" have little basis in science, and some are downright dangerous. Fortunately for us, very few of their flock try to recruit infants and children . . . yet!

CAM Tragedies

Ravi Devgan: Nearly two decades ago, I was contacted by a reporter in Ontario who had identified a poor Mexican Mennonite family who had twins that had major neurologic and mental health issues. They reached out to a physician, Ravi Devgan, who claimed to be able to cure them. Using dangerous injections of sheep fetuses, he defrauded them for over $30,000 [8].

Devgan was sentenced to jail. But, even after his first conviction and the loss of his license, he continued to rip people off from his house in Toronto. He died in prison after his last conviction.

Tyrell Duec: In the spring of 1999, a 13-year-old Saskatchewan boy, Tyrell Dueck garnered headlines around the world because his bone cancer treatment was stopped by his parents. They were convinced by a local chiropractor, lawyer, who was a fundamentalist Christian, and politician that the best treatment was to pray and take him to a quack clinic in Tijuana for treatment. He died of his cancer in July 1999 after the courts said that the parents could basically do what they wanted. His death raised many issues, ethically, morally, and in the courts; it was the death of Tyrell Dueck that sent me on my journey of "quackbusting" [9–11].

Makayla Sault: An 11-year-old girl from the Credit First Nation Reserve in Caldonia, Ontario, became the victim of Brian Clement. He is a notorious Florida-based quack, who runs the *Hippocrates Health Institute*, a facility in West Palm Beach, Florida. The case pitted the McMaster University Pediatric Oncology Department, social service agencies, and the First Nation's chief against each other. The courts finally gave the go-ahead to stop chemotherapy for her leukemia, which had a good chance of putting her into remission.

The case involved more than one Aboriginal girl suffering from treatable leukemia. The State of Florida had originally charged Clement with practicing medicine without a license. The case was quietly dropped in March 2015. One of the puzzling things about Clement is the question of his supplying illegal supplements, which were shipped to the Reserve and other health food stores in Ontario. This was reported to Health Canada, but little seemed to be accomplished. Furthermore, the Aboriginal band sponsored several appearances of Clement to recruit more patients and flog his quackery. Clement continues to flog nonsense treatments and prey on vulnerable people. We can assume that there are many more cases like Makayla in his files [12–18].

Ezekiel Stephan: This case has been in the headlines for six years. It began when a 19-month-old toddler from Alberta died of meningitis. Years ago, thousands of infants and toddlers died of meningitis in North America every year. What makes the 2012 death of Ezekiel especially unusual was the legal case against his parents. His father, David Stephan, and mother, Collet, were charged and convicted in an Alberta Court for failing to provide the necessaries of life in 2016. After years of legal battles and appeals, the case finally reached Canada's Supreme Court in May 2018, where the case was overturned on a technicality. David and Collet have to be retried all over again back in Alberta.

There have been scores of incisive articles, extensive television coverage, and ethical and legal opinions from around the world. The case took years to finally be prosecuted, and the actual trial lasted for weeks. Public opinion, which was largely against the couple from the start, seemed to be opposed due to David Stephan's blogs, television appearances, and especially his own Facebook pages which were basically his way of casting the blame on others. He has never, to this day, told the public that he or his wife had any role in Ezekiel's horrible death.

The most interesting part of the case was David Stephan's direct links to *Truehope Nutritional Support*, a company started by his father Anthony Stephan. It markets natural health products and has withstood Health Canada's challenges for years. David works for the company directly. The company's early days was the focus of our book, *Pig Pills, Inc. The Anatomy of an Academic and Alternative Health Fraud* [19]. The book was co-authored with Marvin Ross and Ron Reinhold.

Truehope's original product, *EmpowerPlus*, made major claims for treating severe mental illness. They marketed it from Alberta, but it has always been made by several companies in the U.S. The reason I mention this company is because the Stephans used them to treat their own children, particularly Ezekiel.

The foundation for the charges and the conviction were because the parents failed to provide the necessaries of life. During the trial, it was revealed that Ezekiel had never been to a medical doctor. He was delivered at home in rural Alberta by a nurse. Ezekiel, like his other siblings, had never received any immunizations.

When Ezekiel became ill with a respiratory condition on 27 February 2012, his health went downhill steadily. Even after he was visited by his grandfather, Anthony Stephan, there was no improvement. He became so "stiff" that he was unable to get into his car seat. He was finally rushed to the *Calgary Children's Hospital* in a coma and was declared "brain dead" on 12 March 2012. The post-mortem showed bacterial meningitis and an empyema (pus in the lung).

Why did the parents fail to recognize how sick he was? Were they entirely to blame? They clearly ignored warning signs that any parent should have recognized. Why did Collet take him to see a naturopath in Lethbridge, but never brought him into the office? It seemed that she just asked the naturopath's front office for *BLAST*, an natural health product containing echinacea.

Of course, his meningitis could have easily been prevented and his life could have been saved if they were caring parents. Instead, they were basically anti-vaccine, anti-medical zealots who instead treated him with olive leaf extract, garlic, onions, pepper, ginger root, and horseradish.

The Crown's evidence was overwhelming, and throughout the trial, David would rant and rave of how bad the Government's case was. It was a giant conspiracy! Evidence was tampered with or withheld! The pathologist was wrong! There was a massive cover-up!

After their conviction by a jury in April 2016, they appealed. The appeal was finally heard in November 2017. David Stephan continued to attack the original conviction with insane rants against the prosecution's case and the jury's decision. He concocted a conspiracy theory about withheld evidence, that Ezekiel did not actually have meningitis or an empyema, and that the ambulance drivers and the staff of the Children's Hospital caused Ezekiel's death because they didn't have the right sized tube when they attempted to intubate him during transport to Calgary.

In May 2018, the case was thrown out by the Supreme Court of Canada in Ottawa. The court ordered a new trial on the original charges. If the Stephans were again convicted, they might actually face more severe consequences.

4. Lessons Learned?

What can we learn from the dangers of CAM and the risks to our children?

- CAM practitioners are sometimes just basically crooks and frauds who have no morals.

- Regulated health professionals who are trained to believe that they have the answers, when they demonstrate no evidence that their treatments works.
- Parents who ignore basic public health measures.

References

1. International Chiropractic Pediatrics Association, a Nonprofit Corporation. Available online: https://icpa4kids.com (accessed on 11 June 2018).
2. The Annals of Quackademic Medicine: Testing Chiropractic in Pregnancy. Available online: https://respectfulinsolence.com/2010/04/09/the-annals-of-quackademic-medicine-testi/ (accessed on 11 June 2018).
3. The Pediatric Section of Chiro.org. Available online: http://www.chiro.org/pediatrics/ (accessed on 11 June 2018).
4. On Vaccination & Chiropractic: When Ideology, History, Perception, Politics and Jurisprudence Collide. Available online: https://www.ncbi.nlm.nih.gov/pmc/articles/PMC3743646/ (accessed on 11 June 2018).
5. Pediatricians Alarmed by Chiropractic Treatments for Babies that 'Border on the Fraudulent'. Available online: http://nationalpost.com/health/pediatricians-alarmed-by-chiropractic-treatments-for-babies-that-border-on-the-fraudulent (accessed on 11 June 2018).
6. ScienceBasedMedicine.org's Response to Sharon Kirkey's Article in National Post, 8 May 2018. Available online: https://sciencebasedmedicine.org/a-canadian-journalist-calls-out-pediatric-chiropractic-and-a-chiropractor-responds/ (accessed on 11 June 2018).
7. Chiropractic Pediatric & Family Conference. Available online: https://www.chiropediatrics.net/live-event-sales-page18924015 (accessed on 11 June 2018).
8. Ravi Devgan, MD Jailed for Defrauding Farmer of $30,000. Available online: https://www.thestar.com/news/gta/2008/02/16/exmd_gets_5_years_for_drug_scam.html (accessed on 11 June 2018).
9. Cancer Patients Go Where Hope Carries Price Tag. Available online: http://www.quackerywatch.com/Cancer/Dueck/gm990325dueck-mexico.html (accessed on 11 June 2018).
10. Arthur, Shafer. Who Decides for the Child? Available online: http://umanitoba.ca/philosophy/ethics/media/Who_decides_for_the_child.pdf (accessed on 11 June 2018).
11. Griffiths, O. *Power & The Glory*. Available online: https://www.amazon.ca/Power-Glory-Griffiths/dp/0968557600 (accessed on 11 June 2018).
12. Walker, C. Makayla Sault, the Girl Who Refused Chemotherapy for Leukemia Dies. *CBC News*, 20 January 2015. Available online: http://www.cbc.ca/news/indigenous/makayla-sault-girl-who-refused-chemo-for-leukemia-dies-1.2829885 (accessed on 11 June 2018).
13. Walker, C. Makayla Sault, Case Reignites Debate over a Minor's Right to Refuse Treatment. *CBC News*, 21 January 2015. Available online: http://www.cbc.ca/news/canada/makayla-sault-case-reignites-debate-over-a-minor-s-right-to-refuse-treatment-1.2920245 (accessed on 11 June 2018).
14. Coyne, J. Canada Lets Makayla Sault Die of Leukemia over Religious Sensitivity. *The New Republic*, 21 January 2015. Available online: https://newrepublic.com/article/120823/canada-lets-makayla-sault-die-leukemia-over-religious-sensitivity (accessed on 11 June 2018).
15. Update: Recent Case Regarding Parent Refusing Chemotherapy for First Nation's Child in Favour of Traditional Medicines: What are the Implications for Health Care Providers? Available online: http://canliiconnects.org/en/commentaries/37105 (accessed on 11 June 2018).
16. Walker, C.; Luke, M. Brian Clement, Hippocrates Health Institute Head, Ordered to Stop Practicing Medicine. *CBC News*, 24 February 2015. Available online: http://www.cbc.ca/news/indigenous/brian-clement-hippocrates-health-institute-head-ordered-to-stop-practising-medicine-1.2968780 (accessed on 11 June 2018).
17. Blackwell, T. Florida Drops Charges against Clinic that Treated Aboriginal Girls with Cancer. *National Post*, 17 March 2015. Available online: http://nationalpost.com/news/world/florida-drops-charges-against-clinic-that-treated-canadian-aboriginal-girls-with-cancer (accessed on 11 June 2018).

18. Walker, C.; Luke, M. Health Canada Investigates Florida Spa Director's Illegal Supplements. *CBC News*, 7 May 2016. Available online: http://www.cbc.ca/news/investigates/supplements-clement-six-nations-1.3570751 (accessed on 11 June 2018).
19. Polevoy, T.; Ross, M.; Reinhold, R. The Anatomy of an Academic and Alternative Health Fraud. Pig Pills, Inc. 2003. Available online: https://www.amazon.ca/dp/B008MHFYEU/ref=cm_sw_r_em_tai_i_c_si0aBbD2A6CB2 (accessed on 11 June 2018).

2

Complementary and Integrative Therapies for Childhood Atopic Dermatitis

Adrienne L. Adler-Neal [1,*], Abigail Cline [1], Travis Frantz [1], Lindsay Strowd [2], Steven R. Feldman [1,2,3,4] and Sarah Taylor [2]

1 Center for Dermatology Research, Department of Dermatology, Wake Forest School of Medicine, Winston-Salem, NC 27101, USA; aecline25@gmail.com (A.C.); tfrantz@wakehealth.edu (T.F.); sfeldman@wakehealth.edu (S.R.F.)
2 Department of Dermatology, Wake Forest School of Medicine, Winston-Salem, NC 27101, USA; lchaney@wakehealth.edu (L.S.); saratayl@wakehealth.edu (S.T.)
3 Department of Pathology, Wake Forest School of Medicine, Winston-Salem, NC 27101, USA
4 Department of Public Health Sciences, Wake Forest School of Medicine, Winston-Salem, NC 27101, USA
* Correspondence: aadler@wakehealth.edu

Abstract: Background: Childhood atopic dermatitis is a chronic inflammatory skin condition that causes significant psychological and financial costs to the individual and society. Treatment regimens may require long-term medication adherence and can be associated with poor patient satisfaction. There is considerable interest in complementary and integrative medicine (CIM) approaches for childhood atopic dermatitis. Objective: To assess the effects of CIM approaches on childhood atopic dermatitis outcomes as defined by randomized, controlled clinical trials. Methods: A PubMed review of CIM-related treatments for pediatric atopic dermatitis was performed, and data related to age, study population, efficacy, treatment regimen, length of treatment, and sample size were included. Results: The search yielded 20 trials related to probiotic/prebiotic treatments for atopic dermatitis, three on the effects of vitamins on children with atopic dermatitis, and two on the effects of Chinese herbal treatments for atopic dermatitis in children and adolescents. The strongest evidence was for supplementation with the probiotics *L. fermentum* and *L. plantarum*. Conclusions: Certain strains of probiotics, specifically *L. plantarum* and *L. fermentum*, may improve clinical severity scores in children with atopic dermatitis. However, additional trials are needed to more thoroughly delineate the effects of additional integrative therapies on childhood atopic dermatitis.

Keywords: integrative medicine; atopic dermatitis; children

---

1. Introduction

Atopic dermatitis (AD) is the most common inflammatory skin condition seen in pediatric populations. Its prevalence in the past twenty years has been steadily increasing, reaching a rate of 13% in the United States [1,2]. A complex constellation of risk factors including irritants, contact and inhaled allergens, stress, and infection contribute to the development and persistence of AD [3]. Clinically, AD is characterized by itching, skin inflammation, skin barrier abnormalities, and increased susceptibility to skin infections [4]. This condition negatively impacts quality of life for affected children and their caregivers and can lead to significant decreases in self-esteem, as well as increased rates of depression, anxiety, and suicidal ideation [5–9].

Despite the existence of effective treatment regimens, poor patient satisfaction with the treatment is common. Less than one third of patients report satisfaction with their current treatment regimens [10]. There is interest in complementary and integrative medicine (CIM) for the treatment of childhood AD, with over 40% of pediatric patients with AD reporting the use of integrative medicine approaches [11]. Recommendations for CIM approaches should be based on evidence. We assessed the effects of CIM on childhood atopic dermatitis outcomes as defined by randomized, controlled clinical trials (RCTs).

2. Methods

A PubMed search included the terms "atopic dermatitis," "children," "pediatrics," "integrative medicine," "complementary medicine," "alternative medicine," "complementary," "integrative," "alternative," "probiotic," "herb," "herbal medicine," "vitamin," and "relaxation". Results were filtered to only include human subjects. Dates included ranged from the earliest entry to January of 2019. Title, abstract, and full review were conducted by one reviewer. We included only randomized controlled trials (RCT) or crossover trials that examined participants less than or equal to eighteen years of age. An exception was made for one study examining Chinese herbal medicine that incorporated individuals 5–21 years of age.

When using the above search terms, anywhere between approximately twenty to eighty trials resulted related to probiotics for the treatment of AD. From those, ten were identified as meeting our study criteria, while the remaining ones cited below were found within the References section of additional articles. For the section related to vitamin supplementation, approximately ninety-five studies resulted from our search, with only one meeting our criteria. An additional two studies were also found from the References section of articles. For studies related to herbal medicine, approximately forty studies were identified on PubMed, two of which fit our classifications.

3. Results

A total of 20 RCTs examined the role of probiotics/prebiotics in the treatment of childhood AD [12–31]. Three RCTs examined the effects of vitamins on children with AD [32–34], and two RCTs delineated the effects of Chinese herbal treatments for AD in children and adolescents (Table 1) [35,36].

Table 1. Probiotics/prebiotics for the treatment of pediatric atopic dermatitis.

Study	Study Type	Treated/ Control (N)	Age Range	Probiotic/Prebiotic Treatment and Daily Dosage	Treatment Length	Outcome Measure	Results
Viljanen et al., 2005	RCT	75/67/66	1.5–11.9 months	*L. rhamnosus GG* (*LGG*) 10^{10} cfu vs. *LGG* 10^{10} cfu, *L. rhamnosus* (*LC705*) 10^{10} cfu, *B. breve* 4×10^8 cfu, *Propionibacterium freudenreichii*, *Shermanii JS* 4×10^9 cfu vs. placebo	4 weeks	SCORAD at 4 weeks	All groups combined showed improvements in SCORAD: −65%. No group differences in changes in SCORAD ($p = 0.27$). In IgE sensitized infants; *LGG* group showed greater reductions in SCORAD (−26.1 points) when compared to placebo (−19.8 points) ($p = 0.04$).
Gruber et al., 2007	RCT	54/48	3–12 months	*LGG* $> 5 \times 10^9$ cfu vs. placebo	12 weeks	SCORAD A, B, and C Subscales at 12 weeks	Probiotic: A (−6.2 points); B (−1.2 points), C (−2.4 points) Placebo: A (−7.9 points), B (−1.6 points), C (−2.4 points) No significant group differences in changes in SCORAD subscales: ($p = 0.60$, 0.27, and 0.52, respectively)
Gore et al., 2012	RCT	35/36/40	3–6 months	*L. paracasei* 10^{10} cfu vs. *B. lactis* 10^{10} cfu vs. placebo	12 weeks	SCORAD at 12 weeks	*L. paracasei*: −51% *B. lactis*: −51% Placebo: −59% No significant differences in changes in SCORAD ($p = 0.7$).
Torii et al., 2011	RCT	26/24	4–15 years	*L. acidophilus* 3×10^{10}cfu vs. placebo	8 weeks	SMS at 8 weeks	Reductions in ADASI score were demonstrated in the probiotic group when compared to placebo ($p < 0.05$).
Farid et al., 2011	RCT	19/21	3 months–6 years	Synbiotic (prebiotic + *L. casei*, *L. rhamnosus*, *S. thermophilus*, *B. breve*, *L. acidophilus*, *B. infantis*, *L. bulgaricus*), 2×10^{10} cfu total dosage vs. placebo	8 weeks	SCORAD at 8 weeks	Synbiotic: −39 points Placebo: −20 points Significant group differences in changes in SCORAD ($p = 0.005$).
Gerasimov et al., 2010	RCT	43/47	12–36 months	*L. acidophilus* and *B. lactis* 10^{10}cfu total dosage vs. placebo	8 weeks	SCORAD at 8 weeks	Probiotic: −14 points Placebo: −8 points Significant group differences in changes in SCORAD ($p = 0.001$). Significant correlation was seen between decreases in CD4 and CD25, and reductions in SCORAD values ($p < 0.05$).
Yesilova et al., 2012	RCT	20/19	1–13 years	*B. bifidum*, *L. acidophilus*, *L. casei*, *L. salivarius*, 4×10^9 cfu total dosage vs. placebo	8 weeks	SCORAD at 8 weeks	Probiotic: −65% Placebo: −46%
						Inflammatory markers	Significant group differences in changes in SCORAD ($p = 0.002$) Significant decreases in IL-6, IFN-γ, and IgE when compared to placebo ($p < 0.01$).
Prakoeswa et al., 2017	RCT	12/10	0–14 years old	*L. plantarum* 10^{10} cfu vs. placebo	12 weeks	SCORAD at 12 weeks	Probiotic: −37 points Placebo: −27 points Significant group differences in changes in SCORAD ($p < 0.001$).

Table 1. *Cont.*

Study	Study Type	Treated/ Control (N)	Age Range	Probiotic/Prebiotic Treatment and Daily Dosage	Treatment Length	Outcome Measure	Results
Han et al., 2012	RCT	44/39	1–13 years	*L. plantarum* 10^{10}cfu vs. placebo	12 weeks	SCORAD at 12 weeks	Probiotic: −9.1 pointes Placebo: −1.8 points Significant group differences in changes in SCORAD ($p = 0.004$). Total eosinophil count was decreased in the probiotic group ($p = 0.023$) as were IFN-γ ($p < 0.001$) and IL-4 ($p = 0.049$).
Yang et al., 2014	RCT	37/34	2–9 years old	*L. casei*, *L. plantarum*, *L. rhamnosus*, and *B. lactis* 2×10^9 cfu of each strain vs. placebo	6 weeks	EASI at 6 weeks	Probiotic: −35% Placebo: −46% No significant group differences in changes in EASI ($p = 0.28$)
Weston et al., 2005	RCT	26/27	6–18 months	*L. fermentum* 2×10^9 cfu vs. placebo	16 weeks	SCORAD at 16 weeks	Probiotic: −17 points ($p = 0.03$). Placebo: −12 points ($p = 0.83$) No data given on intergroup comparison
Wang et al., 2015	RCT	55/53/51/53	1–18 years	*L. paracasei* 2×10^9 cfu vs. *L. fermentum* 2×10^9 cfu vs. *L. paracasei* + *L. fermentum* 4×10^9 cfu vs. placebo	12 weeks	SCORAD at 12 weeks	*L. paracasei*: −25 points *L. fermentum*: −24 points *L. paracasei* + *L. fermentum*: −28 points
						Inflammatory Markers	*Placebo*: −15 points Treatment groups demonstrated lower SCORAD index after treatment when compared to placebo ($p < 0.001$). IL-4 levels decreased after probiotic treatment ($p = 0.04$).
Wu et al., 2012	RCT	27/27	2–14 years	Synbiotic (*L. salivarius* 4×10^9 cfu with prebiotic) vs. prebiotic alone	8 weeks	SCORAD at 8 weeks	Synbiotic: 27 at week 8. Prebiotic: 36 at week 8 Significant group differences in SCORAD at week 8 when controlling for baseline ($p = 0.02$)
Woo et al., 2010	RCT	41/34	2–10 years	*L. sakei* 10^{10} cfu vs placebo	12 weeks	SCORAD at 12 weeks	Probiotic: −31% Placebo: −13%
						Chemokine levels	Significant group differences in changes in SCORAD ($p = 0.01$). Treatment group demonstrated improvements in CCL17 and CCL27 ($p = 0.03$). Levels of cytokines were associated with SCORAD index ($p < 0.001$).
Sistek et al., 2006	RCT	25/24	1–10 years old	*L. rhamnosus* and *B. lactis* 2×10^9 cfu total dosage vs. placebo	12 weeks	SCORAD at 12 weeks	Ratio of probiotic to placebo treatment at treatment endpoint: 0.8 (p = 0.10). In food sensitized children, ratio of probiotic to placebo treatment at treatment endpoint: 0.73 ($p = 0.047$).

Table 1. *Cont.*

Study	Study Type	Treated/ Control (N)	Age Range	Probiotic/Prebiotic Treatment and Daily Dosage	Treatment Length	Outcome Measure	Results
Navarro-Lopez et al., 2018	RCT	23/24	4–17 years old	*B. lactis*, *B. longum*, *L. casei* 10^9 cfu total dosage vs. placebo	12 weeks	SCORAD at 12 weeks	Probiotic: −83% Placebo: −24% Significant group difference in changes in SCORAD ($p < 0.001$)
Passeron et al., 2006	RCT	17/22	2–12 years old	Prebiotic + *L. rhamnosus* 1.2×10^9 cfu vs. prebiotic alone	12 weeks	SCORAD at 12 weeks	Prebiotic + *L. rhamnosus*: −47% Prebiotic: −39% No group differences in changes in SCORAD ($p = 0.54$)
Folster-Holst et al., 2006	RCT	22/25	1–55 months	*LGG* 10^{10}cfu vs. placebo	8 weeks	SCORAD at 8 weeks	Probiotic: −18% Placebo: −24% No significant group differences in changes in SCORAD.
Wu et al., 2017	RCT	30/32	4–48 months	*L. rhamnosus* 350 mg vs. placebo	8 weeks	SCORAD at 8 weeks	Probiotic: = −22 points Placebo: SCORAD = −12 points Significant group differences in SCORAD at week 8 when controlling for baseline ($p = 0.01$).
Shafiei et al., 2011	RCT	18/19	1–36 months	Synbiotic (7 strain probiotic 10^{10} cfu + prebiotic) vs. placebo	12 weeks	SCORAD at 12 weeks	All groups combined showed a significant decrease in SCORAD (−56%; $p < 0.01$). No group differences in changes in SCORAD ($p > 0.05$)

RCT, randomized controlled trial. SCORAD, severity assessment of atopic dermatitis. AD, atopic dermatitis. ADASI, atopic dermatitis area and severity index. SMS, symptom-medication score. EASI, eczema activity, and severity index. CFU, colony-forming unit.

3.1. Probiotics/Prebiotics for the Treatment of Childhood Atopic Dermatitis

Of the 20 RCTs that examined the role of a variety of probiotic/prebiotic mixtures on AD, the most common probiotics used were *L. acidophilus, L. rhamnosus,* and *L. plantarum* (Table 1) [12–31]. A wide array of other probiotics for AD were used (Table 2). The majority of the treatment durations in these studies were between 6 and 12 weeks.

Table 2. Common probiotics used in treating pediatric atopic dermatitis.

Common Probiotics Used for Pediatric Atopic Dermatitis
L. acidophilus
L. plantarum
L. fermentum
L. rhamnosus
L. salivarius
L. sakei
L. casei
B. lactis

Of these, three trials examined children under one year of age [23,25,27]. None of the three trials solely examining children under one year of age showed any improvement in disease severity when compared to placebo. However, a small number of specific probiotic strains were incorporated in these three studies (i.e., *L. paracasei, B. lactis, L. rhamnosus, B. breve, P. freudenreichii,* and *Shermanii JS*), thus limiting the extension of these findings to all probiotic treatments.

Four studies examined *L. acidophilus* (both delivered on its own and in combination with additional probiotics) for the treatment of AD [17,19,21,24]. One RCT of 50 children ages 4–15 compared *L. acidophilus* to placebo treatment [24]. The primary outcome measure was the symptom-medication score (SMS). This score combined the AD Area and Severity Index (ADASI) with the medication score, a marker that represented the amount of steroid ointment used. The treatment length was eight weeks, after which the probiotic group showed greater improvements in the SMS when compared to placebo ($p < 0.05$). No specific information was provided in this article concerning the amount of improvement observed in either group [24]. In an additional RCT, *L. acidophilus* was combined with multiple additional probiotic strains as well as a prebiotic (i.e., synbiotic) and compared with placebo treatment for a duration of 8 weeks in 40 children ages 3 months–6 years [17]. After 8 weeks of treatment, those assigned to the synbiotic group demonstrated a greater decrease in SCORAD index (−39 points) when compared to placebo treatment (−20 points, $p = 0.005$) [17]. *L. acidophilus* treatment also improved the SCORAD index more than placebo did in a separate RCT that treated 90 children ages 12–36 months for 8 weeks with a combination of *L. acidophilus* and *B. lactis* [19]. The treatment group experienced a 14 point reduction in the SCORAD index when compared to an 8 point improvement in the placebo group ($p = 0.001$) [19]. The combination of *L. acidophilus* and *B. lactis* was also associated with decreased CD4 and CD25 values, a factor that correlated with improvements in the SCORAD index ($p < 0.05$) [19]. Further, when *L. acidophilus* was combined with *B. bifidum, L. casei,* and *L. salivarius,* the treatment group exhibited a 65% reduction in the SCORAD index when compared to the 46% reduction observed in the placebo group ($p = 0.002$) [21]. This combination of *L. acidophilus, B. bifidum, L. casei,* and *L. salivarius* also improved inflammatory markers such as IL-6, IFN-γ, and IgE when compared to placebo ($p < 0.01$) [21].

Three RCTs examined the role of *L. plantarum* in treating childhood AD [14,16,22]. In one trial, 12 weeks of treatment with *L. plantarum* in children ages 0–14 improved an average of 37 points in the probiotic group as compared to 27 points in the placebo group ($p < 0.001$) [14]. In an additional RCT, 12 weeks of treatment with *L. plantarum* in children ages 1-13 was associated with a 9-point decrease in the SCORAD index as compared to a 2 point decrease in the placebo group, a group difference that was statistically significant ($p = 0.004$) [22]. Interleukin (IL)-4, interferon (IFN)-γ, and IL-17 were also significantly lower in the probiotic group when compared to placebo. A separate trial combined *L. plantarum* with *L. casei*, *L. rhamnosus*, and *B. lactis* and the effects of six weeks of this regimen were compared with placebo treatment in children 2–9 years old [16]. The probiotic group showed a 35% decrease in Eczema Activity and Severity Index (EASI) scores, whereas the placebo group demonstrated a 46% decrease in EASI scores. There were no significant group differences in changes in EASI scores ($p = 0.28$) [16].

Two RCTs examined *L. fermentum* as a treatment for pediatric AD [18,31]. In the first RCT, 16 weeks of treatment with *L. fermentum* was compared with placebo in 53 children ages 6–18 months old [18]. Probiotic treatment improved SCORAD values an average of 17 points ($p = 0.03$), whereas placebo treatment did not result in statistically significant improvements (−12 points, $p = 0.83$). No statistical data were provided regarding intergroup comparisons of these measures [18]. An additional trial treated children ages 1-18 years with either *L. paracasei*, *L. fermentum*, *L. paracasei* + *L. fermentum*, or placebo for 12 weeks, and the effects on SCORAD index and inflammatory markers (IL-4, IFN-γ, transforming growth factor (TGF)-ß, and tumor necrosis factor (TNF)-α) were measured [31]. SCORAD index improved by 25 points in those treated with *L. paracasei,* 24 points in those treated with *L. fermentum*, 28 points in those given *L. paracasei* + *L. fermentum*, and 15 points in those treated with placebo. All groups demonstrated lower SCORAD indices when compared to placebo and after adjusting for topical steroid use ($p < 0.001$) [31]. There were no group differences in topical steroid use. Treatment with *L. fermentum* and *L. paracasei* also decreased IL-4 levels ($p = 0.04$) [31].

One RCT combined *L. salivarius* with a prebiotic (i.e., synbiotic) and compared it with the use of a prebiotic alone in 54 children ages 2–14 years [28]. Treatment was administered for 8 weeks. At week 8, the synbiotic group demonstrated an average SCORAD index of 27, whereas the placebo group had an average SCORAD index of 36. Significant group differences were observed when controlling for baseline SCORAD values ($p = 0.02$) [20]. One RCT examined *L. sakei* treatment in comparison to placebo in 75 children ages 2–10 years old [29]. The probiotic group demonstrated improvements in SCORAD values (−31%) that were greater than those observed in the placebo group (−13%, $p = 0.01$). The treatment group also demonstrated improvements in cytokine levels, a factor that was associated with improvements in clinical scores ($p < 0.001$) [29].

While four trials incorporated *L. casei* into the probiotic mixture, no RCTs have examined *L. casei* alone. As noted above, *L. casei* was ineffective when combined with *L. plantarum, L. rhamnosus,* and *B. lactis* ($p = 0.28$) [16]. However, *L. casei* was effective when combined with additional strains that may deliver more potent treatment effects (also noted above, i.e., *L. plantarum*, *L. acidophilus*, and *L. salivarius*) ($p < 0.005$) [17,21]. When *L. casei* was combined with *B. lactis* and *B. longum* and examined in 47 individuals 4–17 years of age for 12 weeks, significant improvement in SCORAD values were observed in the treatment group (−83%) when compared to placebo (−24%, $p < 0.001$) [13]. *B. lactis* was also effective when combined with *L. acidophilus* (SCORAD improved by 14 points, $p = 0.001$) and was ineffective when used on its own or when combined with additional strains [12,16,19,23].

Eight trials incorporated the *L. rhamnosus* strain [12,15–17,20,25–27]. Of those, three demonstrated improvements in treatment outcomes when compared to placebo treatment [20]. Specifically, one RCT compared *L. rhamnosus*, *L. rhamnosus* + multiple additional strains, and placebo treatment in 208 children ages 1.5–11.9 months [25]. No group differences were found in the SCORAD index after four weeks of treatment ($p = 0.27$). In an additional trial, 102 children 3–12 months of age were administered *L. rhamonsus* or placebo for 12 weeks and changes in the SCORAD index were measured. Again, no group differences were seen [27]. However, it should be noted that in both of these trials, all of the participants were all under one year of age. In the trial by Yang et al. (discussed above), a probiotic mixture incorporating *L. rhamnosus* demonstrated no efficacy when compared to placebo ($p = 0.28$). In two RCTs, children between the ages of one month and 12 years experienced no benefits of *L. rhamnosus* when compared to a prebiotic treatment alone [15] and when compared to placebo [26]. However, one RCT showed that eight weeks of *L. rhamnosus* treatment in 62 children 4–48 months of age led to improvements in the SCORAD index (−22 points) when compared to placebo (−12 points, $p = 0.01$) [20]. Additionally, L. rhamnosus was combined with B. lactis and showed improvement in children who were food sensitized when compared to placebo (SCORAD ratio of probiotic to placebo treatment was 0.73 ($p = 0.047$) [12]. The strain was also effective when combined with a number of different probiotics and a prebiotic (−39 points) when compared to placebo (−20 points, $p = 0.005$) [17].

Three RCTs listed above included prebiotics with probiotics (i.e., synbiotics) [15,17,28]. Synbiotics had a greater impact on the SCORAD index (39 point improvement) than prebiotics alone (20 point improvement) when the probiotics used was *L. salivarius* ($p = 0.005$) [17]. Treatment with a synbiotic was also more effective than a placebo when the probiotics used were a mixture combining *L. casei, L. rhamnosus, S. thermophilus, B. breve, L. acidophilus, B. infantis*, and *L. bulgaricus* [17]. Prebiotics alone are also effective in improving the SCORAD index (−39%, $p < 0.05$) [15]. In one study not discussed above, 12 weeks of treatment with a synbiotic in 37 children ages 1–36 months old had no effect on SCORAD index when compared to placebo ($p > 0.05$) [30]. However, the probiotic strains used were not listed.

All trials supported the safety of probiotic treatments in children. Few adverse events were observed, and the ones that occurred were mild. One participant reported vomiting after the ingestion of the probiotic [18], while three individuals in another study reported mild abdominal pain after ingestion of a prebiotic and synbiotic [15]. Seventeen participants in an additional study reported side effects such as vomiting, diarrhea, and fever after ingestion of active treatment. However, these side effects were seen in the placebo group as well and no significant group differences were observed [26].

3.2. *Vitamins/Minerals for the Treatment of Childhood Atopic Dermatitis*

Oral pyridoxine, oral zinc sulfate, and topical B12 treatments have been examined in randomized, placebo and vehicle-controlled trials for the treatment of childhood AD (Table 3) [32–34]. Twenty-one patients ages 6 months-18 years treated with topical B12 ointment for 4 weeks demonstrated improvement in SCORAD values at 2 weeks (−3 points) when compared to vehicle (−1 point, $p = 0.01$) and 4 weeks (−4.5 points) when compared to the vehicle (−1.6 points, $p = 0.01$) [33]. Four weeks of treatment with oral pyridoxine in children ages 2–15 and eight weeks of treatment with zinc sulfate in those 1–16 years old showed no effects when compared to placebo/vehicle treatment [32,34]. No significant adverse events were noted as a result of vitamin/mineral ingestion.

3.3. *Chinese Herbs for the Treatment of Childhood Atopic Dermatitis*

Two RCTs examined the role of traditional Chinese herbal medicine (TCHM) in improving the severity of childhood AD (Table 4) [35,36]. One trial incorporated the following herbs into the TCHM mixture: *Flos Ionicerae, Herba menthae, Cortex moutan, Rhizoma atractylodis, and Cortex phellodendri* [35]. Twelve weeks of treatment was compared to placebo in 85 individuals between the ages of 5 and 21 years. TCHM resulted in an improvement of 15% in SCORAD index, while placebo treatment caused an improvement of 18%. There were no group differences in changes in SCORAD values. However, treatment with TCHM did result in a reduction in the total amount of steroids used ($p = 0.02$). A different, crossover trial examined the effects of a TCHM treatment on clinical severity scores in 37 children ages 1–18 years of age [36]. The TCHM mixture incorporates *Ledebouriella seseloides, Potentilla chinensis, Anebia clematidis, Rehmannia glutinosa, Paeonia lactiflora, Lophatherum gracile, Dictamnus dasycarpus, Tribulus terrestris, Glycyrrhiza uralensis, and Schizonepeta tenuifolia*. TCHM treatment was associated with a 51% decrease in erythema scores as compared to a 6.1% decrease during placebo treatment (95% CI for the difference 13.4, 89.7). TCHM treatment was also associated with a 49% decrease in surface damage scores when compared to a 6.2% decrease during placebo treatment (95% CI for the difference 19.2, 97.9) [36]. No adverse events were noted due to TCHM ingestion.

Table 3. Vitamins and minerals for the treatment of pediatric atopic dermatitis.

Study	Study Type	Treated/Control (N)	Age Range	Vitamin/Mineral Treatment	Treatment Time	Outcome Measures	Outcomes
Januchowsi, 2009	RCT	21 patients total	6 months–18 years	Topical B12 vs. placebo	4 weeks	SCORAD at 4 weeks	B12: −4.5 points Placebo: −1.6 points Significant group difference in changes in SCORAD ($p = 0.01$)
Mabin et al., 1995	RCT	19/22	2–15 years	Oral pyridoxine hydrochloride vs. placebo	4 weeks	Skin severity score, daytime itch, nocturnal itch at 4 weeks	No significant differences between groups in any outcomes at the end of treatment. Skin severity score: $p = 0.65$ Daytime itch: $p = 0.72$ Nocturnal itch: $p = 0.33$
Ewing et al., 1991	RCT	25/25	1–16 years	Oral zinc sulfate vs. placebo	8 weeks	Surface area affected, degree of erythema, itch at 8 weeks	No change in disease severity across both groups.

RCT, randomized controlled trial. AD, atopic dermatitis.

Table 4. Chinese herbal treatments for pediatric atopic dermatitis.

Study	Study Type	Treated/Control (N)	Age Range	Chinese Herb Treatment	Treatment Time	Outcome Measures	Outcomes
Hon et al., 2007	RCT	42/43	5–21 years	*Flos ionicerae, Herba menthae, Cortex moutan, Rhizoma atractylodis, and Cortex phellodendri* (TCHM) vs. placebo	12 weeks	SCORAD at 12 weeks	TCHM: −15%
							Placebo: −18%
							No significant group differences in SCORAD
							TCHM group displayed a 1/3rd reduction in the amount of topical corticosteroid used ($p = 0.024$).
Sheehan et al., 1992	Crossover Trial	37	1–18 years	*Ledebouriella seseloides, Potentilla chinensis, Anebia clematidis, Rehmannia glutinosa, Paeonia lactiflora, Lophatherum gracile, Dictamnus dasycarpus, Tribulus terrestris, Glycyrrhiza uralensis, and Schizonepeta tenuifolia* (TCHM) vs. placebo	8 weeks	Extent and severity of erythema and surface damage at 8 weeks	TCHM: 51% decrease in erythema scores and a 49% decrease in surface damage scores
							Placebo: 6.1% decrease in erythema scores and 6.2% decrease in surface damage scores.

RCT, randomized controlled trial. AD, atopic dermatitis. TCHM, traditional Chinese herbal medicine.

4. Discussion

The treatment of pediatric AD can be difficult and may benefit from the combination of allopathic and integrative treatment approaches. To date, probiotics remain the most well-validated CIM approach for treating childhood AD. Appropriate development of the immune system, including the maturation of Th1/Th2 cells in childhood, depends on adequate microbial stimulation [37]. In fact, microbial composition and diversity prevent the shift towards Th2-mediated immunity and the subsequent development of allergic diseases [2,38]. As such, probiotic treatments may improve AD clinical severity through their immunomodulatory effects [29,31]. However, the dosage of probiotic treatments was not standardized across studies and is thus a limitation of the data presented. The strongest evidence exists for treatment with *L. plantarum* and *L. fermentum* in children 12 months of age and older. Specifically, each probiotic was examined separately in two RCTs that demonstrated a reduction in the SCORAD index when *L. plantarum* or *L. fermentum* was delivered alone (i.e., without additional probiotic strains) [14,18,22,31]. Many of the improvements seen were clinically significant since on average, an improvement of 8.7 points on the SCORAD index equates to a one-point improvement on the global severity scale [39]. While one trial did not show any efficacy of *L. plantarum* treatment [16], this study only incorporated six weeks of treatment, while the former RCT's delivered 12 weeks of treatment, potentially highlighting an effect of longer treatment times. This trial also combined *L. plantarum* with potentially less effective probiotic strains (i.e., *L. casei* and *B. lactis*) [16].

Treatment with *L. acidophilus*, *L. salivarius*, *L. paracasei*, and *L. sakei* may also provide benefit when delivered without additional strains. However, each of these bacteria alone has been evaluated in only one RCT [24,28,29,31]. *L. acidophilus* was also effective in improving the SCORAD index when combined with additional strains [19,21]. *L. rhamnosus* may be effective for improving AD-related outcomes [12,15–17,20,25–27]. Multiple studies examining this strain were performed in children less than one year of age, a factor that could have contributed to the lack of efficacy. Further, while three studies showed some improvement, only one of these examined *L. rhamnosus* alone [20]. Future studies are needed to examine the efficacy of *B. lactis* and *L. casei*, as conflicting findings were noted in numerous studies [12,13,16,19,23]. Preliminary evidence suggests that synbiotics may improve AD-related outcomes but demonstrate additional efficacy when combined with an active probiotic [15,17,28]. Limited evidence exists supporting the efficacy of topical B12 ointment [33]. No conclusive evidence exists for the use of TCHM in children with AD [35,36].

Notably, few RCTs have examined the role of mind-body approaches in treating childhood AD. Psychological stress is a key component of an individual's experience with AD and can even exacerbate the disease processes [40]. Interventions that mitigate stress, such as progressive muscle relaxation, mindfulness meditation, and yoga could provide a cost-effective treatment approach in this patient population. However, it remains unknown if mind-body therapies confer benefit in pediatric populations suffering from AD. Outside of probiotic therapies, little to no evidence exists regarding the efficacy of CIM treatments for pediatric AD.

In summary, while CIM approaches hold promise for treating childhood AD and so far are not known to hold many side effects, it remains unknown how these approaches will fit into the broader landscape of traditional AD treatments. Consequently, future clinical trials are needed to comprehensively understand the role of herbal remedies, vitamins, cognitive therapies, relaxation techniques, and additional CIM modalities in treating pediatric AD.

Author Contributions: Conceptualization, A.L.A.-N. and S.R.F.; methodology, A.L.A.-N., S.R.F., T.F., and A.C.; writing—original draft preparation, A.L.A.-N.; writing—review and editing, A.L.A.-N., S.R.F., A.C., T.F., S.T., and L.S.

References

1. Silverberg, J.I. Public Health Burden and Epidemiology of Atopic Dermatitis. *Dermatol. Clin.* **2017**, *35*, 283–289. [CrossRef] [PubMed]
2. Yao, T.C.; Chang, C.J.; Hsu, Y.H.; Huang, J.L. Probiotics for allergic diseases: Realities and myths. *Pediatr. Allergy Immunol.* **2010**, *21*, 900–919. [CrossRef] [PubMed]
3. Kantor, R.; Silverberg, J.I. Environmental risk factors and their role in the management of atopic dermatitis. *Expert Rev. Clin. Immunol.* **2017**, *13*, 15–26. [CrossRef] [PubMed]
4. Ahn, C.; Huang, W. Clinical Presentation of Atopic Dermatitis. *Adv. Exp. Med. Biol.* **2017**, *1027*, 39–46. [PubMed]
5. Kim, S.H.; Hur, J.; Jang, J.Y.; Park, H.S.; Hong, C.H.; Son, S.J.; Chang, K.J. Psychological Distress in Young Adult Males with Atopic Dermatitis: A Cross-Sectional Study. *Medicine (Baltimore)* **2015**, *94*, e949. [CrossRef] [PubMed]
6. Ronnstad, A.T.M.; Halling-Overgaard, A.S.; Hamann, C.R.; Skov, L.; Egeberg, A.; Thyssen, J.P. Association of atopic dermatitis with depression, anxiety, and suicidal ideation in children and adults: A systematic review and meta-analysis. *J. Am. Acad. Dermatol.* **2018**, *79*, 448–456. [CrossRef]
7. Chernyshov, P.V. Stigmatization and self-perception in children with atopic dermatitis. *Clin. Cosmet. Investig. Dermatol.* **2016**, *9*, 159–166. [CrossRef]
8. Beattie, P.E.; Lewis-Jones, M.S. A comparative study of impairment of quality of life in children with skin disease and children with other chronic childhood diseases. *Br. J. Dermatol.* **2006**, *155*, 145–151. [CrossRef]
9. Yang, E.J.; Beck, K.M.; Sekhon, S.; Bhutani, T.; Koo, J. The impact of pediatric atopic dermatitis on families: A review. *Pediatr. Dermatol.* **2019**, *36*, 66–71. [CrossRef]
10. Paller, A.S.; McAlister, R.O.; Doyle, J.J.; Jackson, A. Perceptions of physicians and pediatric patients about atopic dermatitis, its impact, and its treatment. *Clin. Pediatr. (Phila)* **2002**, *41*, 323–332. [CrossRef]
11. Hughes, R.; Ward, D.; Tobin, A.M.; Keegan, K.; Kirby, B. The use of alternative medicine in pediatric patients with atopic dermatitis. *Pediatr. Dermatol.* **2007**, *24*, 118–120. [CrossRef] [PubMed]
12. Sistek, D.; Kelly, R.; Wickens, K.; Stanley, T.; Fitzharris, P.; Crane, J. Is the effect of probiotics on atopic dermatitis confined to food sensitized children? *Clin. Exp. Allergy* **2006**, *36*, 629–633. [CrossRef] [PubMed]
13. Navarro-Lopez, V.; Ramirez-Bosca, A.; Ramon-Vidal, D.; Ruzafa-Costas, B.; Genoves-Martinez, S.; Chenoll-Cuadros, E.; Carrion-Gutierrez, M.; Horga de la Parte, J.; Prieto-Merino, D.; Codoner-Cortes, F.M. Effect of Oral Administration of a Mixture of Probiotic Strains on SCORAD Index and Use of Topical Steroids in Young Patients With Moderate Atopic Dermatitis: A Randomized Clinical Trial. *JAMA Dermatol.* **2018**, *154*, 37–43. [CrossRef] [PubMed]
14. Prakoeswa, C.R.S.; Herwanto, N.; Prameswari, R.; Astari, L.; Sawitri, S.; Hidayati, A.N.; Indramaya, D.M.; Kusumowidagdo, E.R.; Surono, I.S. Lactobacillus plantarum IS-10506 supplementation reduced SCORAD in children with atopic dermatitis. *Benef. Microbes.* **2017**, *8*, 833–840. [CrossRef]
15. Passeron, T.; Lacour, J.P.; Fontas, E.; Ortonne, J.P. Prebiotics and synbiotics: Two promising approaches for the treatment of atopic dermatitis in children above 2 years. *Allergy* **2006**, *61*, 431–437. [CrossRef] [PubMed]
16. Yang, H.J.; Min, T.K.; Lee, H.W.; Pyun, B.Y. Efficacy of Probiotic Therapy on Atopic Dermatitis in Children: A Randomized, Double-blind, Placebo-controlled Trial. *Allergy Asthma Immunol. Res.* **2014**, *6*, 208–215. [CrossRef] [PubMed]
17. Farid, R.; Ahanchian, H.; Jabbari, F.; Moghiman, T. Effect of a new synbiotic mixture on atopic dermatitis in children: A randomized-controlled trial. *Iran J. Pediatr.* **2011**, *21*, 225–230.
18. Weston, S.; Halbert, A.; Richmond, P.; Prescott, S.L. Effects of probiotics on atopic dermatitis: A randomised controlled trial. *Arch. Dis. Child.* **2005**, *90*, 892–897. [CrossRef]
19. Gerasimov, S.V.; Vasjuta, V.V.; Myhovych, O.O.; Bondarchuk, L.I. Probiotic supplement reduces atopic dermatitis in preschool children: A randomized, double-blind, placebo-controlled, clinical trial. *Am. J. Clin. Dermatol.* **2010**, *11*, 351–361. [CrossRef]

20. Wu, Y.J.; Wu, W.F.; Hung, C.W.; Ku, M.S.; Liao, P.F.; Sun, H.L.; Lu, K.H.; Sheu, J.N.; Lue, K.H. Evaluation of efficacy and safety of Lactobacillus rhamnosus in children aged 4-48 months with atopic dermatitis: An 8-week, double-blind, randomized, placebo-controlled study. *J. Microbiol. Immunol. Infect.* **2017**, *50*, 684–692. [CrossRef]
21. Yesilova, Y.; Calka, O.; Akdeniz, N.; Berktas, M. Effect of probiotics on the treatment of children with atopic dermatitis. *Ann. Dermatol.* **2012**, *24*, 189–193. [CrossRef] [PubMed]
22. Han, Y.; Kim, B.; Ban, J.; Lee, J.; Kim, B.J.; Choi, B.S.; Hwang, S.; Ahn, K.; Kim, J. A randomized trial of Lactobacillus plantarum CJLP133 for the treatment of atopic dermatitis. *Pediatr. Allergy Immunol.* **2012**, *23*, 667–673. [CrossRef] [PubMed]
23. Gore, C.; Custovic, A.; Tannock, G.W.; Munro, K.; Kerry, G.; Johnson, K.; Peterson, C.; Morris, J.; Chaloner, C.; Murray, C.S.; et al. Treatment and secondary prevention effects of the probiotics Lactobacillus paracasei or Bifidobacterium lactis on early infant eczema: Randomized controlled trial with follow-up until age 3 years. *Clin. Exp. Allergy* **2012**, *42*, 112–122. [CrossRef] [PubMed]
24. Torii, S.; Torii, A.; Itoh, K.; Urisu, A.; Terada, A.; Fujisawa, T.; Yamada, K.; Suzuki, H.; Ishida, Y.; Nakamura, F.; et al. Effects of oral administration of Lactobacillus acidophilus L-92 on the symptoms and serum markers of atopic dermatitis in children. *Int. Arch. Allergy Immunol.* **2011**, *154*, 236–245. [CrossRef]
25. Viljanen, M.; Savilahti, E.; Haahtela, T.; Juntunen-Backman, K.; Korpela, R.; Poussa, T.; Tuure, T.; Kuitunen, M. Probiotics in the treatment of atopic eczema/dermatitis syndrome in infants: A double-blind placebo-controlled trial. *Allergy* **2005**, *60*, 494–500. [CrossRef]
26. Folster-Holst, R.; Muller, F.; Schnopp, N.; Abeck, D.; Kreiselmaier, I.; Lenz, T.; von Ruden, U.; Schrezenmeir, J.; Christophers, E.; Weichenthal, M. Prospective, randomized controlled trial on Lactobacillus rhamnosus in infants with moderate to severe atopic dermatitis. *Br. J. Dermatol.* **2006**, *155*, 1256–1261. [CrossRef]
27. Gruber, C.; Wendt, M.; Sulser, C.; Lau, S.; Kulig, M.; Wahn, U.; Werfel, T.; Niggemann, B. Randomized, placebo-controlled trial of Lactobacillus rhamnosus GG as treatment of atopic dermatitis in infancy. *Allergy* **2007**, *62*, 1270–1276. [CrossRef]
28. Wu, K.G.; Li, T.H.; Peng, H.J. Lactobacillus salivarius plus fructo-oligosaccharide is superior to fructo-oligosaccharide alone for treating children with moderate to severe atopic dermatitis: A double-blind, randomized, clinical trial of efficacy and safety. *Br. J. Dermatol.* **2012**, *166*, 129–136. [CrossRef]
29. Woo, S.I.; Kim, J.Y.; Lee, Y.J.; Kim, N.S.; Hahn, Y.S. Effect of Lactobacillus sakei supplementation in children with atopic eczema-dermatitis syndrome. *Ann. Allergy Asthma Immunol.* **2010**, *104*, 343–348. [CrossRef]
30. Shafiei, A.; Moin, M.; Pourpak, Z.; Gharagozlou, M.; Aghamohammadi, A.; Sajedi, V.; Soheili, H.; Sotoodeh, S.; Movahedi, M. Synbiotics could not reduce the scoring of childhood atopic dermatitis (SCORAD): A randomized double blind placebo-controlled trial. *Iran J. Allergy Asthma Immunol.* **2011**, *10*, 21–28.
31. Wang, I.J.; Wang, J.Y. Children with atopic dermatitis show clinical improvement after Lactobacillus exposure. *Clin. Exp. Allergy* **2015**, *45*, 779–787. [CrossRef] [PubMed]
32. Ewing, C.I.; Gibbs, A.C.; Ashcroft, C.; David, T.J. Failure of oral zinc supplementation in atopic eczema. *Eur. J. Clin. Nutr.* **1991**, *45*, 507–510. [PubMed]
33. Januchowski, R. Evaluation of topical vitamin B(12) for the treatment of childhood eczema. *J. Altern. Complement. Med.* **2009**, *15*, 387–389. [CrossRef] [PubMed]
34. Mabin, D.C.; Hollis, S.; Lockwood, J.; David, T.J. Pyridoxine in atopic dermatitis. *Br. J. Dermatol.* **1995**, *133*, 764–767. [CrossRef] [PubMed]
35. Hon, K.L.; Leung, T.F.; Ng, P.C.; Lam, M.C.; Kam, W.Y.; Wong, K.Y.; Lee, K.C.; Sung, Y.T.; Cheng, K.F.; Fok, T.F.; et al. Efficacy and tolerability of a Chinese herbal medicine concoction for treatment of atopic dermatitis: A randomized, double-blind, placebo-controlled study. *Br. J. Dermatol.* **2007**, *157*, 357–363. [CrossRef]
36. Sheehan, M.P.; Atherton, D.J. A controlled trial of traditional Chinese medicinal plants in widespread non-exudative atopic eczema. *Br. J. Dermatol.* **1992**, *126*, 179–184. [CrossRef]
37. Martinez, F.D.; Holt, P.G. Role of microbial burden in aetiology of allergy and asthma. *Lancet* **1999**, *354* (Suppl. 2), SII12–SII15. [CrossRef]
38. Singh, M.; Ranjan Das, R. Probiotics for allergic respiratory diseases–Putting it into perspective. *Pediatr. Allergy Immunol.* **2010**, *21*, e368–e376. [CrossRef]

39. Schram, M.E.; Spuls, P.I.; Leeflang, M.M.; Lindeboom, R.; Bos, J.D.; Schmitt, J. EASI, (objective) SCORAD and POEM for atopic eczema: Responsiveness and minimal clinically important difference. *Allergy* **2012**, *67*, 99–106. [CrossRef]
40. Arndt, J.; Smith, N.; Tausk, F. Stress and atopic dermatitis. *Curr. Allergy Asthma Rep.* **2008**, *8*, 312–317. [CrossRef]

3

Sleeping without Prescription: Management of Sleep Disorders in Children with Autism with Non-Pharmacological Interventions and Over-the-Counter Treatments

Dario Esposito [1,†], Arianna Belli [1,†], Raffaele Ferri [2] and Oliviero Bruni [3,*]

1 Child Neurology and Psychiatry Unit, Department of Human Neurosciences, Sapienza University of Rome, 00185 Rome, Italy; dario.esposito@uniroma1.it (D.E.); arianna.belli@uniroma1.it (A.B.)
2 Sleep Research Centre, Oasi Research Institute–IRCCS, 94018 Troina, Italy; rferri@oasi.en.it
3 Department of Developmental and Social Psychology, Sapienza University of Rome, 00185 Rome, Italy
* Correspondence: oliviero.bruni@uniroma1.it
† These authors contributed equally to this work.

Abstract: Autism Spectrum Disorders (ASD) are lifelong neurodevelopmental conditions characterized by abnormal social interaction, communication, and behavior. Sleep disturbances represent a common comorbidity in children and adolescents with ASD, with prevalence ranging from 50 to 80%. It has been proved that sleep disruption worsens the symptoms of autism and results in challenging behaviors. Improving sleep should therefore be a primary therapeutic goal. Treatment options range from lifestyle modifications to pharmacological therapy. Several reviews have been written on pharmacological treatments, but very few on the beneficial effects of non-pharmacological interventions, over-the-counter drugs, and nutritional supplements. This study consists of a narrative review of the literature, presenting the available evidence on the following treatments: sleep education, behavioral interventions, complementary and alternative medicine (special mattresses and blankets, massage, aromatherapy, yoga, physical activity), and commonly used over-the-counter medications and supplements (antihistamines, melatonin, tryptophan, carnosine, iron, vitamins, and herbal remedies). For some treatments—such as melatonin and behavioral interventions—effectiveness in ASD is well established in the literature, while other interventions appear of benefit in clinical practice, even if specific studies in children and adolescents with ASD are lacking. Conversely, other treatments only seem to show anecdotal evidence supporting their use.

Keywords: autism; sleep; non-pharmacological; behavioral; complementary and alternative medicine; antihistamines; melatonin; supplement; herbal medicine; over-the-counter

1. Introduction

Autism Spectrum Disorders (ASD) are a group of lifelong, heterogeneous neurodevelopmental conditions, characterized by early-onset deficits in social interaction and communication, and restricted, repetitive interests and behaviors [1].

Sleep disturbances represent a common comorbidity in children with ASD, with prevalence ranging from 50 to 80% [2]. One of the main complaints of parents of children with ASD is insomnia, which indeed is a major reason of medical consultation [3]. Sleep disturbances reported in ASD children also include parasomnias, sleep disordered breathing, sleep-related movement disorders, and excessive daytime sleepiness [4]. Emotional dysregulation, fixation on daytime events, inability to understand social cues related to sleep, anxiety, hyperarousal, and sensory processing issues are some core neurobehavioral features of ASD that may contribute to sleep disorders [5]. Furthermore, challenging behaviors may lead to ineffective or even harmful bedtime routines that are not conducive to good sleep [6]. It has been proven that sleep disruption in such children worsens the symptoms of autism [7]. Shorter sleep duration has been shown to predict greater social communication impairment, higher rates of stereotypic behaviors, and more non-functional routines [8]. Conversely, it is well established that aggressive behavior independently predicts sleep problems in children with ASD [9].

Treating these conditions should therefore be a primary therapeutic goal, given their significant impact on quality of life of patients and their families. Treatment options range from lifestyle modifications and behavioral interventions to pharmacological therapies [4]. In a stepwise approach to sleep disturbances in children with ASD—before administering prescription drugs—sleep education, behavioral interventions and over-the-counter (OTC) medications are advisable [10]. Parents generally consider behavioral interventions preferable to medication and equally effective [11]. Some non-prescription drugs—such as some antihistamines and melatonin—are among the most used substances for managing insomnia in children [12]. Complementary and Alternative Medicine (CAM) is also widely used for children with ASD [13,14], or other mental issues, given that the majority of parents perceive these therapies as a helpful and holistic therapeutic approach [15].

However, the potential of sleep hygiene and behavioral interventions is poorly understood and often underestimated by clinicians and families [16]. Moreover, some non-prescription treatments have been thoroughly studied in recent years, showing new and promising evidence for treating sleep disturbances in ASD. However, there is insufficient evidence to draw conclusions on the efficacy of other widespread remedies for sleep problems and it has been reported that only less than 20% of CAM interventions was recommended by medical doctors in the pediatric psychiatric care [13].

With regard to prescription sleep medications (e.g., α2-receptor agonists, benzodiazepines, Z-drugs, antipsychotics, and antidepressants), they should be considered to be an additional treatment option to improve sleep in children when non-pharmacological interventions are unsuccessful [17]. However, none of these sleep-promoting drugs is approved by the Food and Drug Administration (FDA) for children and adolescents with ASD. Off-label prescription in children is possible, but clinicians are often discouraged to use these molecules by their relevant potential side effects (e.g., movement disorders, hormonal and metabolic dysregulation, autonomic dysfunction).

Several reviews have been written on the pharmacological treatment of sleep disorders in autistic children [18–20], but few on the beneficial effects of non-pharmacological interventions, OTC treatments, and nutritional supplements. The aim of this narrative review is to evaluate the available evidence on these treatments of sleep disorders in children with ASD, to provide a useful guide to manage their sleep disorders.

We have specifically focused on the pediatric autistic population for several reasons that make this group unique and different from adults with ASD: the heavy impact of sleep disruption on neurodevelopment during infancy and childhood, the relative lack of psychotropic medications approved for the treatment of sleep disorders in pediatric age, and the distinctive therapeutic needs of patients in developmental age (e.g., parental intervention in applying sleep hygiene and behavioral techniques, and specific nutritional deficits).

2. Materials and Methods

This study consists of a narrative review of the literature. Extensive literature searches were conducted from 8 March 2020 to 30 April 2020 using PubMed and Web of Science core collection databases. Data for this work come from original articles, official guidelines, and previous reviews, published from the inception of databases up to 30 April 2020. The following keywords and search terms were used in different combinations: autism, autism spectrum disorder, or ASD, sleep, sleep disorders, sleep disturbances, sleep problems, insomnia, children, adolescents, behavioral sleep interventions, parent-based interventions, alternative medicine treatments, non-pharmacological treatments, alternative medicine interventions, educational program, sleep education, parent education, sleep hygiene, sport, physical activity, over-the-counter medications, non-prescription drugs, melatonin, antihistamine, supplements, vitamins, iron, tryptophan, amino acids, herbal medicine, phytotherapy.

The reference lists of the articles retrieved through this preliminary search were examined as well, and some of them were also included in our review based on their relevance to our topic. Two authors (A.B. and D.E.) independently performed the search and screening of papers, resolving any disagreement by consensus.

Only articles in English and Italian have been selected. We retained all types of study designs and we only excluded studies with a small sample size, given the scarcity of studies on certain topics (such as alternative medicine treatments for sleep disturbances in children with ASD).

Whenever it was possible, we considered studies including children with ASD only, but investigations related to other populations were retained as well, if specific data on children with ASD were lacking.

3. Non-pharmacological Interventions

As a general tenet of pediatric practice, non-pharmacological intervention is the preferred first treatment option before initiation of pharmacologic therapies [17]. Even if sleep medications are popular treatment options for the ease of delivery (taking a pill), as well as the rapid improvement often experienced [21], they have some notable limitations, such as their short- and long-term side effects and the lack of efficacy in some disorders [22]. Accordingly, the latest guidelines for the treatment of insomnia and disrupted sleep behavior in children and adolescents with ASD, published by the American Academy of Neurology [20], recommend parent counseling to implement good sleep habits and behavioral techniques as a first-line approach. Furthermore, when there is a decision to start a pharmacologic treatment, behavioral interventions and good sleep hygiene practices should always be associated [20,23–25]. In other words, sleep problems in children should be approached in a stepwise fashion, with increasing intensity on a case-by-case basis when lower level strategies appear ineffective [10] (Table 1).

Table 1. Stepwise approach to sleep disturbances in children. Adapted from Howlett et al. (2020) [10].

Level 1	Sleep education and implementation of healthy sleep practices
Level 2	Specific behavioral strategies
Level 3	Medications

3.1. Parent-Based Sleep Education

Parent sleep education has been found to be effective in the general pediatric population [17], and in small samples of children with ASD [26–29]. A 2017 meta-synthesis of previously published systematic reviews [30] showed that parent-based sleep education programs have strong positive effects on some sleep problems of children with ASD—specifically self-settling and night awakenings—and moderate or weak positive effects on all the other sleep domains.

Nevertheless, it should be taken into account that the different possible ways of delivering sleep education may affect its outcome. A randomized controlled trial (RCT) in which parents of autistic children were given a standardized sleep education pamphlet on insomnia showed no improvement in sleep-onset latency (SOL), total sleep time (TST), wake time after sleep onset (WASO), and fragmentation of sleep [26]. Conversely, another study reported that group versus individualized sleep education did not influence the outcome in a cohort of autistic children: improvements in sleep-onset delay and other outcomes related to child and family functioning were reported regardless of the mode of education [27]. Recently, a trial was carried out to compare online and face-to-face sleep education in families of ASD children [31]. Both interventions positively impacted parent ratings of their children's sleep behavior and parental quality of life and fatigue, even if actigraphy data showed no improvement in objective measures of sleep (i.e., TST, sleep efficiency (SE), and number of awakenings). Overall, the study demonstrated that an online parental sleep education program was as effective as a face-to-face intervention. Instead, the online program showed even better results in some areas, such as greater reduction of parental fatigue.

According to a recent review of parent training programs associated with other behavioral interventions for children with ASD [32], this kind of treatments have the potential to reduce sleep problems such as initiating and maintaining sleep, early-morning and night awakenings, and bedtime resistance.

However, more research is needed about parental education and sleep hygiene in children with ASD, especially considering that in most studies, sleep hygiene modifications were part of a multimodal intervention, including behavioral or pharmacological treatments [16,22,32,33]. The most common and evidence-based pediatric sleep practice recommendations have been reviewed [34] and recently organized in a mnemonic tool—"ABCs of SLEEPING"—[10], whose characteristics are summarized in Table 2.

Table 2. Evidence-based pediatric sleep practice recommendations of the 'ABCs of SLEEPING' mnemonic. Adapted from Howlett et al. (2020) and Allen et al. (2016) [10,34].

Practice Areas	Recommendations	Level of Empirical Support [1]
Age-appropriate Bedtime, wake-times, and naps with Consistency	- Consistency of bedtimes, wake-times, and naps - Bedtime no later than 9 p.m. - Age-appropriate amount of sleep [2]	Strong Moderate Moderate
Schedules and routines	- Consistent and relaxing bedtime routine - Daytime activities should not interfere with sleep	Strong Moderate
Location	- Dark, cool, and quiet sleep location; limit distractions - Activities in bedroom restricted to quiet play and sleep	Limited Limited
No Electronics in the bedroom or before bed	- No electronics in bedroom - Do not use electronics within a 1 h before bedtime	Strong Limited
Exercise and diet	- Physical activity on a daily basis - Well-balanced and healthy diet	Equivocal Limited
Positivity and relaxation	- Positive living atmosphere, free of conflict - Child should feel relaxed and calm before bed	Moderate Limited
Independence falling asleep	- Encourage falling asleep and staying asleep without parent help	Strong
Needs met during the day ... equals Great sleep	- Satisfy emotional and physiological needs during daytime	Moderate

[1] levels of empirical support as defined by Allen et al. (2016) [34]. [2] see Paruthi [35].

3.2. Behavioral Interventions

Behavioral interventions include specific strategies, based on principles of learning and behavior with the aim of developing positive sleep-related habits, as well as relaxation and self-soothing skills [36].

These interventions may be classified as antecedent approaches (such as bedtime fading, stimulus fading, scheduled awakenings) and consequence-based interventions (i.e., standard and graduated extinction) [37]. The main behavioral strategies applied in the literature and in clinical practice are described below:

- Extinction. Also known as "planned ignoring", it is the most widely studied behavioral strategy, in which the caregiver ignores all the "undesirable sleep behaviors"—such as crying—after placing the child in bed, so as to remove reinforcement for these behaviors and promote self-settling [38]. This approach (standard extinction) has been found to reduce several sleep problems among children with ASD, including night-time awakenings, co-sleeping, sleep latency, and bedtime resistance [39–41]. Variants of extinction are "gradual extinction" and "extinction with parental presence". Gradual extinction differs from the standard because the parents ignore bedtime disruption just for a predetermined amount of time, before engaging with the child [40]. Gradual extinction has also been found to reduce sleep disturbances and co-sleeping; however, more research is needed on this behavioral strategy [40]. According to the strategy of extinction with parental presence, the caregiver remains in the child's room with little or no interaction [42].

- Extinction. Also known as "planned ignoring", it is the most widely studied behavioral strategy, in which the caregiver ignores all the "undesirable sleep behaviors"—such as crying—after placing the child in bed, so as to remove reinforcement for these behaviors and promote self-settling [38]. This approach (standard extinction) has been found to reduce several sleep problems among children with ASD, including night-time awakenings, co-sleeping, sleep latency, and bedtime resistance [39–41]. Variants of extinction are "gradual extinction" and "extinction with parental presence". Gradual extinction differs from the standard because the parents ignore bedtime disruption just for a predetermined amount of time, before engaging with the child [40]. Gradual extinction has also been found to reduce sleep disturbances and co-sleeping; however, more research is needed on this behavioral strategy [40]. According to the strategy of extinction with parental presence, the caregiver remains in the child's room with little or no interaction [42].
- Scheduled awakenings. Strategy used to reduce episodes of disorders of arousal, such as sleep terrors, which requires the child to be awoken before the usual occurrence of the sleep terror episode, in order to reduce the fearful response [37,42]. This behavioral intervention has also been proven to be effective in increasing TST [42].
- Bedtime fading. Putting children to bed before the time they effectively fall asleep (sleep-onset time) increases the chances of bedtime resistance. Therefore, in this procedure the child is initially put to bed 30 min later than his/her average sleep-onset time. Then bedtime is gradually anticipated by 30 min every few days, until reaching the desired bedtime [40].
- Stimulus fading. This strategy involves the parent gradually increasing the distance between himself/herself and the child, until he/she can fall asleep, so as to specifically reduce co-sleeping [43].
- Chronotherapy. Bedtime is gradually delayed over time, to "re-set" the circadian rhythm and improve early-morning awakenings, sleep latency and night awakenings [40].
- Bedtime "pass". A bedtime pass is a card or any equivalent object given to the child at bedtime that may be exchanged for one "free trip out of bed" or other forms of parental consolation after bedtime. If the bedtime pass has already been used, the parent should rapidly take the child back to bed. This kind of intervention can be used to teach the child to self-soothe and stay in bed in case of difficult sleep onset or frequent night awakenings [5,18].
- Positive reinforcement. This type of intervention uses rewards to promote the desired behaviors. Rewards are typically provided for the child upon awakening in the morning [44–46], though sometimes reinforcements may be provided during the sleep-onset period in the form of social attention for demonstrating sleep compatible behaviors [47].
- Cognitive strategies. Group of techniques targeting the non-productive sleep-related beliefs of the child (e.g., the belief that he/she cannot improve his/her sleep), often including also coping strategies, such as teaching relaxation skills [42,48].

The successful application of behavioral approaches requires both knowledgeable psychologists or clinicians, able to teach the appropriate techniques, and motivated caregivers, who should implement these strategies consistently, despite being often challenging [17]. Therefore, it is often easier and more acceptable for parents to associate sleep education with behavioral gradual interventions (such as gradual extinction and fading), rather than abrupt approaches (e.g., standard extinction techniques) [25].

Clearly, the involvement of caregivers in the implementation of these interventions is fundamental, considering that they are usually parent-mediated [25]. Nevertheless, a recent pilot study [49] evaluated the effects of personalized behavioral sleep treatment in adolescents with high-functioning ASD, suggesting that treatment components (such as psychoeducation, relaxing bedtime routine, sleep checklist or relaxation techniques) directed towards verbal adolescents with ASD may be beneficial in addition to the more common parent-mediated sleep interventions.

Among the sleep problems addressed in the literature, behavioral interventions are the most often used to treat night awakenings, followed by bedtime disturbances [22]. On the other hand, the most common treatments employed in the literature are multi-component interventions, most often including parent psychoeducation to improve healthy sleep practices, graduated extinction, and reinforcement [22,30,42]. Notably, most of the behavioral interventions described in the literature have only minor or no difference from the techniques used with typically developing children [42].

The National Autism Center guidelines [50] considers behavioral approaches in the "emerging evidence strength" category. In particular, according to a 2017 review [30], behavioral interventions have very strong effect ranking for morning awakening, co-sleeping, and self-settling, and a moderate effect ranking on night awakenings. However, the examined papers showed high heterogeneity across study outcomes [30]. Furthermore, most of the studies evaluating behavioral interventions included only a small number of participants or showed low methodological quality, therefore limiting the ability to draw accurate conclusions about their effectiveness in children and adolescents with ASD [39,42].

Notably, among the different behavioral techniques, the choice of a specific one should be guided by the parents' preferences [51], given that there is no conclusive evidence that one approach is more effective than another [52].

3.3. Other Interventions

3.3.1. Weighted Blankets and Vests

Weighted blankets and vests are a widespread non-traditional treatment for sleep disturbances in children with ASD. The rational of their use is providing proprioceptive deep pressure stimulation to the child, which is postulated to result in an increased parasympathetic tone, leading to improved arousal modulation, decreased anxiety, heart rate, and cortisol, thus promoting sleep [53,54]. Despite their popularity, to the extent of our knowledge, only one study assessed the effectiveness of weighted blankets in treating sleep problems in the pediatric population with ASD. This RCT evaluated sleep with both objective and subjective methods (actigraphy and parent-reported sleep diaries); behavioral outcomes of the interventions were assessed as well. No difference was found in any sleep measure and behavioral outcome between the weighted-blanket group and the standard-blanket group. Nevertheless, the weighted blanket was favored by parents and children on subjective preference measures [55]. The above-mentioned trial found no serious adverse event associated with weighted-blanket use. Yet, in 2010 a report highlighted potential safety issues of weighted blankets and vests, following the death of an autistic child because of inappropriate use of a weighted blanket [53]. In conclusion, to date there is no evidence of efficacy and safety for the use of weighted blankets and vests as a treatment of sleep disturbances in autistic children [55].

3.3.2. Sound-To-Sleep (STS) Mattress

In 2017, a preliminary randomized crossover study [56] examined efficacy and tolerability of a mattress-based technology—the STS system—in the treatment of sleep problems in 45 autistic children (aged 2.5–12.9 years). The STS mattress technology embeds sound and synched vibrations, allowing the user to both hear and feel sounds that they choose to play. The authors of this article suggested that this system may activate the parasympathetic nervous system, thus promoting sleep and relaxation. After two weeks of use, the STS system resulted in improvements in parent-reported sleep quality, and actigraphy-derived sleep duration and efficiency, with good tolerance and reported ease of use.

3.3.3. Massage

The use of massage in autistic children with sleep problems is based on theoretical grounds similar to those supporting the use of weighted blankets and the above-mentioned mattress-based technologies. A systematic review evaluating non-traditional approaches to sleep problems in children with autism [54] has included the findings of four studies investigating the effect of different types of massage therapy (Qigong massage, Thai massage, and parent-provided massage). One study [57] reported the association of massage therapy with a decrease in challenging behaviors at bedtime. Another study [58] found improvements in night-time awakenings and SOL for patients receiving Qigong massage. It should be taken into account, though, that both studies included a small number of participants (20 and 15 children, respectively). A third study [59] reported an improvement in sleep behavior associated with Thai massage in a larger sample, but no specific aspect of sleep behavior was described. The fourth and last reviewed article [60] claimed an improvement of sleep behavior following Qigong massage, but sleep was measured in the context of a broader sensory assessment, making it difficult to assess whether sleep behavior specifically improved. Therefore, we can only conclude that there is weak evidence on the effects of massage therapy on sleep of autistic children.

3.3.4. Aromatherapy

Only one clinical trial was carried out to evaluate the effects of aromatherapy on sleep in children with ASD [61]. During this study, aromatherapy with 2% lavender oil was administered via foot and leg massage to 12 school-aged children. SOL, sleep duration, and night awakenings where then recorded by observers who checked the children every 30 min. No difference was found in any sleep measure between the nights with and without aromatherapy suggesting no effect on sleep.

3.3.5. Yoga

A recent RCT assessed the efficacy of a structured yoga intervention for sleep, gastrointestinal and behavioral problems in a cohort of 64 ASD children aged 5 to 16 years [62]. The participants were subdivided into two groups, one followed the usual school curriculum, while the other was taught yoga for 70 min/day during a three months period. A pre- and post-intervention questionnaire, including 15 questions about sleep, was completed by the caregivers. A significant improvement in sleep quality in all the investigated sleep domains was found in children following the structured yoga intervention.

3.3.6. Sport and Physical Activity

Several studies examined physical activity as a variable that might influence sleep in autistic children. An observational study [63] conducted on 10 children with ASD demonstrated that activity level, as measured by actigraphy, was significantly correlated with sleep quality, as evaluated by a parent-reported questionnaire. Moreover, interventional studies were conducted to assess the impact of different physical activities on sleep quality in children with autism. Recently, an RCT [64] evaluated the effects of a basketball skill training delivered twice weekly for 12 weeks. The intervention was found to be effective in improving all sleep parameters considered (SE, SOL, sleep duration, and WASO).

A pilot study [65] with 10 participants also examined the influence of aerobic exercise and motor skills training on sleep in young patients with ASD. Children took part in thrice-weekly trainings and their sleep was both subjectively (parent-reported sleep logs and questionnaires) and objectively (sleep EEG) assessed. An improvement in SE, SOL, and WASO was found during the nights following the training. Nevertheless, such improvements were not found at the end of the 3-week period of the intervention.

In two small-sample studies, aquatic interventions have also been examined. In the first one [66], 1 h of aquatic exercise, 2 times per week, seemed to improve sleep latency and duration in 8 children aged 6–10 years. Conversely, in the second study [67], the authors found that in their sample of 40 autistic children, only those with a specific profile—high sensory sensitivity and avoidance and low autism severity—showed decreased sleep disturbance after the intervention.

In conclusion, there is mixed evidence about the effect of physical activity and specific sports on sleep disturbances in autistic children.

4. Oral Over-the-Counter Medicines

Sleep pills should be considered to be an additional treatment option to improve sleep in children when non-pharmacological interventions are unsuccessful [17]. However, in children with ASD pharmacological treatment is sometimes convenient as a first-line strategy together with non-pharmacological approaches, given the greater severity of sleep disturbances in these patients [25]. Both prescription hypnotic drugs and OTC sleep-promoting agents might be useful in clinical practice. Due to the scarcity of controlled studies, there is no sleep medication approved by the FDA and only one—prolonged-release melatonin for the treatment of insomnia—approved by the EMA for children and adolescents with ASD. Sleep-promoting agents are therefore widely prescribed off-label, the most commonly used off-label medications being sedating antihistamines (e.g., diphenhydramine or hydroxyzine), melatonin, α2-receptor agonists (e.g., clonidine), benzodiazepines, pyrimidine derivatives (e.g., zaleplon and zolpidem), antipsychotics (e.g., risperidone and quetiapine), and sedating antidepressants (e.g., trazodone and mirtazapine) [68].

Some of the above-mentioned agents—i.e., antihistamines and melatonin—are available over the counter in many countries all over the world. Non-prescription medications—including OTC drugs, nutritional supplements, and herbal remedies—are indeed widespread therapies for sleep disturbances in children, as they are generally easily accessible and well accepted by caregivers. Furthermore, oral non-prescription treatments are often considered to be a "safe choice" by clinicians, as they usually have less significant side effects in comparison to some prescription hypnotic drugs—such as antipsychotics and antidepressants [12,69].

Here we describe the oral non-prescription treatments and nutritional supplements most commonly used for sleep problems in children with ASD: melatonin, antihistamines, tryptophan, carnosine, vitamin D, iron, other multivitamin and mineral supplements, and herbal remedies.

4.1. Melatonin

Melatonin (N-acetyl-5-methoxytryptamine) is a serotonin-derived neurohormone produced by the pineal gland. Its secretion mainly happens during darkness—beginning in the evening and peaking between 2:00 and 4:00 a.m.—and is suppressed by the light [70]. Among its many biological functions (antioxidant properties, anti-inflammatory effects, involvement in early development of neurons and glia), melatonin plays a key role in establishing and regulating the circadian rhythm and has a hypnotic function, via the activation of melatonin receptors MT1 (mainly involved in REM sleep), MT2 (mainly involved in NREM sleep), or both [71,72].

Having well-known chronobiotic and sleep-inducing properties and being perceived as a "natural" substance (due to its endogenous production), melatonin is one of the most frequently prescribed drugs in children and adolescents with sleep problems [12,73,74]. More specifically, a large Australian survey reported that melatonin was prescribed in children with autism and comorbid sleep problems by 85.2% of pediatricians [12]. Initial dosages in children usually range from 1 to 3 mg/night (up to 5 mg/night in adolescents), administered 30–60 min before bedtime. If no improvements are noted, dosage can be titrated by 1–3 mg every 1–2 weeks up to a maximum dose of 10 mg. However, the clinician should consider that patients who have not responded to 6 mg/night are less likely to benefit from a higher dosage [20,75]. No serious adverse events have been associated with melatonin use. The most often reported side effects in children include headache, morning drowsiness, increased enuresis, dizziness, diarrhea, rash and hypothermia [76–78]. Earlier morning awakenings were sometimes reported in children supplemented with melatonin [76].

The administration of exogenous melatonin has been proven to anticipate sleep onset [79,80], without altering sleep architecture [71]. It should be taken into account, though, that the timing of administration is critical in determining the effectiveness of treatment. When used as a sleep inductor (i.e., for sleep-onset insomnia), melatonin should be administered about 30 min before the desired time of sleep [75]. By contrast, when used as a chronobiotic (i.e., for delayed sleep phase syndrome), the maximum effect on phase advance is obtained with administration 3 to 5 h before dim light melatonin onset (DLMO) for the dosage of 0.5 mg of melatonin [81]. DLMO is not predictable using sleep diaries, actigraphy, or polysomnography. However, it can be determined in home settings by measuring melatonin in saliva (collected from a cotton plug chewed for 1–2 min every hour from 7–8 p.m. to 11–12 p.m.) before starting melatonin treatment [82]. Conversely, if disrupted sleep is the main concern, melatonin treatment is usually ineffective in improving maintenance of sleep [71].

Melatonin is of special interest in ASD, in view of the abnormal central and peripheral serotonin neurobiology reported in these conditions [83,84]. In individuals with ASD, several studies reported abnormal levels of daytime or night-time melatonin, compared to typically developing controls [85–88], and nocturnal excretion in urine of 6-sulphatoxymelatonin (a melatonin metabolite) was found to correlate negatively with the severity of autistic symptoms [85]. Furthermore, children with ASD and comorbid sleep-onset delay showed genetic abnormalities in the metabolic pathway of melatonin more frequently than the general population [89].

A recent meta-synthesis [30] summarized the findings of eight systematic reviews on management of sleep disorders in children with ASD, five of which [88,90–93] included studies evaluating the effectiveness of melatonin. Two reviews included not only studies on melatonin, but also studies on other interventions for sleep disorders [90,91]. Both concluded that among the evaluated treatments, supplemental melatonin appears to have the strongest evidence supporting its use. Of the three reviews that focused on melatonin [88,92,93], one [88] was a systematic review and meta-analysis on melatonin-related findings in autistic individuals, including 18 studies on melatonin as a treatment for sleep. These studies reported improvements in SOL, night-time awakenings, and TST. Five of the studies were double-blind, placebo-controlled crossover trials and were included in a meta-analysis: significant improvements in sleep duration and latency were found, but no significant change in the number of night awakenings. Another research group [93] evaluated the effectiveness of melatonin on sleep disorders within the framework of a broader assessment of pharmacological therapies for individuals with pervasive developmental disorders, concluding that the use of melatonin may be considered for the treatment of sleep problems of these patients. Similarly, the third review [92] aimed to assess the efficacy and safety of supplemental melatonin for disordered sleep in persons with ASD. Seven studies, of the 12 identified, included children with ASD. The authors concluded that the available literature supports the use of melatonin for sleep disturbances in autistic patients, given its beneficial effects and its few and minor side effects. Finally, the overall findings of the meta-synthesis showed that melatonin had strong evidence of positive effect on SOL, TST, bedtime resistance, and co-sleeping, whereas its effectiveness was ranked as moderate in improving the longest sleep episode, night awakenings, nocturnal activity, parasomnias, sleep disordered breathing, sleep anxiety, and sleep problems not otherwise specified. Only a weak effect was found for SE, as several the studies yield negative results for this parameter [30].

Not included in the above-mentioned meta-synthesis, but of interest for its design, is a study conducted on a large sample of autistic children and adolescents over a period of 12 weeks [94]. This RCT showed that controlled-release melatonin at the dosage of 3 mg/night (1 mg immediately released and 2 mg released over a 6 h period), alone or in combination with cognitive-behavioral therapy (CBT), is effective in improving SOL, TST, WASO, and number of awakenings, as measured by actigraphy, with moderate-to-large effect sizes. Furthermore, the authors highlighted that the combination treatment group (CBT + melatonin) had higher rates of patients completing the treatment schedule and of patients obtaining clinically significant changes in sleep measures. This seems to suggest a greater effectiveness of melatonin when administered in association with a cognitive-behavioral intervention, at least in the short term.

From a practical point of view, in some children with autism a major limitation for melatonin treatment is the loss of efficacy after an initial good response [25]. Often, patients in whom the benefits of melatonin disappear after some time have been shown to have a slow metabolism of melatonin, due to a single nucleotide polymorphism in the CYP1A2 gene [95]. This may result in increased melatonin levels during daytime and, consequently, in the loss of the circadian melatonin rhythm, thus explaining the fading of effectiveness of exogenous melatonin over time [96]. As a consequence of these findings, there is now a greater understanding that low (0.5 mg), rather than high doses can work for some children, with diminishing effects for doses over 6 mg [25].

Table 3 summarizes some clinical tips on the use of melatonin, proposed during an expert consensus conference [71].

Table 3. Recommendations for prescribing melatonin in children with ASD. Adapted from Bruni et al. (2015) [71].

Consider melatonin in children with	Sleep-onset insomnia and/or difficulty awakening up in the morning.
Measure ...	DLMO when possible before starting the treatment.
Minimum age for administration	Administration after 6 months of age is generally considered safe.
Time of administration in children	- If used as sleep inductor: 30 min before bedtime.
	- If used as chronobiotic: 2–3 h before DLMO or 3–4 h before actual sleep-onset time.
Dosage	If used as a sleep inductor: - start with 1–3 mg (up to 5 mg in adolescents);
	- if needed, increase by 1–3 mg every 1–2 week until effect (maximum 3 mg if < 40 kg; up to 5–6 mg if > 40 kg (see text)).
	If used as chronobiotic: - start with a low dose of 0.2–0.5 mg; - if needed, increase by 0.2–0.5 mg every week until effect; - if no response after 1 week: increase dose by 1 mg every week until effect; - when 1 mg is effective: try lower dose.
Treatment duration	- Treatment duration should be tailored to the specific patient but in general should not be less than 1 month;
	Stopping successful treatment too early may result in relapse of insomnia.
	- Treatment can be withdrawn just before puberty (around 12 years of age) or shortly thereafter.
	- Stop melatonin treatment once a year for one week (preferably in summer) after a normal sleep cycle is established.
When melatonin treatment is not effective/loses effectiveness over time	- Check timing of administration.
	- Be aware that loss of efficacy of melatonin treatment is most likely caused by slow melatonin metabolism: in some cases, dose reduction is warranted instead of dose escalation.
	- Reconsider diagnosis: look for neuropsychiatric and medical comorbidities and treat them.
	- Concomitant medications can influence melatonin metabolism:
	e.g., ciprofloxacin, cimetidine, fluvoxamine (inhibitors) or carbamazepine, insulin, omeprazole (inducers).
If sleep maintenance problems after start of melatonin treatment	Melatonin dose is probably too high.

DLMO = Dim Light Melatonin Onset.

Recently, several studies have been published about the efficacy and safety of pediatric prolonged-release melatonin (PedPRM) in children with ASD. A randomized, double-blind controlled trial [97] in 125 subjects aged 2–17.5 years with ASD or Smith-Magenis syndrome showed that PedPRM mini-tablets (from 2 to 10 mg) significantly improved TST and SOL, with clinically relevant effect sizes. These improvements were well established after the first 3 weeks of treatment and then maintained throughout the entire duration of the study (13 weeks). Notably, 41% of participants responded initially to the low-dose (2 mg) PedPRM and did not require dose escalation; whereas, among the patients requiring a dose increase to the 5 mg PedPRM, half of them responded well, while the other half was eligible for further dose escalation to 10 mg. The authors did not report earlier morning awakenings in the PedPRM-treated group, differently from children treated with immediate-release melatonin [76]. There was no sign of tolerance development. Beside the decreased overall sleep disturbance, children's externalized disruptive behaviors and caregivers' quality of life also improved with PedPRM versus placebo [98]. The same authors then followed part of the subjects who completed the previous study up to 104 weeks of treatment, to assess long-term efficacy and safety of PedPRM [99,100]. They concluded that the improvements were maintained throughout the treatment period, and that children showed also longer uninterrupted sleep period and reduction in mid-sleep awakenings [99]. With regard to the tolerability profile, PedPRM seemed to be generally safe, the most frequent adverse reactions being fatigue (6.3%)—often reported after dose escalation and quickly resolved by decreasing the dose, sleepiness (6.3%) and mood swings (4.2%). There was no evidence of delayed growth or pubertal development and the discontinuation of PedPRM was not associated with withdrawal effects nor rebound insomnia.

4.2. Antihistamines

Histamine, together with other neurotransmitters (such as acetylcholine, norepinephrine, serotonin and orexin), is a major "wake-promoting" agent [101–104]. The histaminergic neurons in the central nervous system (CNS) are localized within the tuberomammillary nucleus in the posterior hypothalamus, which has therefore been described as a "wakefulness center". These neurons project mainly to the H1 and H3 receptors of the orexin-rich perifornical hypothalamus and the cholinergic neurons in the basal forebrain. The discharge activity of this histaminergic system is highest during attentive vigilance, while it is strongly reduced during quiet wakefulness, and completely suppressed during drowsiness, NREM, and REM sleep [104]. Differently from the past, antihistamine drugs are now considered to be inverse agonists of histamine receptors, instead of pure antagonists (H1-H4) [105–107]. Regarding the treatment of sleep problems, the first-generation ("sedating" and non-selective) H1-antihistamines are the most commonly used agents for pediatric insomnia [69,108], thanks to their ability to pass the blood–brain barrier and their minimal effects on sleep architecture (reduced duration of REM sleep) [103,109,110]. These include ethanolamines (such as diphenhydramine) and piperazine derivatives (such as hydroxyzine), the most frequently used medications, as well as others, such as trimeprazine and niaprazine.

Not all antihistamine drugs are sold OTC in all countries, as the drug markets are differently regulated in the different nations. Nevertheless, considering that the most widely used antihistamine—diphenhydramine—is a non-prescription drug in the US, we decided to include this class of medications in our review.

The common doses recommended by manufacturers and/or by experimental studies for these drugs are summarized in Table 4.

Table 4. Recommended dosages of some commonly used antihistamines for treating sleep disorders in children.

Antihistamine	Dosage	Effects on Sleep	Refs
Diphenhydramine	0.5 mg/kg up to 25 mg/day	↓ SOL; ↓ arousal threshold	[111,112]
Hydroxyzine	0.5–1 mg/kg/day	↓ SOL; ↓ arousal threshold	[113]
Niaprazine	1 mg/kg/day	↓ SOL; ↓ arousal threshold; effect on sleep maintenance (e.g., ↑ TST)	[114,115]
Most common side effects: daytime drowsiness, gastrointestinal disturbances (vomiting, constipation), paradoxical excitation, anti-cholinergic effects [25].			

↓ = decrease; ↑ = increase.

Despite that the use of antihistamines is widespread in the pediatric population, randomized controlled studies in children are lacking [18], and this is even more true in ASD [19]. The most often used antihistamine drug, diphenhydramine hydrochloride, has generally been studied in adults [114,116]. For adults, the usual dosage ranges from 25 to 50 mg/day while in children, the recommended dosage is 0.5 mg/kg/day up to a maximum of 25 mg/day. However, only one study investigated the effectiveness of this medication in children with sleep disorders aged 2 to 12 years [111], reporting reduced SOL and night awakenings. On the contrary, a more recent RCT [112] in children younger than 2 years showed that diphenhydramine was not more effective than placebo neither in reducing awakenings nor in improving parental satisfaction of their children's sleep. Also, hydroxyzine [113], and niaprazine [114,115] have been used to treat sleep disturbances in children: their usual dosage and effects on sleep are reported in Table 4. A randomized double-blind placebo-controlled trial [117] was conducted to test the efficacy of the antihistamine trimeprazine on sleep disturbances of infants aged 6 to 27 months, showing that this compound is clinically ineffective in treating this condition.

Other antihistamine compounds often used as sleep-inducing medications in adults include doxylamine, pyrilamine, cyproheptadine, and promethazine [107], even though they are more rarely used to treat pediatric insomnia.

As mentioned above, first-generation antihistamines cross the blood–brain barrier, therefore their most common adverse reactions at therapeutic dosage involve the CNS: fatigue, sedation, and sleepiness or, paradoxically, irritability, hyperactivity, and seizures. Notably, tolerance to these drugs can develop quickly, leading to dramatic hyperarousal as well as hyperactivity [118]. In the pediatric population, they might also affect learning: according to some authors [119], the use of a sedating antihistamine (diphenhydramine) can reduce learning abilities of atopic children if compared to second-generation (non-sedating) antihistamines or placebo. First-generation H1-antihistamines may interact also with other receptors, causing several other adverse reactions: anti-muscarinic effects (mydriasis, dry eyes, dry mouth, constipation, and urinary hesitancy and retention); anti-serotonin effects (increased appetite and weight gain); anti-alpha-adrenergic effects (dizziness and orthostatic hypotension) [109,110]. Some authors reported severe adverse reactions after the administration of diphenhydramine, including catatonic stupor, anxiety, visual hallucinations, and more rarely, respiratory insufficiency and seizures [120,121]. On the other hand, hydroxyzine is thought to be safer, with no fatal case reported [122]. An overdose of first-generation antihistamines is potentially lethal in children, due to cardiorespiratory arrest, anticholinergic syndrome (flushed skin, hallucinations, seizures, hypertension, fever), and CNS function suppression symptoms, such as lethargy, altered consciousness, and coma. Notably, infants and children often exhibit initial paradoxical hyperarousal, hallucinations, and seizures before progressing to coma [110,123].

Due to the lack of robust evidence and the relatively significant safety issues [25], antihistamines should not be used as a first-line approach for the pharmacological treatment of sleep disturbances in children and adolescents with ASD without comorbidities that would justify their use.

4.3. Tryptophan/5-Hydroxytryptophan

Tryptophan or L-tryptophan (Trp) is an essential amino acid, necessary for the biosynthesis of proteins. After ingestion, it participates in many metabolic pathways where it is converted into different bioactive molecules (such as serotonin, melatonin, kynurenine, and the vitamin niacin) [124]. 5-hydroxytryptophan (5-HTP) is the intermediate metabolite in the biosynthesis of serotonin from Trp and it easily crosses the blood–brain barrier. It is obtained from hydroxylation of Trp by the enzyme Trp-hydroxylase. As this is the rate-limiting step in serotonin synthesis, therapeutic doses of 5-HTP effectively increase the biosynthesis of serotonin in the CNS [25,125].

The mechanisms through which Trp/5-HTP influence sleep appear to be multiple and not completely understood. It is well established that by increasing the CNS concentration of serotonin, 5-HTP provides substrates for melatonin production and enhances serotonin-mediated regulation of sleep. The serotonergic system—in the past considered slow wave sleep-inducing but later regarded as wake-promoting—might actually have different effects on sleep that depend on its degree and timing of activation. Serotonin may indeed directly inhibit sleep, but subsequently induce a cascade of physiological processes that enhance sleep, mediated by yet to be identified sleep-promoting factors [126,127].

Trp at doses of 1 g/day or more has been shown to increase TST and decrease sleep latency and arousal after sleep onset in adults with insomnia [128,129]. It has not an opioid-like effect and does not prevent desired arousal from sleep, causing none [130] to negligible alterations of the physiological sleep architecture (minimal decrease in REM sleep and increase in NREM sleep) [131]. In subjects with neuropsychiatric syndromes and self-reported sleep disturbances, Trp given at bedtime (dosages from 1.2 g to 3 g) was found to increase the amount of slow wave sleep, without altering the amount of REM sleep [132]. Furthermore, Trp dietary intake in the general population has recently been shown to be positively associated with self-reported sleep duration [133]. As for 5-HTP, its use in healthy humans has been shown to increase REM sleep at dosages ranging from 200 to 600 mg/day [134].

Trp and 5-HTP appear to be safe and have few and mild side effects. However, in consideration of the possibility of serotonin syndrome, Trp and 5-HTP should not be used in patients currently treated with many antidepressants (such as monoamine oxidase inhibitors, SSRI, or tricyclic antidepressants) [135]. Tremor, nausea, and dizziness have been reported in association with Trp, but almost exclusively when taken at high doses (70–200 mg/kg/day) or in association with SSRI [136]. As for 5-HTP, some patients experience nausea and vomiting when taking it, especially at the beginning of treatment, but such symptoms are benign and usually transitory. It is suggested, to avoid them, to initiate the therapy at low doses and increase them gradually if necessary [135]. Reports of cases of eosinophilia-myalgia syndrome (EMS) in patients taking L-Trp in 1989 should not raise concerns about the use of Trp or 5-HTP as dietary supplements. Investigations found out that a contaminant, rather than Trp itself, had caused this illness: a new bacterial strain, used by a single manufacturer in the fermentation process of Trp, together with insufficient purification of the product, were responsible for the EMS epidemic [137]. Trp was temporarily banned from the market by the FDA, until 2005. Since then, Trp-containing products are available and commonly used as dietary supplements. After 1989, 5-HTP has become popular in place of Trp. Because of its biochemical similarity to Trp, 5-HTP has been under vigilance for its safety, but no ascertained cases of toxicity have emerged, even though 5-HTP is widely used worldwide. Extensive analyses of several sources of 5-HTP did not find toxic contaminants or any other significant impurity [137].

In the pediatric population, Trp and 5-HTP supplementation proved to be effective in reducing NREM parasomnias [138,139]. A clinical trial [139], conducted on 165 children and adolescents diagnosed with primary NREM parasomnia, compared the outcome of patients taking Trp (dose range: 500–4500 mg/day, mean dose of 2400 mg/day) with that of patients who chose not to be supplemented: an improvement in parasomnias was found in 84% of children using Trp, whereas only 47% of children not using it experienced a reduction in parasomnia symptoms ($p < 0.001$). Another clinical trial [138] proved that in a group of 45 children with sleep terrors, those taking 5-HTP (2 mg/kg/day at bedtime) not only improved their symptoms in a significantly greater proportion than those not being supplemented, but also maintained the improvements at the 6-month follow-up.

Furthermore, Trp seems to reduce night awakenings in children and adolescents. In a pilot study [140] on children aged 7 to 17 years, melatonin supplementation ("ME group") was compared to melatonin + vitamin B6 + Trp supplementation ("MET group"): after two months of supplementation, a statistically significant reduction of the number of night awakenings was found in the "MET group", but not in the "ME group". Similar results were found by another study [141] conducted on a large sample of younger children (748 patients aged 12 to 48 months) that had to undergo audiologic testing requiring the child to be asleep. A solution containing melatonin, Trp and vitamin B6 proved to be significantly more effective than melatonin alone in reducing the number of tests that had to be repeated due to awakening of the child. Such findings suggest the potential benefits of Trp in improving disrupted sleep in the pediatric population.

Interestingly, morning Trp ingestion seems to also have an influence on sleep onset and termination in children. A Japanese study [142] conducted on a large cohort investigated the relationship between dietary tryptophan intake at breakfast and some sleep characteristics, subjectively assessed using questionnaires. It was found that among preschoolers, those who reported a very short SOL, also reported a significantly higher Trp intake at breakfast than those who reported a very long SOL (mean Trp intake at breakfast: 440 mg versus 302 mg). Furthermore, in the same study the amount of Trp taken at breakfast seemed to inversely correlate with the frequency of difficulties in falling asleep and in waking up.

Nevertheless, Trp appears to improve sleep in children also when administered during night-time. In a clinical trial [143] conducted on 30 infants with sleep problems, participants were given tryptophan-enriched cereals and sleep-promoting formula milk with high levels of Trp at supper. The actigraphic evaluation of their sleep showed statistically significant improvements in sleep time, time spent in the crib and SE, if compared to the same parameters recorded during a control week. Such findings, while proving the effectiveness of Trp on children's sleep, leave uncertainties on the role played by the timing of its assumption.

As for children with ASD, experimental studies investigating the effects on sleep of Trp/5-HTP supplementation are lacking. However, data from metabolomic studies suggest alterations of the Trp metabolism in children affected by ASD [144–146]. More specifically, in these patients Trp appears to be preferentially transformed in metabolites of the kynurenine pathway, at the expense of the serotonin-melatonin pathway [146], thus potentially playing a crucial role in the pathogenesis of sleep disruption.

4.4. Carnosine

Carnosine or L-carnosine is a dipeptide composed by alanine and histidine, which acts as an antitoxic and neuroprotective agent in the nervous system and muscles [147]. Its circulating levels have been shown to be lower in autistic patients than controls [148,149] and recent studies suggest that high oxidative stress might contribute to the worsening of sleep disorders and behavioral symptoms in ASD individuals [88,150]. Some authors [151], therefore, suggested that 800 mg/day of carnosine might improve communication and behavior of autistic children.

As a consequence of this background, in a recent controlled trial [152], the effects of carnosine supplementation on children with ASD were tested. A cohort of 43 children with ASD, aged between 4 and 16 years, was randomized to 500 mg of L-carnosine or placebo, administered once daily for 2 months. The authors then monitored the effects of this treatment on sleep parameters and core autistic symptoms, through parent-report questionnaires. At the end of the supplementation period, significant improvements were observed in sleep duration, parasomnias, and total sleep disorders scores in the carnosine group, even though no effect size was provided. On the other hand, in disagreement with the previously cited study [151], the supplementation was found to have no effect on autism severity. No significant adverse reaction was reported by these authors.

4.5. Iron

Iron is the most abundant metal in the CNS and is crucial for various metabolic pathways within the brain. Its homeostasis in cerebral cells is therefore accurately regulated, so that the brain is less affected by acute diseases that reduce peripheral iron levels (e.g., acute anemia) in comparison with other organs. However, chronic imbalance of iron homeostasis can affect several cellular processes in which iron is involved: catecholamine synthesis and reuptake, serotonin synthesis, affinity, and expression of dopaminergic D2 receptors, mitochondrial efficiency, and myelination of neurons [153]. Furthermore, it has been shown [154] that iron deficiency—especially in the early stages of brain development—can lead to structural brain damages of several regions, such as hippocampus, basal nuclei, and cerebellum.

In recent years, the association between iron deficiency and sleep disorders has received growing attention in the scientific literature [155]. Low levels of iron have been associated with restless legs syndrome/periodic limb movement disorder (RLS/PLMD) [156] and RLS-induced insomnia [157,158], parasomnias [159], sleep disordered breathing [160], attention deficit and hyperactivity disorder (ADHD) [161], and "restless sleep disorder", a newly proposed diagnosis [162].

The prevalence of iron deficiency peaks in children [163], and even more in those with ASD. This might be also due to their frequently narrow food preference, which could lead to inadequate intake of iron and substances modulating its bioavailability ("enhancers", such as vitamin C or citrate; or "inhibitors", such as calcium and fibers) [164–166]. During the first stages of iron deficiency, ferritin levels—reflecting the iron stores—drop faster, while hemoglobin remains normal. As a consequence, measuring serum ferritin is suggested to detect non-anemic iron deficiency, especially in children with ASD and sleep disorders [18,167,168], even if false increases in ferritin levels are possible because ferritin is an acute-phase reactant [169].

However, it should be noted that data correlating ferritin concentration with sleep parameters in autistic children are unclear and further research is needed. Some authors [170] described in a group of 102 children (68 with ASD, 16 with developmental delay, and 18 controls) an association between low serum ferritin levels and sleep fragmentation with reduced SE, but a cause/effect relationship could not be confirmed. Moreover, in a retrospective study [171] enrolling 53 children with ASD, it was found that serum ferritin was significantly lower in patients with ASD and poor SE, compared to those with good SE, as measured by polysomnography. This study also reported that PLMD was significantly more frequent in children with ASD than in controls, but there was no significant difference in ferritin levels between autistic patients with and without PLMD. In another study [172], the effect of iron supplementation in 33 children with ASD and restless sleep was investigated. After 8 weeks of treatment with 6 mg/kg/day of elemental iron, the children's restlessness in bed improved significantly, as well as mean ferritin levels (from 16 μg/L to 29 μg/L), hemoglobin, and mean corpuscular volume. However, no correlation was found between restless sleep scores—as measured by two sleep questionnaires—and serum ferritin concentration. No improvement was described in other sleep parameters either.

As has been shown, only limited data are currently available for children with ASD. Nevertheless, many authors suggest the administration of iron supplements in this population when low ferritin levels (below 30–50 ng/mL) and poor sleep quality are both present [20,25,164]. The recommended initial dose in the pediatric age is usually 1–2 mg/kg/day of elemental iron divided in 2–3 doses between meals; the clinician may then titrate up to 6 mg/kg/day, in order to reach a serum ferritin concentration of 30–50 ng/mL or more [20,173]. Follow-up visits should be scheduled within 2–3 months of oral iron initiation, to check ferritin levels and to identify potential hinders to iron absorption and adherence to therapy [167]. Notably, the elemental iron should not be administered with milk or dairy products, nor with anti-acids, H2-receptors antagonists, and proton-pump inhibitors, which can affect iron absorption [166]. Compliance to therapy—especially in the pediatric age—has been shown to be the main problem for iron supplementation in children with RLS [167]. Indeed, many factors can affect adherence to treatment: poor palatability, frequent gastrointestinal side effects—such as constipation—[20,174], difficulty in swallowing pills, or teeth staining for liquid preparations [175].

4.6. Vitamin D

In healthy individuals, vitamin D, a fat-soluble pro-hormone, is mainly obtained by endogenous production taking place in the skin through the action of B band ultraviolet (UVB) solar radiation on a precursor molecule. A smaller amount of vitamin D also comes from dietary intake and supplementation. Vitamin D is then hydroxylated to 25-hydroxyvitamin D (25(OH)D) in the liver, and subsequently converted into the metabolically active form 1,25-dihydroxyvitamin D (calcitriol), primarily in the kidneys [176]. Maintaining calcium homeostasis and bone health are traditionally known as the main roles of vitamin D; however, there is growing evidence that vitamin D contributes to sleep regulation too and two mechanism have been proposed. First, similarly to other neuroactive steroids, vitamin D can modulate neuronal excitability via its receptors (VDR) in the brain. Several studies reported vitamin D to bind VDR in many sleep-regulating areas of the CNS (such as the anterior and posterior hypothalamus), thus potentially modulating their activation. Second, it has been found that the tryptophan hydroxylase-2 (TPH2) gene is regulated by a sequence of DNA known as the vitamin D response element. Vitamin D can therefore induce the expression of this brain enzyme and, consequently, the production of 5-HTP, precursor of serotonin and melatonin [177]. Furthermore, vitamin D has also been linked to the pathophysiology of RLS [178] through two main mechanisms: dopaminergic dysfunction and iron dysregulation. VDR are indeed highly expressed in the midbrain, in particular in the substantia nigra, supporting dopaminergic neurons survival by increasing glutathione and reducing oxidative stress in experimental models [179–181]. Moreover, it has been demonstrated that low vitamin D levels are often associated with iron deficiency in children, even if there is no clear etiological explanation for this correlation [182].

A prospective study on a large French pediatric cohort suggested an association between low serum levels of 25(OH)D in the cord blood and an increased risk of being a persistent short sleeper in preschool age [183]. However, another observational study [184] did not confirm the association between cord blood vitamin D deficiency and any sleep parameter, neither objectively nor subjectively assessed, at the age of 2 years. Nevertheless, the same study found that children with vitamin D deficiency at the age of 2 years had significantly shorter night sleep duration and total sleep duration—measured both subjectively and objectively—than those with normal vitamin D levels ($p < 0.05$). Furthermore, a clinical trial conducted in older Chinese children (age range 8–14 years) showed that 25(OH)D serum levels are positively correlated with sleep duration and that insufficiency/deficiency of vitamin D (25(OH)D $\leq$ 20 ng/mL) is independently associated with an increased probability of insufficient sleep [185].

In children with ASD—to our knowledge—no adequate interventional study has been carried out to investigate the effects of vitamin D supplementation on sleep. Despite that, in recent years an increasing number of studies have shown lower serum levels of vitamin D in children with ASD than in neurotypical children [186,187]. Consequently, it might be useful to assess vitamin D levels in autistic children with sleep disturbances [18]. A fairly large consensus exists that when a vitamin D deficiency is found, an appropriate dosage for supplementation in all infants and most children is 400–600 international units (IU)/day, i.e., approximately 10–15 μg/day. [188]. However, some authors reported that vitamin D blood levels are more relevant than the administered dose in improving sleep quality, with the most beneficial effects on sleep being obtained for 25(OH)D hematic concentrations of 60–80 ng/mL [189].

4.7. Multivitamin and Mineral Supplements

Based on the finding that plasma levels of many vitamins and minerals are often lower in children with ASD than in neurotypical children, a placebo-controlled trial was conducted in which multivitamin and mineral supplements were administered for 3 months to autistic children, aged 3 to 8 years [190]. At the end of the study period, many domains of health and behavior of the children, including sleep, were assessed by means of a parent-report questionnaire. Compared to the placebo group, the group taking the supplement had slightly better scores in the sleep domain of the questionnaire ($p < 0.05$). However, the small sample size and the lack of detailed sleep assessment before and after supplementation make the evidence provided by this study quite weak. A similar study was conducted later on a larger group of children and adults with ASD [191], but the sleep scores of the questionnaire showed no statistically significant difference between the placebo group and multivitamin and mineral supplement group. These findings suggest that to date, there is no evidence supporting the use of multivitamin and mineral supplements for the treatment of sleep disturbances in autistic children and adolescents.

4.8. Herbal Remedies

The use of herbal remedies as an alternative treatment for sleep disturbances is widespread because these products are readily accessible over the counter and generally perceived to be safe [192]. However, there is limited scientific support of the efficacy and safety of many herbs traditionally known for their sedative effects [125,193]. We will here review the evidence available for valerian, lemon balm, passionflower, lavender, St. John's Wort, and chamomile.

Valerian (*Valeriana* spp.) is the most studied herbal remedy for insomnia. Extracts from its roots are commonly used for their sedative and anxiolytic effects and it has indeed been shown that they may modulate cortical excitability in humans [194]. As for other herbal remedies, the therapeutic effects of valerian may rise both from the individual effects of each of its constituents (volatile sesquiterpenes, valepotriates and amino acids) and from their reciprocal interactions on the gamma aminobutyric acid (GABA) and adenosine systems [195,196]. As a sedative, valerian is usually administered 30 to 60 min before bedtime, with an average daily dose of 912 mg (ranging from 300 to 3645 mg/day in different studies) [125,197]. Results of clinical trials testing the effects on sleep of different species of valerian (*officinalis*, *edulis*, *wallichii* or unspecified) are conflicting and controversial. In 2015, a meta-analysis [197] including 12 RCT described no significant difference between valerian supplements and placebo in improving SOL, sleep duration, SE, WASO, or sleep quality. Nevertheless, a recent systematic review [193] including 17 studies—nine of which did not appear in the meta-analysis cited above—reported mixed findings: several trials showed improvements in sleep quality and other subjective parameters of sleep after administration of valerian [198–200], while other studies did not find any significant effect [201–203]. However, many of these trials had relevant limitations, such as the lack of objective measures of sleep parameters or small samples. Regarding adverse effects of valerian, gastrointestinal upset, contact allergies, headache, restless sleep, and mydriasis have rarely been reported [125]. One study [204] signaled a significantly greater incidence of diarrhea in subjects treated with valerian; however, this has not been confirmed by other studies [197].

Lemon balm (*Melissa officinalis*) is a perennial herb alleged to have hypnotic properties [205]. In healthy volunteers, the administration of 240 mg/day of *Melissa officinalis* extract, together with 360 mg of *Valeriana officinalis* root extract, before bedtime, improved sleep quality with a statistically significant difference over placebo [206]. In patients with mild-to-moderate anxiety and sleep disturbances, 600 mg of lemon balm leaf extract were found to reduce anxiety-related insomnia [207] and in menopausal women 160 mg of *Melissa officinalis* extract, associated with 320 mg/day of *Valeriana officinalis*, reduced symptoms of sleep disorders [200]. The effectiveness and tolerability of a combined valerian/lemon balm preparation on dyssomnia were investigated in children as well [208]. In this study, conducted on a large sample of patients younger than 12 years, dosages were patient-tailored, up to 640 mg/day of valerian and 320 mg/day of lemon balm, and the treatment lasted for 4 weeks (+/−1 week). In total, 80.9% of the patients who suffered from dyssomnia experienced an improvement and the supplement was judged to have a good tolerability in 96.7% of them. However, it should be noticed that symptoms were subjectively assessed by parents without a standardized and validated questionnaire and that the study was not placebo-controlled. Another clinical trial, aiming to assess the action of different herbal preparations on parent-reported sleep bruxism in children, reported mixed findings: Melissa officinalis resulted effective when symptoms were assessed through a Visual Analogue Scale, but ineffective, when the sleep diaries were considered [209].

Passiflora incarnata, commonly known as passionflower, has a history of use for the treatment of anxiety and insomnia symptoms [210]. An experimental study showed that passionflower can positively affect sleep regulation by modulating the expression of several circadian clock genes [211]. However, its exact mechanism of action is not entirely known. A recent RCT investigated the effects of passionflower extract tea on polysomnographic sleep parameters in a large sample of adults with insomnia, finding a significant increase in TST—but not in SE and WASO—in the passionflower group compared to the placebo group [212].

Lavender (*Lavandula*) has been studied in recent years for its effects on anxiety and sleep in adults. In 2010, in a RCT [213], 80 mg of oral lavender oil supplements (silexan) administered for 6 weeks were shown to be as effective as a common benzodiazepine (lorazepam) in adults with generalized anxiety disorder, improving both anxiety scores and subjectively reported sleep quality. Moreover, two other RCT [214,215] confirmed the anxiolytic effect of 80 mg/day of silexan for 10 weeks, also suggesting its effectiveness in reducing anxiety-related disturbed sleep, as measured by the Pittsburgh Sleep Quality Index (PSQI). Finally, in 2012 a phase II open-label trial on patients with post-traumatic stress disorder or somatization disorder [216], showed an improvement in morning tiredness and night awakenings, as reported in their sleep diaries, after 6 weeks of treatment with 80 mg/day of silexan. The main adverse reactions reported were mild or moderate gastrointestinal complaints.

St. John's Wort (*Hypericum perforatum*) is a flowering herb used for a variety of clinical conditions, such as depression, anxiety, and sleep disorders. The most active components are thought to be hyperforin and hypericin, although other components have bioactivity [125]. A major role is apparently held by hyperforin, which inhibits the reuptake of serotonin, norepinephrine, dopamine, GABA, and L-glutamate [217,218], even if further research is needed to clarify the mechanisms of action of *Hypericum* [219]. No published clinical trial specifically investigated the effects of St. John's Wort on sleep disturbances. However, it has been reported that in adults, 900 mg of St. John's Wort decreased scores of the sleep problem scale [220] and increased REM sleep latency [221] compared with placebo. Side effects associated with St. John's Wort during clinical trials included gastrointestinal complaints, dizziness, fatigue, anxiety, photosensitivity and headaches [125]. However, the main concern about St. John's Wort use is the possibility of severe drug interactions, mediated by the CYP450 and intestinal P-glycoprotein induction and by its serotonin-promoting effects.

German chamomile (*Matricaria recutita*) is a member of the daisy plant family, widely used as a natural remedy for a variety of mild clinical problems, among which insomnia. Sedative effects of German chamomile are mild and may be due to a benzodiazepine-like compound found in the flowerhead, the flavonoid apigenin, which binds the benzodiazepine receptors [192]. Although chamomile has a popular reputation of being a relaxing and sleep-facilitating compound, clinical studies are scarce. A study on elderly people who were administered chamomile extract (400 mg/day) for 28 days reported improvements in general sleep quality and SOL assessed by the PSQI [222], while another study on sleep-disturbed postpartum women found a mild improvement only in self-reported "physical symptoms-related sleep inefficiency" after 2 weeks of chamomile tea, but not after 4 weeks [223]. Moreover, in a randomized, double-blind, placebo-controlled pilot trial with subjects suffering from primary chronic insomnia, no significant differences over placebo were found in Insomnia Severity Index (ISI) and PSQI following the administration of 540 mg/day of chamomile for 28 days [224].

To the extent of our knowledge, no study has evaluated the clinical effectiveness of the above-mentioned herbal remedies on sleep disturbances in children with ASD [54].

5. Conclusions

Sleep disturbances in children with ASD are a challenging issue for patients, families, and clinicians. Non-pharmacological and oral non-prescription treatments are widely used to treat these conditions. Despite that, the available evidence on the subject is limited and often controversial. We reviewed the literature concerning these therapeutic approaches, to provide practitioners with a comprehensive guide.

The first step in approaching sleep problems in children and adolescents with ASD should always be parent counseling to implement good sleep habits and behavioral techniques. We have reported above the mnemonic tool "ABCs of SLEEPING" summarizing several evidence-based sleep hygiene practices, and the most studied behavioral interventions for sleep in children, such as standard and gradual extinction, positive reinforcement, and bedtime fading. Notably, the behavioral approach to use should be chosen according to the parents' preferences, given that there is no conclusive evidence that one technique is more effective than another, and that caregivers motivation is crucial to the success of these interventions. Furthermore, when there is a decision to start a pharmacologic treatment, behavioral interventions and good sleep hygiene practices should be always maintained.

With regard to the other non-pharmacological interventions reviewed (weighted blankets and vests, mattress-based technologies, massage, aromatherapy, yoga, sports, and physical activity), no strong evidence recommending their use to improve sleep in children and adolescents with

ASD is available. However, promising results come from a small number of clinical trials using mattress-based technologies, yoga therapy, massage, and physical activity, showing at the same time no significant adverse effect. While awaiting further well-designed studies on larger samples, some of these interventions might be reasonable options in specific cases, even though we recommend that clinicians inform parents of the lack of strong evidence, if asked for their opinion on these interventions.

Among the oral non-prescription sleep-promoting agents reviewed above, melatonin is one of the most used and studied substances in children with ASD, given their often-abnormal melatonin plasma levels. Melatonin has been shown to be both effective and relatively safe and has, indeed, strong evidence of positive effect on SOL, TST, bedtime resistance, and co-sleeping, while it has only moderate or lower effects in improving other sleep problems, such as frequent night awakenings. Furthermore, a greater effectiveness of melatonin has also been suggested when administered in association with a cognitive-behavioral intervention. Recently, a prolonged-release formulation of melatonin has been approved for use in children with ASD. Advantages of this treatment compared to immediate-release melatonin are improvements in sleep disruption, night-time and early-morning awakenings, as well as in disruptive behaviors. In long-term studies (up to 104 weeks) no significant adverse event has been reported, excluding also relevant consequences on pubertal growth.

As for sedating antihistamines, despite their widespread use as sleep-inducing agents in the pediatric population, there is limited evidence of their effectiveness in improving sleep in children, and no evidence at all for children and adolescents with ASD. Moreover, the frequent and quickly developing tolerance to these molecules, as well as their relatively significant safety issues, make antihistamines unsuitable medications for a first-line approach to sleep disturbances in autistic children and adolescents. Nevertheless, their use may be appropriate in patients that do not benefit from first-line treatment strategies, as well as in those with comorbid allergic symptoms.

Regarding tryptophan and its metabolite 5-HTP, the alterations of their metabolism found in patients with autism make these molecules a reasonable treatment option for autistic children with comorbid sleep problems, especially for those experiencing parasomnias and frequent night awakenings; tryptophan and 5-HTP have indeed been found to improve such symptoms in neurotypical children. Other positive aspects of this supplement seem to be the relative absence of side effects and the lack of development of tolerance with long-term use.

As for carnosine, it has shown promising, yet preliminary results in improving sleep in a small sample of autistic children and adolescents; further research is needed to confirm the effectiveness of this molecule as a treatment for sleep disorders in children with and without ASD.

We also reviewed the increasing evidence linking iron deficiency to sleep disorders: even if this topic has been thoroughly investigated in the pediatric age, the data currently available on children with ASD are scarce. Nevertheless, some authors suggest checking serum ferritin levels in autistic children with sleep disturbances and to administer oral iron supplements when low ferritin levels and poor sleep quality—especially restlessness in sleep—are both present.

As for vitamin D, even if no clinical trial has proven beneficial effects of this molecule on sleep in the pediatric population with ASD, there is sufficient evidence that vitamin D deficiency in children is associated with bad sleep. It is, therefore, often suggested to monitor serum 25(OH)D level in all children and adolescents with ASD and comorbid sleep disorder and to supplement them if vitamin D deficiency is found.

Tentative treatments with multivitamin and mineral supplements for sleep problems have also been carried out, based on the finding of low plasma levels of many vitamins and minerals in children with ASD, but the available evidence does not support this kind of treatment.

Concerning herbal remedies, to the extent of our knowledge, no study has evaluated the clinical effectiveness of valerian, lemon balm, passionflower, lavender, St. John's Wort, and chamomile on sleep disturbances in children with ASD. Moreover, even in other populations the evidence is limited and often mixed. Promising results in improving sleep have been found by some studies on adults and neurotypical children using valerian—alone or in association with lemon balm-, passionflower, and lavender oil. Nevertheless, well-designed, placebo-controlled clinical trials on larger samples are needed to confirm such findings. Therefore, the use of these substances—alone or as an adjunctive therapy—in the autistic pediatric population should be guided by clinical experience and parents should be provided with information about their known efficacy, safety profile, and possible interactions with other treatments—especially for St. John's Wort, the use of which should be discouraged, given the relevant safety concerns.

In conclusion, whereas for some non-pharmacological interventions and oral non-prescription treatments effectiveness on sleep disturbances in ASD children and adolescents has been ascertained, for other remedies—despite their common use—further and rigorous research is needed.

Author Contributions: Conceptualization, O.B., A.B. and D.E.; methodology, O.B.; validation, O.B. and R.F.; investigation, A.B. and D.E.; data curation, A.B. and D.E.; writing—original draft preparation, A.B. and D.E.; writing—review and editing, O.B. and R.F.; visualization, A.B. and D.E.; supervision, O.B. and R.F.; project administration, O.B. All authors have read and agreed to the published version of the manuscript.

Acknowledgments: In this section you can acknowledge any support given which is not covered by the author contribution or funding sections. This may include administrative and technical support, or donations in kind (e.g., materials used for experiments).

References

1. Lai, M.-C.; Lombardo, M.V.; Baron-Cohen, S. Autism. *Lancet* **2014**, *383*, 896–910. [CrossRef]
2. Carmassi, C.; Palagini, L.; Caruso, D.; Masci, I.; Nobili, L.; Vita, A.; Dell'Osso, L. Systematic Review of Sleep Disturbances and Circadian Sleep Desynchronization in Autism Spectrum Disorder: Toward an Integrative Model of a Self-Reinforcing Loop. *Front. Psychiatry* **2019**, *10*, 366. [CrossRef]
3. Souders, M.C.; Zavodny, S.; Eriksen, W.; Sinko, R.; Connell, J.; Kerns, C.; Schaaf, R.; Pinto-Martin, J. Sleep in Children with Autism Spectrum Disorder. *Curr. Psychiatry Rep.* **2017**, *19*, 34. [CrossRef]
4. Klukowski, M.; Wasilewska, J.; Lebensztejn, D. Sleep and gastrointestinal disturbances in autism spectrum disorder in children. *Dev. Period. Med.* **2015**, *19*, 157–161.
5. Grigg-Damberger, M.; Ralls, F. Treatment strategies for complex behavioral insomnia in children with neurodevelopmental disorders. *Curr. Opin. Pulm. Med.* **2013**, *19*, 616–625. [CrossRef] [PubMed]
6. Henderson, K. Policies and Practices Used by States to Serve Children with Autism Spectrum Disorders. *J. Disabil. Policy Stud.* **2011**, *22*, 106–115. [CrossRef]
7. Sikora, D.M.; Johnson, K.; Clemons, T.; Katz, T. The relationship between sleep problems and daytime behavior in children of different ages with autism spectrum disorders. *Pediatrics* **2012**, *130* (Suppl. 2), S83–S90. [CrossRef] [PubMed]
8. Cohen, S.; Conduit, R.; Lockley, S.W.; Rajaratnam, S.M.; Cornish, K.M. The relationship between sleep and behavior in autism spectrum disorder (ASD): A review. *J. Neurodev. Disord.* **2014**, *6*, 44. [CrossRef]
9. Shui, A.M.; Katz, T.; Malow, B.A.; Mazurek, M.O. Predicting sleep problems in children with autism spectrum disorders. *Res. Dev. Disabil.* **2018**, *83*, 270–279. [CrossRef]
10. Howlett, M.; Jemcov, A.; Adams, A.; Corkum, P. ABCs of SLEEPING tool: Improving access to care for pediatric insomnia. *Clin. Pract. Pediatr. Psychol.* **2020**, *8*, 1–12. [CrossRef]
11. Goodday, A.; Corkum, P.; Smith, I.M. Parental Acceptance of Treatments for Insomnia in Children with Attention-Deficit/Hyperactivity Disorder, Autistic Spectrum Disorder, and their Typically Developing Peers. *Child. Health Care* **2014**, *43*, 54–71. [CrossRef]
12. Heussler, H.; Chan, P.; Price, A.M.H.; Waters, K.; Davey, M.J.; Hiscock, H. Pharmacological and non-pharmacological management of sleep disturbance in children: An Australian Paediatric Research Network survey. *Sleep Med.* **2013**, *14*, 189–194. [CrossRef] [PubMed]
13. Whitehouse, A.J.O. Complementary and alternative medicine for autism spectrum disorders: Rationale, safety and efficacy. *J. Paediatr. Child. Health* **2013**, *49*, E438–E442. [CrossRef] [PubMed]

14. Brondino, N.; Fusar-Poli, L.; Rocchetti, M.; Provenzani, U.; Barale, F.; Politi, P. Complementary and Alternative Therapies for Autism Spectrum Disorder. *Evid. Based Complement. Alternat. Med.* **2015**, *2015*, 258589. [CrossRef]
15. Wang, C.; Preisser, J.; Chung, Y.; Li, K. Complementary and alternative medicine use among children with mental health issues: Results from the National Health Interview Survey. *BMC Complement. Altern. Med.* **2018**, *18*, 241. [CrossRef]
16. Keogh, S.; Bridle, C.; Siriwardena, N.A.; Nadkarni, A.; Laparidou, D.; Durrant, S.J.; Kargas, N.; Law, G.R.; Curtis, F. Effectiveness of non-pharmacological interventions for insomnia in children with Autism Spectrum Disorder: A systematic review and meta-analysis. *PLoS ONE* **2019**, *14*, e0221428. [CrossRef]
17. Williams Buckley, A.; Hirtz, D.; Oskoui, M.; Armstrong, M.J.; Batra, A.; Bridgemohan, C.; Coury, D.; Dawson, G.; Donley, D.; Findling, R.L.; et al. Practice guideline: Treatment for insomnia and disrupted sleep behavior in children and adolescents with autism spectrum disorder: Report of the Guideline Development, Dissemination, and Implementation Subcommittee of the American Academy of Neurology. *Neurology* **2020**, *94*, 392–404. [CrossRef]
18. Bruni, O.; Angriman, M.; Melegari, M.G.; Ferri, R. Pharmacotherapeutic management of sleep disorders in children with neurodevelopmental disorders. *Expert Opin. Pharmacother.* **2019**, *20*, 2257–2271. [CrossRef]
19. Relia, S.; Ekambaram, V. Pharmacological Approach to Sleep Disturbances in Autism Spectrum Disorders with Psychiatric Comorbidities: A Literature Review. *Med. Sci.* **2018**, *6*, 95. [CrossRef]
20. Blackmer, A.B.; Feinstein, J.A. Management of Sleep Disorders in Children with Neurodevelopmental Disorders: A Review. *Pharmacotherapy* **2016**, *36*, 84–98. [CrossRef]
21. Malow, B.; MacDonald, L.; Fawkes, D.; Alder, M.; Katz, T. Teaching Children with Autism Spectrum Disorder How to Sleep Better: A Pilot Educational Program for Parents. *Clin. Pract. Pediatr. Psychol.* **2016**, *4*. [CrossRef]
22. Carnett, A.; Hansen, S.; McLay, L.; Neely, L.; Lang, R. Quantitative-Analysis of Behavioral Interventions to Treat Sleep Problems in Children with Autism. *Dev. Neurorehabil.* **2019**, 1–14. [CrossRef] [PubMed]
23. Jan, J.E.; Owens, J.A.; Weiss, M.D.; Johnson, K.P.; Wasdell, M.B.; Freeman, R.D.; Ipsiroglu, O.S. Sleep hygiene for children with neurodevelopmental disabilities. *Pediatrics* **2008**, *122*, 1343–1350. [CrossRef] [PubMed]
24. Honaker, S.M.; Meltzer, L.J. Bedtime Problems and Night Awakenings in Young Children: An Update of the Evidence. *Paediatr. Respir. Rev.* **2014**, *15*, 333–339. [CrossRef]
25. Bruni, O.; Angriman, M.; Calisti, F.; Comandini, A.; Esposito, G.; Cortese, S.; Ferri, R. Practitioner Review: Treatment of chronic insomnia in children and adolescents with neurodevelopmental disabilities. *J. Child. Psychol. Psychiatry* **2018**, *59*, 489–508. [CrossRef]
26. Adkins, K.W.; Molloy, C.; Weiss, S.K.; Reynolds, A.; Goldman, S.E.; Burnette, C.; Clemons, T.; Fawkes, D.; Malow, B.A. Effects of a standardized pamphlet on insomnia in children with autism spectrum disorders. *Pediatrics* **2012**, *130* (Suppl. 2), S139–S144. [CrossRef]
27. Malow, B.A.; Adkins, K.W.; Reynolds, A.; Weiss, S.K.; Loh, A.; Fawkes, D.; Katz, T.; Goldman, S.E.; Madduri, N.; Hundley, R.; et al. Parent-based sleep education for children with autism spectrum disorders. *J. Autism Dev. Disord.* **2014**, *44*, 216–228. [CrossRef]
28. Johnson, C.R.; Turner, K.S.; Foldes, E.; Brooks, M.M.; Kronk, R.; Wiggs, L. Behavioral parent training to address sleep disturbances in young children with autism spectrum disorder: A pilot trial. *Sleep Med.* **2013**, *14*, 995–1004. [CrossRef]
29. Papadopoulos, N.; Sciberras, E.; Hiscock, H.; Williams, K.; McGillivray, J.; Mihalopoulos, C.; Engel, L.; Fuller-Tyszkiewicz, M.; Bellows, S.T.; Marks, D.; et al. Sleeping sound with autism spectrum disorder (ASD): Study protocol for an efficacy randomised controlled trial of a tailored brief behavioural sleep intervention for ASD. *BMJ Open* **2019**, *9*, e029767. [CrossRef]
30. Cuomo, B.M.; Vaz, S.; Lee, E.A.L.; Thompson, C.; Rogerson, J.M.; Falkmer, T. Effectiveness of Sleep-Based Interventions for Children with Autism Spectrum Disorder: A Meta-Synthesis. *Pharmacotherapy* **2017**, *37*, 555–578. [CrossRef]
31. Roberts, C.A.; Smith, K.C.; Sherman, A.K. Comparison of Online and Face-to-Face Parent Education for Children with Autism and Sleep Problems. *J. Autism Dev. Disord.* **2019**, *49*, 1410–1422. [CrossRef] [PubMed]
32. Kirkpatrick, B.; Louw, J.S.; Leader, G. Efficacy of parent training incorporated in behavioral sleep interventions for children with autism spectrum disorder and/or intellectual disabilities: A systematic review. *Sleep Med.* **2019**, *53*, 141–152. [CrossRef] [PubMed]

33. McLay, L.K.; France, K.G.; Knight, J.; Blampied, N.M.; Hastie, B. The effectiveness of function-based interventions to treat sleep problems, including unwanted co-sleeping, in children with autism. *Behav. Interv.* **2019**, *34*, 30–51.
34. Allen, S.L.; Howlett, M.D.; Coulombe, J.A.; Corkum, P.V. ABCs of SLEEPING: A review of the evidence behind pediatric sleep practice recommendations. *Sleep Med. Rev.* **2016**, *29*, 1–14. [CrossRef] [PubMed]
35. Paruthi, S.; Brooks, L.J.; D'Ambrosio, C.; Hall, W.A.; Kotagal, S.; Lloyd, R.M.; Malow, B.A.; Maski, K.; Nichols, C.; Quan, S.F.; et al. Recommended Amount of Sleep for Pediatric Populations: A Consensus Statement of the American Academy of Sleep Medicine. *J. Clin. Sleep Med.* **2016**, *12*, 785–786. [CrossRef]
36. Owens, J.A.; Mindell, J.A. Pediatric insomnia. *Pediatr. Clin. N. Am.* **2011**, *58*, 555–569. [CrossRef]
37. Turner, K.S.; Johnson, C.R. Behavioral Interventions to Address Sleep Disturbances in Children with Autism Spectrum Disorders: A Review. *Top. Early Child. Spec. Educ.* **2013**, *33*, 144–152. [CrossRef]
38. Weiskop, S.; Matthews, J.; Richdale, A. Treatment of sleep problems in a 5-year-old boy with autism using behavioural principles. *Autism* **2001**, *5*, 209–221. [CrossRef]
39. Herrmann, S. Counting Sheep: Sleep Disorders in Children with Autism Spectrum Disorders. *J. Pediatr Health Care* **2016**, *30*, 143–154. [CrossRef]
40. Vriend, J.L.; Corkum, P.V.; Moon, E.C.; Smith, I.M. Behavioral interventions for sleep problems in children with autism spectrum disorders: Current findings and future directions. *J. Pediatr Psychol.* **2011**, *36*, 1017–1029. [CrossRef]
41. Weiskop, S.; Richdale, A.; Matthews, J. Behavioural treatment to reduce sleep problems in children with autism or fragile X syndrome. *Dev. Med. Child. Neurol.* **2005**, *47*, 94–104. [CrossRef] [PubMed]
42. Rigney, G.; Ali, N.S.; Corkum, P.V.; Brown, C.A.; Constantin, E.; Godbout, R.; Hanlon-Dearman, A.; Ipsiroglu, O.; Reid, G.J.; Shea, S.; et al. A systematic review to explore the feasibility of a behavioural sleep intervention for insomnia in children with neurodevelopmental disorders: A transdiagnostic approach. *Sleep Med. Rev.* **2018**, *41*, 244–254. [CrossRef] [PubMed]
43. Schreck, K.A. Behavioral treatments for sleep problems in autism: Empirically supported or just universally accepted? *Behav. Interv.* **2001**, *16*, 265–278. [CrossRef]
44. Didden, R.; Curfs, L.M.; Sikkema, S.P.; de Moor, J. Functional assessment and treatment of sleeping problems with developmentally disabled children: Six case studies. *J. Behav. Ther. Exp. Psychiatry* **1998**, *29*, 85–97. [CrossRef]
45. Curfs, L.M.; Didden, R.; Sikkema, S.P.; De Die-Smulders, C.E. Management of sleeping problems in Wolf-Hirschhorn syndrome: A case study. *Genet. Couns.* **1999**, *10*, 345–350. [PubMed]
46. Bramble, D. Rapid-acting treatment for a common sleep problem. *Dev. Med. Child. Neurol.* **1997**, *39*, 543–547.
47. Allen, K.D.; Kuhn, B.R.; DeHaai, K.A.; Wallace, D.P. Evaluation of a behavioral treatment package to reduce sleep problems in children with Angelman Syndrome. *Res. Dev. Disabil.* **2013**, *34*, 676–686. [CrossRef]
48. Kodak, T.; Piazza, C.C. Assessment and behavioral treatment of feeding and sleeping disorders in children with autism spectrum disorders. *Child. Adolesc. Psychiatr. Clin. N. Am.* **2008**, *17*, 887–905. [CrossRef]
49. Van Deurs, J.R.; McLay, L.K.; France, K.G.; Blampied, N.M.; Lang, R.B.; Hunter, J.E. Behavioral Sleep Intervention for Adolescents with Autism Spectrum Disorder: A Pilot Study. *Adv. Neurodev. Disord.* **2019**, *3*, 397–410. [CrossRef]
50. National Autism Center. *National Standards Report—Addressing the Need for Evidence-Based Practice Guidelines for Autism Spectrum Disorders*; National Autism Center: Randolph, MA, USA, 2009; pp. 1–3.
51. Wiggs, L.; France, K. Behavioural treatments for sleep problems in children and adolescents with physical illness, psychological problems or intellectual disabilities. *Sleep Med. Rev.* **2000**, *4*, 299–314. [CrossRef]
52. Angriman, M.; Caravale, B.; Novelli, L.; Ferri, R.; Bruni, O. Sleep in children with neurodevelopmental disabilities. *Neuropediatrics* **2015**, *46*, 199–210. [CrossRef] [PubMed]
53. Creasey, N.; Finlay, F. Question 2: Do weighted blankets improve sleep in children with an autistic spectrum disorder? *Arch. Dis. Child.* **2013**, *98*, 919–920. [CrossRef] [PubMed]
54. McLay, L.-L.K.; France, K. Empirical research evaluating non-traditional approaches to managing sleep problems in children with autism. *Dev. Neurorehabil.* **2016**, *19*, 123–134. [CrossRef] [PubMed]
55. Gringras, P.; Green, D.; Wright, B.; Rush, C.; Sparrowhawk, M.; Pratt, K.; Allgar, V.; Hooke, N.; Moore, D.; Zaiwalla, Z.; et al. Weighted blankets and sleep in autistic children–a randomized controlled trial. *Pediatrics* **2014**, *134*, 298–306. [CrossRef] [PubMed]

56. Frazier, T.W.; Krishna, J.; Klingemier, E.; Beukemann, M.; Nawabit, R.; Ibrahim, S. A Randomized, Crossover Trial of a Novel Sound-to-Sleep Mattress Technology in Children with Autism and Sleep Difficulties. *J. Clin. Sleep Med.* **2017**, *13*, 95–104. [CrossRef] [PubMed]
57. Escalona, A.; Field, T.; Singer-Strunck, R.; Cullen, C.; Hartshorn, K. Brief report: Improvements in the behavior of children with autism following massage therapy. *J. Autism Dev. Disord.* **2001**, *31*, 513–516. [CrossRef]
58. Silva, L.M.T.; Cignolini, A.; Warren, R.; Budden, S.; Skowron-Gooch, A. Improvement in sensory impairment and social interaction in young children with autism following treatment with an original Qigong massage methodology. *Am. J. Chin. Med.* **2007**, *35*, 393–406. [CrossRef]
59. Piravej, K.; Tangtrongchitr, P.; Chandarasiri, P.; Paothong, L.; Sukprasong, S. Effects of Thai traditional massage on autistic children's behavior. *J. Altern. Complement. Med.* **2009**, *15*, 1355–1361. [CrossRef]
60. Silva, L.M.T.; Schalock, M.; Ayres, R.; Bunse, C.; Budden, S. Qigong massage treatment for sensory and self-regulation problems in young children with autism: A randomized controlled trial. *Am. J. Occup. Ther.* **2009**, *63*, 423–432. [CrossRef]
61. Williams, T.I. Evaluating Effects of Aromatherapy Massage on Sleep in Children with Autism: A Pilot Study. *Evid. Based Complement. Altern. Med.* **2006**, *3*, 373–377. [CrossRef]
62. Narasingharao, K.; Pradhan, B.; Navaneetham, J. Efficacy of Structured Yoga Intervention for Sleep, Gastrointestinal and Behaviour Problems of ASD Children: An Exploratory Study. *J. Clin. Diagn. Res.* **2017**, *11*, VC01–VC06. [CrossRef] [PubMed]
63. Wachob, D.; Lorenzi, D.G. Brief Report: Influence of Physical Activity on Sleep Quality in Children with Autism. *J. Autism Dev. Disord.* **2015**, *45*, 2641–2646. [CrossRef] [PubMed]
64. Tse, C.Y.A.; Lee, H.P.; Chan, K.S.K.; Edgar, V.B.; Wilkinson-Smith, A.; Lai, W.H.E. Examining the impact of physical activity on sleep quality and executive functions in children with autism spectrum disorder: A randomized controlled trial. *Autism* **2019**, *23*, 1699–1710. [CrossRef] [PubMed]
65. Brand, S.; Jossen, S.; Holsboer-Trachsler, E.; Pühse, U.; Gerber, M. Impact of aerobic exercise on sleep and motor skills in children with autism spectrum disorders—A pilot study. *Neuropsychiatr. Dis. Treat.* **2015**, *11*, 1911–1920. [CrossRef]
66. Oriel, K.N.; Kanupka, J.W.; DeLong, K.S.; Noel, K. The Impact of Aquatic Exercise on Sleep Behaviors in Children With Autism Spectrum Disorder: A Pilot Study. *Focus Autism Dev. Disabil.* **2016**, *31*, 254–261. [CrossRef]
67. Lawson, L.M.; Little, L. Feasibility of a Swimming Intervention to Improve Sleep Behaviors of Children with Autism Spectrum Disorder. *Ther. Recreat. J.* **2017**, *51*. [CrossRef]
68. Pelayo, R.; Yuen, K. Pediatric sleep pharmacology. *Child. Adolesc. Psychiatr. Clin. N. Am.* **2012**, *21*, 861–883. [CrossRef]
69. Owens, J.A.; Rosen, C.L.; Mindell, J.A. Medication use in the treatment of pediatric insomnia: Results of a survey of community-based pediatricians. *Pediatrics* **2003**, *111*, e628–e635. [CrossRef]
70. Kennaway, D.J. Melatonin and development: Physiology and pharmacology. *Semin. Perinatol.* **2000**, *24*, 258–266. [CrossRef]
71. Bruni, O.; Alonso-Alconada, D.; Besag, F.; Biran, V.; Braam, W.; Cortese, S.; Moavero, R.; Parisi, P.; Smits, M.; Van der Heijden, K.; et al. Current role of melatonin in pediatric neurology: Clinical recommendations. *Eur. J. Paediatr. Neurol.* **2015**, *19*, 122–133. [CrossRef]
72. Gobbi, G.; Comai, S. Differential Function of Melatonin MT1 and MT2 Receptors in REM and NREM Sleep. *Front. Endocrinol.* **2019**, *10*, 87. [CrossRef]
73. Owens, J.A.; Rosen, C.L.; Mindell, J.A.; Kirchner, H.L. Use of pharmacotherapy for insomnia in child psychiatry practice: A national survey. *Sleep Med.* **2010**, *11*, 692–700. [CrossRef] [PubMed]
74. Hartz, I.; Furu, K.; Bratlid, T.; Handal, M.; Skurtveit, S. Hypnotic drug use among 0–17 year olds during 2004–2011: A nationwide prescription database study. *Scand. J. Public Health* **2012**, *40*, 704–711. [CrossRef] [PubMed]
75. Cortese, S.; Wang, F.; Angriman, M.; Masi, G.; Bruni, O. Sleep Disorders in Children and Adolescents with Autism Spectrum Disorder: Diagnosis, Epidemiology, and Management. *CNS Drugs* **2020**, *34*, 415–423. [CrossRef]

76. Gringras, P.; Gamble, C.; Jones, A.P.; Wiggs, L.; Williamson, P.R.; Sutcliffe, A.; Montgomery, P.; Whitehouse, W.P.; Choonara, I.; Allport, T.; et al. Melatonin for sleep problems in children with neurodevelopmental disorders: Randomised double masked placebo controlled trial. *BMJ* **2012**, *345*, e6664. [CrossRef] [PubMed]
77. Andersen, I.M.; Kaczmarska, J.; McGrew, S.G.; Malow, B.A. Melatonin for insomnia in children with autism spectrum disorders. *J. Child. Neurol.* **2008**, *23*, 482–485. [CrossRef] [PubMed]
78. Wasdell, M.B.; Jan, J.E.; Bomben, M.M.; Freeman, R.D.; Rietveld, W.J.; Tai, J.; Hamilton, D.; Weiss, M.D. A randomized, placebo-controlled trial of controlled release melatonin treatment of delayed sleep phase syndrome and impaired sleep maintenance in children with neurodevelopmental disabilities. *J. Pineal Res.* **2008**, *44*, 57–64. [CrossRef]
79. Wirz-Justice, A.; Armstrong, S.M. Melatonin: Nature's soporific? *J. Sleep Res.* **1996**, *5*, 137–141.
80. Van Geijlswijk, I.M.; Korzilius, H.P.L.M.; Smits, M.G. The use of exogenous melatonin in delayed sleep phase disorder: A meta-analysis. *Sleep* **2010**, *33*, 1605–1614. [CrossRef]
81. Burgess, H.J.; Revell, V.L.; Molina, T.A.; Eastman, C.I. Human phase response curves to three days of daily melatonin: 0.5 mg versus 3.0 mg. *J. Clin. Endocrinol. Metab.* **2010**, *95*, 3325–3331. [CrossRef]
82. Keijzer, H.; Smits, M.G.; Peeters, T.; Looman, C.W.N.; Endenburg, S.C.; Gunnewiek, J.M.T.K. Evaluation of salivary melatonin measurements for Dim Light Melatonin Onset calculations in patients with possible sleep-wake rhythm disorders. *Clin. Chim. Acta* **2011**, *412*, 1616–1620. [CrossRef] [PubMed]
83. Harrington, R.A.; Lee, L.-C.; Crum, R.M.; Zimmerman, A.W.; Hertz-Picciotto, I. Serotonin hypothesis of autism: Implications for selective serotonin reuptake inhibitor use during pregnancy. *Autism Res.* **2013**, *6*, 149–168. [CrossRef] [PubMed]
84. Daly, E.; Ecker, C.; Hallahan, B.; Deeley, Q.; Craig, M.; Murphy, C.; Johnston, P.; Spain, D.; Gillan, N.; Gudbrandsen, M.; et al. Response inhibition and serotonin in autism: A functional MRI study using acute tryptophan depletion. *Brain* **2014**, *137*, 2600–2610. [CrossRef] [PubMed]
85. Tordjman, S.; Anderson, G.M.; Pichard, N.; Charbuy, H.; Touitou, Y. Nocturnal excretion of 6-sulphatoxymelatonin in children and adolescents with autistic disorder. *Biol. Psychiatry* **2005**, *57*, 134–138. [CrossRef] [PubMed]
86. Goldman, S.E.; Adkins, K.W.; Calcutt, M.W.; Carter, M.D.; Goodpaster, R.L.; Wang, L.; Shi, Y.; Burgess, H.J.; Hachey, D.L.; Malow, B.A. Melatonin in children with autism spectrum disorders: Endogenous and pharmacokinetic profiles in relation to sleep. *J. Autism Dev. Disord.* **2014**, *44*, 2525–2535. [CrossRef]
87. Melke, J.; Goubran Botros, H.; Chaste, P.; Betancur, C.; Nygren, G.; Anckarsäter, H.; Rastam, M.; Ståhlberg, O.; Gillberg, I.C.; Delorme, R.; et al. Abnormal melatonin synthesis in autism spectrum disorders. *Mol. Psychiatry* **2008**, *13*, 90–98. [CrossRef]
88. Rossignol, D.A.; Frye, R.E. Melatonin in autism spectrum disorders: A systematic review and meta-analysis. *Dev. Med. Child. Neurol.* **2011**, *53*, 783–792. [CrossRef]
89. Veatch, O.J.; Pendergast, J.S.; Allen, M.J.; Leu, R.M.; Johnson, C.H.; Elsea, S.H.; Malow, B.A. Genetic variation in melatonin pathway enzymes in children with autism spectrum disorder and comorbid sleep onset delay. *J. Autism Dev. Disord.* **2015**, *45*, 100–110. [CrossRef]
90. Malow, B.A.; Byars, K.; Johnson, K.; Weiss, S.; Bernal, P.; Goldman, S.E.; Panzer, R.; Coury, D.L.; Glaze, D.G. Sleep Committee of the Autism Treatment Network A practice pathway for the identification, evaluation, and management of insomnia in children and adolescents with autism spectrum disorders. *Pediatrics* **2012**, *130* (Suppl. 2), S106–S124. [CrossRef]
91. Hollway, J.A.; Aman, M.G. Pharmacological treatment of sleep disturbance in developmental disabilities: A review of the literature. *Res. Dev. Disabil.* **2011**, *32*, 939–962. [CrossRef]
92. Guénolé, F.; Godbout, R.; Nicolas, A.; Franco, P.; Claustrat, B.; Baleyte, J.-M. Melatonin for disordered sleep in individuals with autism spectrum disorders: Systematic review and discussion. *Sleep Med. Rev.* **2011**, *15*, 379–387. [CrossRef] [PubMed]
93. Sung, M.; Fung, D.S.S.; Cai, Y.; Ooi, Y.P. Pharmacological management in children and adolescents with pervasive developmental disorder. *Aust. N. Z. J. Psychiatry* **2010**, *44*, 410–428. [CrossRef] [PubMed]
94. Cortesi, F.; Giannotti, F.; Sebastiani, T.; Panunzi, S.; Valente, D. Controlled-release melatonin, singly and combined with cognitive behavioural therapy, for persistent insomnia in children with autism spectrum disorders: A randomized placebo-controlled trial. *J. Sleep Res.* **2012**, *21*, 700–709. [CrossRef] [PubMed]

95. Braam, W.; Keijzer, H.; Struijker Boudier, H.; Didden, R.; Smits, M.; Curfs, L. CYP1A2 polymorphisms in slow melatonin metabolisers: A possible relationship with autism spectrum disorder? *J. Intellect. Disabil. Res.* **2013**, *57*, 993–1000. [CrossRef]
96. Braam, W.; van Geijlswijk, I.; Keijzer, H.; Smits, M.G.; Didden, R.; Curfs, L.M.G. Loss of response to melatonin treatment is associated with slow melatonin metabolism. *J. Intellect. Disabil. Res.* **2010**, *54*, 547–555. [CrossRef]
97. Gringras, P.; Nir, T.; Breddy, J.; Frydman-Marom, A.; Findling, R.L. Efficacy and Safety of Pediatric Prolonged-Release Melatonin for Insomnia in Children with Autism Spectrum Disorder. *J. Am. Acad. Child. Adolesc. Psychiatry* **2017**, *56*, 948–957.e4. [CrossRef]
98. Schroder, C.M.; Malow, B.A.; Maras, A.; Melmed, R.D.; Findling, R.L.; Breddy, J.; Nir, T.; Shahmoon, S.; Zisapel, N.; Gringras, P. Pediatric Prolonged-Release Melatonin for Sleep in Children with Autism Spectrum Disorder: Impact on Child Behavior and Caregiver's Quality of Life. *J. Autism Dev. Disord.* **2019**, *49*, 3218–3230. [CrossRef]
99. Maras, A.; Schroder, C.M.; Malow, B.A.; Findling, R.L.; Breddy, J.; Nir, T.; Shahmoon, S.; Zisapel, N.; Gringras, P. Long-Term Efficacy and Safety of Pediatric Prolonged-Release Melatonin for Insomnia in Children with Autism Spectrum Disorder. *J. Child. Adolesc. Psychopharmacol.* **2018**, *28*, 699–710. [CrossRef]
100. Malow, B.A.; Findling, R.L.; Schroder, C.M.; Maras, A.; Breddy, J.; Nir, T.; Zisapel, N.; Gringras, P. Sleep, Growth, and Puberty After 2 Years of Prolonged-Release Melatonin in Children with Autism Spectrum Disorder. *J. Am. Acad. Child. Adolesc. Psychiatry* **2020**. [CrossRef]
101. Brown, R.E.; Stevens, D.R.; Haas, H.L. The physiology of brain histamine. *Prog. Neurobiol.* **2001**, *63*, 637–672. [CrossRef]
102. Eriksson, K.S.; Sergeeva, O.; Brown, R.E.; Haas, H.L. Orexin/hypocretin excites the histaminergic neurons of the tuberomammillary nucleus. *J. Neurosci.* **2001**, *21*, 9273–9279. [CrossRef] [PubMed]
103. Stahl, S.M. Selective histamine H1 antagonism: Novel hypnotic and pharmacologic actions challenge classical notions of antihistamines. *CNS Spectr.* **2008**, *13*, 1027–1038. [CrossRef]
104. Thakkar, M.M. Histamine in the regulation of wakefulness. *Sleep Med. Rev.* **2011**, *15*, 65–74. [CrossRef]
105. Shirley, D.W.; Sterrett, J.; Haga, N.; Durham, C. The therapeutic versatility of antihistamines: A comprehensive review. *Nurse Pract.* **2020**, *45*, 8–21. [CrossRef] [PubMed]
106. Fitzsimons, R.; Van der Poel, L.-A.; Thornhill, W.; Du Toit, G.; Shah, N.; Brough, H.A. Antihistamine use in children. *Arch. Dis. Child. Educ. Pract. Ed.* **2015**, *100*, 122–131. [CrossRef]
107. Simons, F.E.R.; Simons, K.J. H1 antihistamines: Current status and future directions. *World Allergy Organ. J.* **2008**, *1*, 145–155. [CrossRef] [PubMed]
108. Schnoes, C.J.; Kuhn, B.R.; Workman, E.F.; Ellis, C.R. Pediatric prescribing practices for clonidine and other pharmacologic agents for children with sleep disturbance. *Clin. Pediatr.* **2006**, *45*, 229–238. [CrossRef] [PubMed]
109. Church, M.K.; Maurer, M.; Simons, F.E.R.; Bindslev-Jensen, C.; Van Cauwenberge, P.; Bousquet, J.; Holgate, S.T.; Zuberbier, T. Global Allergy and Asthma European Network Risk of first-generation H(1)-antihistamines: A GA(2)LEN position paper. *Allergy* **2010**, *65*, 459–466. [CrossRef] [PubMed]
110. Kalpaklioglu, F.; Baccioglu, A. Efficacy and safety of H1-antihistamines: An update. *Antiinflamm. Antiallergy Agents Med. Chem.* **2012**, *11*, 230–237. [CrossRef]
111. Russo, R.M.; Gururaj, V.J.; Allen, J.E. The effectiveness of diphenhydramine HCl in pediatric sleep disorders. *J. Clin. Pharmacol.* **1976**, *16*, 284–288. [CrossRef]
112. Merenstein, D.; Diener-West, M.; Halbower, A.C.; Krist, A.; Rubin, H.R. The Trial of Infant Response to Diphenhydramine: The TIRED Study—A Randomized, Controlled, Patient-Oriented Trial. *Arch. Pediatr. Adolesc. Med.* **2006**, *160*, 707–712. [CrossRef] [PubMed]
113. Sezer, T.; Alehan, F. Chloral hydrate versus hydroxyzine HCL for sedation prior to pediatric sleep EEG recording. *Int. J. Neurosci.* **2013**, *123*, 719–723. [CrossRef] [PubMed]
114. Montanari, G.; Schiaulini, P.; Covre, A.; Steffan, A.; Furlanut, M. Niaprazine vs. chlordesmethyldiazepam in sleep disturbances in pediatric outpatients. *Pharmacol. Res.* **1992**, *25* (Suppl. 1), 83–84. [CrossRef]
115. Ottaviano, S.; Giannotti, F.; Cortesi, F. The effect of niaprazine on some common sleep disorders in children. A double-blind clinical trial by means of continuous home-videorecorded sleep. *Child. Nerv. Syst.* **1991**, *7*, 332–335. [CrossRef] [PubMed]

116. Teutsch, G.; Mahler, D.L.; Brown, C.R.; Forrest, W.H.; James, K.E.; Brown, B.W. Hypnotic efficacy of diphenhydramine, methapyrilene, and pentobarbital. *Clin. Pharmacol. Ther.* **1975**, *17*, 195–201. [CrossRef] [PubMed]
117. France, K.G.; Blampied, N.M.; Wilkinson, P. A multiple-baseline, double-blind evaluation of the effects of trimeprazine tartrate on infant sleep disturbance. *Exp. Clin. Psychopharmacol.* **1999**, *7*, 502–513. [CrossRef]
118. Gringras, P. When to use drugs to help sleep. *Arch. Dis. Child.* **2008**, *93*, 976–981. [CrossRef]
119. Vuurman, E.F.; Van Veggel, L.M.; Uiterwijk, M.M.; Leutner, D.; O'Hanlon, J.F. Seasonal allergic rhinitis and antihistamine effects on children's learning. *Ann. Allergy* **1993**, *71*, 121–126. [CrossRef]
120. Dinndorf, P.A.; McCabe, M.A.; Frierdich, S. Risk of abuse of diphenhydramine in children and adolescents with chronic illnesses. *J. Pediatr.* **1998**, *133*, 293–295. [CrossRef]
121. Sutter, A.I.M.; Lemiengre, M.; Campbell, H.; Mackinnon, H.F. Antihistamines for the common cold. *Cochrane Database Syst. Rev.* **2003**, CD001267. [CrossRef]
122. Magera, B.E.; Betlach, C.J.; Sweatt, A.P.; Derrick, C.W. Hydroxyzine intoxication in a 13-month-old child. *Pediatrics* **1981**, *67*, 280–283. [PubMed]
123. Anagnostou, K.; Swan, K.; Brough, H. The use of antihistamines in children. *Paediatr. Child. Health* **2016**. [CrossRef]
124. Friedman, M. Analysis, Nutrition, and Health Benefits of Tryptophan. *Int. J. Tryptophan Res.* **2018**, *11*, 1178646918802282. [CrossRef]
125. Meolie, A.L.; Rosen, C.; Kristo, D.; Kohrman, M.; Gooneratne, N.; Aguillard, R.N.; Fayle, R.; Troell, R.; Townsend, D.; Claman, D.; et al. Oral nonprescription treatment for insomnia: An evaluation of products with limited evidence. *J. Clin. Sleep Med.* **2005**, *1*, 173–187. [CrossRef] [PubMed]
126. Monti, J.M. Serotonin control of sleep-wake behavior. *Sleep Med. Rev.* **2011**, *15*, 269–281. [CrossRef]
127. Imeri, L.; Mancia, M.; Bianchi, S.; Opp, M.R. 5-Hydroxytryptophan, but not L-tryptophan, alters sleep and brain temperature in rats. *Neuroscience* **2000**, *95*, 445–452. [CrossRef]
128. Hartmann, E.; Spinweber, C.L. Sleep induced by L-tryptophan. Effect of dosages within the normal dietary intake. *J. Nerv. Ment. Dis.* **1979**, *167*, 497–499. [CrossRef]
129. Schneider-Helmert, D.; Spinweber, C.L. Evaluation of L-tryptophan for treatment of insomnia: A review. *Psychopharmacology* **1986**, *89*, 1–7. [CrossRef]
130. Spinweber, C.L. L-tryptophan administered to chronic sleep-onset insomniacs: Late-appearing reduction of sleep latency. *Psychopharmacology* **1986**, *90*, 151–155. [CrossRef]
131. Hartmann, E. Editorial: L-tryptophan: A possible natural hypnotic substance. *JAMA* **1974**, *230*, 1680–1681. [CrossRef]
132. Bergonzi, P.; Capocchi, G.; Chiurulla, C.; Mennuni, G.; Tempesta, E. Tryptophan and sleep in subjects with neuropsychiatric syndromes. *Riv. Neurol.* **1973**, *43*, 403–409. [PubMed]
133. Lieberman, H.R.; Agarwal, S.; Fulgoni, V.L. Tryptophan Intake in the US Adult Population Is Not Related to Liver or Kidney Function but Is Associated with Depression and Sleep Outcomes. *J. Nutr.* **2016**, *146*, 2609S–2615S. [CrossRef] [PubMed]
134. Wyatt, R.J.; Zarcone, V.; Engelman, K.; Dement, W.C.; Snyder, F.; Sjoerdsma, A. Effects of 5-hydroxytryptophan on the sleep of normal human subjects. *Electroencephalogr. Clin. Neurophysiol.* **1971**, *30*, 505–509. [CrossRef]
135. Birdsall, T.C. 5-Hydroxytryptophan: A clinically-effective serotonin precursor. *Altern. Med. Rev.* **1998**, *3*, 271–280.
136. Fernstrom, J.D. Effects and side effects associated with the non-nutritional use of tryptophan by humans. *J. Nutr.* **2012**, *142*, 2236S–2244S. [CrossRef] [PubMed]
137. Das, Y.T.; Bagchi, M.; Bagchi, D.; Preuss, H.G. Safety of 5-hydroxy-L-tryptophan. *Toxicol. Lett.* **2004**, *150*, 111–122. [CrossRef]
138. Bruni, O.; Ferri, R.; Miano, S.; Verrillo, E. L -5-Hydroxytryptophan treatment of sleep terrors in children. *Eur. J. Pediatr.* **2004**, *163*, 402–407. [CrossRef]
139. Van Zyl, L.T.; Chung, S.A.; Shahid, A.; Shapiro, C.M. L-Tryptophan as Treatment for Pediatric Non-Rapid Eye Movement Parasomnia. *J. Child. Adolesc. Psychopharmacol.* **2018**, *28*, 395–401. [CrossRef]
140. Bravaccio, C.; Terrone, G.; Rizzo, R.; Gulisano, M.; Tosi, M.; Curatolo, P.; Emberti Gialloreti, L. Use of nutritional supplements based on melatonin, tryptophan and vitamin B6 (Melamil Tripto®) in children with primary chronic headache, with or without sleep disorders: A pilot study. *Minerva Pediatr.* **2020**, *72*, 30–36. [CrossRef]

141. Della Volpe, A.; Lucia, A.D.; Pirozzi, C.; Pastore, V. Comparative Study between the use of Melatonin and A Solution with Melatonin, Tryptophan, and Vitamin B6 as an Inducer of Spontaneous Sleep in Children During an Auditory Response Test: An Alternative to Commonly Used Sedative Drugs. *J. Int. Adv. Otol.* **2017**, *13*, 69–73. [CrossRef]
142. Harada, T.; Hirotani, M.; Maeda, M.; Nomura, H.; Takeuchi, H. Correlation between breakfast tryptophan content and morning-evening in Japanese infants and students aged 0–15 yrs. *J. Physiol. Anthropol.* **2007**, *26*, 201–207. [CrossRef]
143. Cubero, J.; Chanclón, B.; Sánchez, S.; Rivero, M.; Rodríguez, A.B.; Barriga, C. Improving the quality of infant sleep through the inclusion at supper of cereals enriched with tryptophan, adenosine-5′-phosphate, and uridine-5′-phosphate. *Nutr. Neurosci.* **2009**, *12*, 272–280. [CrossRef] [PubMed]
144. Yap, I.K.S.; Angley, M.; Veselkov, K.A.; Holmes, E.; Lindon, J.C.; Nicholson, J.K. Urinary metabolic phenotyping differentiates children with autism from their unaffected siblings and age-matched controls. *J. Proteome Res.* **2010**, *9*, 2996–3004. [CrossRef]
145. Boccuto, L.; Chen, C.-F.; Pittman, A.R.; Skinner, C.D.; McCartney, H.J.; Jones, K.; Bochner, B.R.; Stevenson, R.E.; Schwartz, C.E. Decreased tryptophan metabolism in patients with autism spectrum disorders. *Mol. Autism* **2013**, *4*, 16. [CrossRef] [PubMed]
146. Gevi, F.; Zolla, L.; Gabriele, S.; Persico, A.M. Urinary metabolomics of young Italian autistic children supports abnormal tryptophan and purine metabolism. *Mol. Autism* **2016**, *7*, 47. [CrossRef] [PubMed]
147. Guiotto, A.; Calderan, A.; Ruzza, P.; Borin, G. Carnosine and carnosine-related antioxidants: A review. *Curr. Med. Chem.* **2005**, *12*, 2293–2315. [CrossRef] [PubMed]
148. Ming, X.; Stein, T.P.; Barnes, V.; Rhodes, N.; Guo, L. Metabolic perturbance in autism spectrum disorders: A metabolomics study. *J. Proteome Res.* **2012**, *11*, 5856–5862. [CrossRef]
149. Bala, K.A.; Doğan, M.; Mutluer, T.; Kaba, S.; Aslan, O.; Balahoroğlu, R.; Çokluk, E.; Üstyol, L.; Kocaman, S. Plasma amino acid profile in autism spectrum disorder (ASD). *Eur. Rev. Med. Pharmacol. Sci.* **2016**, *20*, 923–929.
150. Villafuerte, G.; Miguel-Puga, A.; Rodríguez, E.M.; Machado, S.; Manjarrez, E.; Arias-Carrión, O. Sleep deprivation and oxidative stress in animal models: A systematic review. *Oxid. Med. Cell Longev.* **2015**, *2015*, 234952. [CrossRef]
151. Chez, M.G.; Buchanan, C.P.; Aimonovitch, M.C.; Becker, M.; Schaefer, K.; Black, C.; Komen, J. Double-blind, placebo-controlled study of L-carnosine supplementation in children with autistic spectrum disorders. *J. Child. Neurol.* **2002**, *17*, 833–837. [CrossRef]
152. Mehrazad-Saber, Z.; Kheirouri, S.; Noorazar, S.-G. Effects of L-Carnosine Supplementation on Sleep Disorders and Disease Severity in Autistic Children: A Randomized, Controlled Clinical Trial. *Basic Clin. Pharmacol. Toxicol.* **2018**, *123*, 72–77. [CrossRef] [PubMed]
153. Hare, D.J.; Ayton, S.; Bush, A.I.; Lei, P. A delicate balance: Iron metabolism and diseases of the brain. *Front. Aging Neurosci.* **2013**, *5*. [CrossRef]
154. Marques, A.H.; O'Connor, T.G.; Roth, C.; Susser, E.; Bjørke-Monsen, A.-L. The influence of maternal prenatal and early childhood nutrition and maternal prenatal stress on offspring immune system development and neurodevelopmental disorders. *Front. Neurosci.* **2013**, *7*. [CrossRef] [PubMed]
155. Leung, W.; Singh, I.; McWilliams, S.; Stockler, S.; Ipsiroglu, O.S. Iron deficiency and sleep—A scoping review. *Sleep Med. Rev.* **2020**, *51*. [CrossRef] [PubMed]
156. Earley, C.J.; Allen, R.P.; Beard, J.L.; Connor, J.R. Insight into the pathophysiology of restless legs syndrome. *J. Neurosci. Res.* **2000**, *62*, 623–628. [CrossRef]
157. Sloand, J.A.; Shelly, M.A.; Feigin, A.; Bernstein, P.; Monk, R.D. A double-blind, placebo-controlled trial of intravenous iron dextran therapy in patients with ESRD and restless legs syndrome. *Am. J. Kidney Dis.* **2004**, *43*, 663–670. [CrossRef]
158. Allen, R.P.; Adler, C.H.; Du, W.; Butcher, A.; Bregman, D.B.; Earley, C.J. Clinical efficacy and safety of IV ferric carboxymaltose (FCM) treatment of RLS: A multi-centred, placebo-controlled preliminary clinical trial. *Sleep Med.* **2011**, *12*, 906–913. [CrossRef]
159. Kotagal, S. Treatment of dyssomnias and parasomnias in childhood. *Curr. Treat. Options Neurol.* **2012**, *14*, 630–649. [CrossRef]
160. Kerstein, R.; Stimpson, P.; Caulfield, H.; Ellis, G. Iron deficiency and sleep disordered breathing in children–cause or effect? *Int. J. Pediatr. Otorhinolaryngol.* **2009**, *73*, 275–280. [CrossRef]

161. Konofal, E.; Lecendreux, M.; Deron, J.; Marchand, M.; Cortese, S.; Zaïm, M.; Mouren, M.C.; Arnulf, I. Effects of iron supplementation on attention deficit hyperactivity disorder in children. *Pediatr. Neurol.* **2008**, *38*, 20–26. [CrossRef]
162. DelRosso, L.M.; Bruni, O.; Ferri, R. Restless sleep disorder in children: A pilot study on a tentative new diagnostic category. *Sleep* **2018**, *41*. [CrossRef] [PubMed]
163. Georgieff, M.K. Iron assessment to protect the developing brain. *Am. J. Clin. Nutr.* **2017**, *106*, 1588S–1593S. [CrossRef]
164. Dosman, C.F.; Drmic, I.E.; Brian, J.A.; Senthilselvan, A.; Harford, M.; Smith, R.; Roberts, S.W. Ferritin as an indicator of suspected iron deficiency in children with autism spectrum disorder: Prevalence of low serum ferritin concentration. *Dev. Med. Child. Neurol.* **2006**, *48*, 1008–1009. [CrossRef] [PubMed]
165. Gunes, S.; Ekinci, O.; Celik, T. Iron deficiency parameters in autism spectrum disorder: Clinical correlates and associated factors. *Ital. J. Pediatr.* **2017**, *43*, 86. [CrossRef] [PubMed]
166. Clénin, G.E. The treatment of iron deficiency without anaemia (in otherwise healthy persons). *Swiss Med. Wkly.* **2017**, *147*, w14434. [CrossRef] [PubMed]
167. DelRosso, L.M.; Chan, J.H.M.; Wrede, J.E.; Lockhart, C.T.; Yi, T.; Ferri, R. Determinants of ferritin response to oral iron supplementation in children with sleep movement disorders. *Sleep* **2020**, *43*. [CrossRef]
168. Oatley, H.; Borkhoff, C.M.; Chen, S.; Macarthur, C.; Persaud, N.; Birken, C.S.; Maguire, J.L.; Parkin, P.C.; Targ, K. Screening for Iron Deficiency in Early Childhood Using Serum Ferritin in the Primary Care Setting. *Pediatrics* **2018**, *142*. [CrossRef]
169. Panagiotou, J.P.; Douros, K. Clinicolaboratory Findings and Treatment of Iron-Deficiency Anemia in Childhood. *Pediatr. Hematol. Oncol.* **2004**, *21*, 519–532. [CrossRef]
170. Lane, R.; Kessler, R.; Buckley, A.W.; Rodriguez, A.; Farmer, C.; Thurm, A.; Swedo, S.; Felt, B. Evaluation of Periodic Limb Movements in Sleep and Iron Status in Children with Autism. *Pediatr. Neurol.* **2015**, *53*, 343–349. [CrossRef]
171. Youssef, J.; Singh, K.; Huntington, N.; Becker, R.; Kothare, S.V. Relationship of serum ferritin levels to sleep fragmentation and periodic limb movements of sleep on polysomnography in autism spectrum disorders. *Pediatr. Neurol.* **2013**, *49*, 274–278. [CrossRef]
172. Dosman, C.F.; Brian, J.A.; Drmic, I.E.; Senthilselvan, A.; Harford, M.M.; Smith, R.W.; Sharieff, W.; Zlotkin, S.H.; Moldofsky, H.; Roberts, S.W. Children with autism: Effect of iron supplementation on sleep and ferritin. *Pediatr. Neurol.* **2007**, *36*, 152–158. [CrossRef] [PubMed]
173. Munzer, T.; Felt, B. The Role of Iron in Pediatric Restless Legs Syndrome and Periodic Limb Movements in Sleep. *Semin. Neurol.* **2017**, *37*, 439–445. [CrossRef] [PubMed]
174. Picchietti, D.L. Should oral iron be first-line therapy for pediatric restless legs syndrome and periodic limb movement disorder? *Sleep Med.* **2017**, *32*, 220–221. [CrossRef] [PubMed]
175. DelRosso, L.; Bruni, O. Treatment of pediatric restless legs syndrome. In *Advances in Pharmacology*; Elsevier: Amsterdam, The Netherlands, 2019; Volume 84, pp. 237–253. ISBN 978-0-12-816758-8.
176. Holick, M.F. Vitamin D deficiency. *N. Engl. J. Med.* **2007**, *357*, 266–281. [CrossRef] [PubMed]
177. Muscogiuri, G.; Barrea, L.; Scannapieco, M.; Di Somma, C.; Scacchi, M.; Aimaretti, G.; Savastano, S.; Colao, A.; Marzullo, P. The lullaby of the sun: The role of vitamin D in sleep disturbance. *Sleep Med.* **2019**, *54*, 262–265. [CrossRef]
178. Wali, S.; Alsafadi, S.; Abaalkhail, B.; Ramadan, I.; Abulhamail, B.; Kousa, M.; Alshamrani, R.; Faruqui, H.; Faruqui, A.; Alama, M.; et al. The Association Between Vitamin D Level and Restless Legs Syndrome: A Population-Based Case-Control Study. *J. Clin. Sleep Med.* **2018**, *14*, 557–564. [CrossRef]
179. Lima, L.A.R.; Lopes, M.J.P.; Costa, R.O.; Lima, F.A.V.; Neves, K.R.T.; Calou, I.B.F.; Andrade, G.M.; Viana, G.S.B. Vitamin D protects dopaminergic neurons against neuroinflammation and oxidative stress in hemiparkinsonian rats. *J. Neuroinflamm.* **2018**, *15*, 249. [CrossRef]
180. Nakamura, K.; Wang, W.; Kang, U.J. The Role of Glutathione in Dopaminergic Neuronal Survival. *J. Neurochem.* **1997**, *69*, 1850–1858. [CrossRef] [PubMed]
181. Orme, R.P.; Bhangal, M.S.; Fricker, R.A. Calcitriol imparts neuroprotection in vitro to midbrain dopaminergic neurons by upregulating GDNF expression. *PLoS ONE* **2013**, *8*, e62040. [CrossRef]
182. Jin, H.J.; Lee, J.H.; Kim, M.K. The prevalence of vitamin D deficiency in iron-deficient and normal children under the age of 24 months. *Blood Res.* **2013**, *48*, 40–45. [CrossRef]

183. Yong, C.Y.; Reynaud, E.; Forhan, A.; Dargent-Molina, P.; Heude, B.; Charles, M.-A.; Plancoulaine, S.; Annesi-Maesano, I.; Bernard, J.Y.; Botton, J.; et al. Cord-blood vitamin D level and night sleep duration in preschoolers in the EDEN mother-child birth cohort. *Sleep Med.* **2019**, *53*, 70–74. [CrossRef] [PubMed]
184. Deng, Y.; Wang, G.; Ye, X.; Jiang, Y.; Lin, Q.; Dong, S.; Song, Y.; Zhu, L.; Meng, M.; Li, W.; et al. The association between 25-hydroxyvitamin D levels and children's sleep-wake patterns: A prospective cohort study. *Sleep Med.* **2020**, *67*, 207–214. [CrossRef] [PubMed]
185. Gong, Q.-H.; Li, S.-X.; Li, H.; Chen, Q.; Li, X.-Y.; Xu, G.-Z. 25-Hydroxyvitamin D Status and Its Association with Sleep Duration in Chinese Schoolchildren. *Nutrients* **2018**, *10*, 1013. [CrossRef] [PubMed]
186. Wang, T.; Shan, L.; Du, L.; Feng, J.; Xu, Z.; Staal, W.G.; Jia, F. Serum concentration of 25-hydroxyvitamin D in autism spectrum disorder: A systematic review and meta-analysis. *Eur. Child. Adolesc. Psychiatry* **2016**, *25*, 341–350. [CrossRef]
187. Bivona, G.; Gambino, C.M.; Iacolino, G.; Ciaccio, M. Vitamin D and the nervous system. *Neurol. Res.* **2019**, *41*, 827–835. [CrossRef]
188. Bouillon, R. Comparative analysis of nutritional guidelines for vitamin D. *Nat. Rev. Endocrinol.* **2017**, *13*, 466–479. [CrossRef]
189. Gominak, S.C.; Stumpf, W.E. The world epidemic of sleep disorders is linked to vitamin D deficiency. *Med. Hypotheses* **2012**, *79*, 132–135. [CrossRef]
190. Adams, J.B.; Holloway, C. Pilot study of a moderate dose multivitamin/mineral supplement for children with autistic spectrum disorder. *J. Altern. Complement. Med.* **2004**, *10*, 1033–1039. [CrossRef]
191. Adams, J.B.; Audhya, T.; McDonough-Means, S.; Rubin, R.A.; Quig, D.; Geis, E.; Gehn, E.; Loresto, M.; Mitchell, J.; Atwood, S.; et al. Effect of a vitamin/mineral supplement on children and adults with autism. *BMC Pediatr.* **2011**, *11*, 111. [CrossRef]
192. Gyllenhaal, C.; Merritt, S.L.; Peterson, S.D.; Block, K.I.; Gochenour, T. Efficacy and safety of herbal stimulants and sedatives in sleep disorders. *Sleep Med. Rev.* **2000**, *4*, 229–251. [CrossRef]
193. Guadagna, S.; Barattini, D.F.; Rosu, S.; Ferini-Strambi, L. Plant Extracts for Sleep Disturbances: A Systematic Review...Vitafoods 2019 in Geneva. *Evid.-Based Complement. Altern. Med.* **2020**, 1–9. [CrossRef] [PubMed]
194. Mineo, L.; Concerto, C.; Patel, D.; Mayorga, T.; Paula, M.; Chusid, E.; Aguglia, E.; Battaglia, F. Valeriana officinalis Root Extract Modulates Cortical Excitatory Circuits in Humans. *Neuropsychobiology* **2017**, *75*, 46–51. [CrossRef] [PubMed]
195. Houghton, P.J. The scientific basis for the reputed activity of Valerian. *J. Pharm. Pharmacol.* **1999**, *51*, 505–512. [CrossRef] [PubMed]
196. Müller, C.E.; Schumacher, B.; Brattström, A.; Abourashed, E.A.; Koetter, U. Interactions of valerian extracts and a fixed valerian-hop extract combination with adenosine receptors. *Life Sci.* **2002**, *71*, 1939–1949. [CrossRef]
197. Leach, M.J.; Page, A.T. Herbal medicine for insomnia: A systematic review and meta-analysis. *Sleep Med. Rev.* **2015**, *24*, 1–12. [CrossRef] [PubMed]
198. Leathwood, P.D.; Chauffard, F.; Heck, E.; Munoz-Box, R. Aqueous extract of valerian root (*Valeriana officinalis* L.) improves sleep quality in man. *Pharmacol. Biochem. Behav.* **1982**, *17*, 65–71. [CrossRef]
199. Herrera-Arellano, A.; Luna-Villegas, G.; Cuevas-Uriostegui, M.; Alvarez, L.; Vargas-Pineda, G.; Zamilpa, A.; Tortoriello, J. Polysomnographic Evaluation of the Hypnotic Effect of Valeriana edulis Standardized Extract in Patients Suffering from Insomnia. *Planta Medica* **2001**, *67*, 695–699. [CrossRef]
200. Taavoni, S.; Nazem ekbatani, N.; Haghani, H. Valerian/lemon balm use for sleep disorders during menopause. *Complement. Ther. Clin. Pract.* **2013**, *19*, 193–196. [CrossRef]
201. Oxman, A.D.; Flottorp, S.; Håvelsrud, K.; Fretheim, A.; Odgaard-Jensen, J.; Austvoll-Dahlgren, A.; Carling, C.; Pallesen, S.; Bjorvatn, B. A Televised, Web-Based Randomised Trial of an Herbal Remedy (Valerian) for Insomnia. *PLoS ONE* **2007**, *2*, e1040. [CrossRef]
202. Cuellar, N.G.; Ratcliffe, S.J. Does valerian improve sleepiness and symptom severity in people with restless legs syndrome? *Altern. Ther. Health Med.* **2009**, *15*, 22–28.
203. Barton, D.L.; Atherton, P.J.; Bauer, B.A.; Moore, D.F.; Mattar, B.I.; Lavasseur, B.I.; Rowland, K.M.; Zon, R.T.; Lelindqwister, N.A.; Nagargoje, G.G.; et al. The use of Valeriana officinalis (Valerian) in improving sleep in patients who are undergoing treatment for cancer: A phase III randomized, placebo-controlled, double-blind study (NCCTG Trial, N01C5). *J. Support. Oncol.* **2011**, *9*, 24–31. [CrossRef] [PubMed]

204. Jacobs, B.P.; Bent, S.; Tice, J.A.; Blackwell, T.; Cummings, S.R. An Internet-Based Randomized, Placebo-Controlled Trial of Kava and Valerian for Anxiety and Insomnia. *Medicine* **2005**, *84*, 197–207. [CrossRef] [PubMed]
205. Świąder, K.; Wijaya, C.H.; Startek, K. The therapeutic properties of Lemon balm (*Melissa officinalis* L.): Reviewing novel findings and medical indications. *J. Appl. Bot. Food Qual.* **2019**, *92*, 327–335. [CrossRef]
206. Cerny, A.; Schmid, K. Tolerability and efficacy of valerian/lemon balm in healthy volunteers (a double-blind, placebo-controlled, multicentre study). *Fitoterapia* **1999**, *70*, 221–228. [CrossRef]
207. Cases, J.; Ibarra, A.; Feuillère, N.; Roller, M.; Sukkar, S.G. Pilot trial of Melissa officinalis L. leaf extract in the treatment of volunteers suffering from mild-to-moderate anxiety disorders and sleep disturbances. *Med. J. Nutr. Metab.* **2011**, *4*, 211–218. [CrossRef]
208. Müller, S.F.; Klement, S. A combination of valerian and lemon balm is effective in the treatment of restlessness and dyssomnia in children. *Phytomedicine* **2006**, *13*, 383–387. [CrossRef]
209. Tavares-Silva, C.; Holandino, C.; Homsani, F.; Luiz, R.R.; Prodestino, J.; Farah, A.; De Lima, J.P.; Simas, R.C.; Castilho, C.V.V.; Leitão, S.G.; et al. Homeopathic medicine of Melissa officinalis combined or not with Phytolacca decandra in the treatment of possible sleep bruxism in children: A crossover randomized triple-blinded controlled clinical trial. *Phytomedicine* **2019**, *58*, 152869. [CrossRef]
210. Dhawan, K.; Dhawan, S.; Sharma, A. Passiflora: A review update. *J. Ethnopharmacol.* **2004**, *94*, 1–23. [CrossRef]
211. Toda, K.; Hitoe, S.; Takeda, S.; Shimizu, N.; Shimoda, H. Passionflower Extract Induces High-amplitude Rhythms without Phase Shifts in the Expression of Several Circadian Clock Genes in Vitro and in Vivo. *Int. J. Biomed. Sci.* **2017**, *13*, 84–92.
212. Lee, J.; Jung, H.-Y.; Lee, S.I.; Choi, J.H.; Kim, S.-G. Effects of Passiflora incarnata Linnaeus on polysomnographic sleep parameters in subjects with insomnia disorder: A double-blind randomized placebo-controlled study. *Int. Clin. Psychopharmacol.* **2020**, *35*, 29–35. [CrossRef]
213. Woelk, H.; Schläfke, S. A multi-center, double-blind, randomised study of the Lavender oil preparation Silexan in comparison to Lorazepam for generalized anxiety disorder. *Phytomedicine* **2010**, *17*, 94–99. [CrossRef] [PubMed]
214. Kasper, S.; Gastpar, M.; Müller, W.E.; Volz, H.-P.; Möller, H.-J.; Dienel, A.; Schläfke, S. Silexan, an orally administered Lavandula oil preparation, is effective in the treatment of "subsyndromal" anxiety disorder: A randomized, double-blind, placebo controlled trial. *Int. Clin. Psychopharmacol.* **2010**, *25*, 277–287. [CrossRef] [PubMed]
215. Kasper, S.; Anghelescu, I.; Dienel, A. Efficacy of orally administered Silexan in patients with anxiety-related restlessness and disturbed sleep–A randomized, placebo-controlled trial. *Eur. Neuropsychopharmacol.* **2015**, *25*, 1960–1967. [CrossRef] [PubMed]
216. Uehleke, B.; Schaper, S.; Dienel, A.; Schlaefke, S.; Stange, R. Phase II trial on the effects of Silexan in patients with neurasthenia, post-traumatic stress disorder or somatization disorder. *Phytomed. Int. J. Phytother. Phytopharmacol.* **2012**, *19*, 665–672. [CrossRef]
217. Nathan, P. The experimental and clinical pharmacology of St John's Wort (*Hypericum perforatum* L.). *Mol. Psychiatry* **1999**, *4*, 333–338. [CrossRef]
218. Müller, W.E.; Singer, A.; Wonnemann, M.; Hafner, U.; Rolli, M.; Schäfer, C. Hyperforin represents the neurotransmitter reuptake inhibiting constituent of hypericum extract. *Pharmacopsychiatry* **1998**, *31*, 16–21. [CrossRef]
219. Nathan, P.J. Hypericum perforatum (St John's Wort): A non-selective reuptake inhibitor? A review of the recent advances in its pharmacology. *J. Psychopharmacol.* **2001**, *15*, 47–54. [CrossRef]
220. Al-Akoum, M.; Maunsell, E.; Verreault, R.; Provencher, L.; Otis, H.; Dodin, S. Effects of Hypericum perforatum (St. John's wort) on hot flashes and quality of life in perimenopausal women: A randomized pilot trial. *Menopause* **2009**, *16*, 307–314. [CrossRef]
221. Sharpley, A.L.; McGavin, C.L.; Whale, R.; Cowen, P.J. Antidepressant-like effect of Hypericum perforatum (St John's wort) on the sleep polysomnogram. *Psychopharmacology* **1998**, *139*, 286–287. [CrossRef]
222. Adib-Hajbaghery, M.; Mousavi, S.N. The effects of chamomile extract on sleep quality among elderly people: A clinical trial. *Complement. Ther. Med.* **2017**, *35*, 109–114. [CrossRef]

223. Chang, S.M.; Chen, C.-H. Effects of an intervention with drinking chamomile tea on sleep quality and depression in sleep disturbed postnatal women: A randomized controlled trial. *J. Adv. Nurs.* **2016**, *72*, 306–315. [CrossRef] [PubMed]

224. Zick, S.M.; Wright, B.D.; Sen, A.; Arnedt, J.T. Preliminary examination of the efficacy and safety of a standardized chamomile extract for chronic primary insomnia: A randomized placebo-controlled pilot study. *BMC Complement. Altern. Med.* **2011**, *11*, 78. [CrossRef] [PubMed]

4

Immersive Virtual Reality for Pediatric Pain

Andrea Stevenson Won [1], Jakki Bailey [2], Jeremy Bailenson [2], Christine Tataru [2], Isabel A. Yoon [2] and Brenda Golianu [2,*]

1 Department of Communication, Cornell University, 417 Mann Library Building, Ithaca, NY 14853, USA; a.s.won@cornell.edu
2 Department of Anesthesiology and Perioperative Medicine, Stanford University, 300 Pasteur Dr. H3580A, Stanford, CA 94305, USA; jakki7@stanford.edu (J.B.); bailenso@stanford.edu (J.B.); ctataru5@stanford.edu (C.T.); iayoon@stanford.edu (I.A.Y.)
* Correspondence: bgolianu@stanford.edu

Abstract: Children must often endure painful procedures as part of their treatment for various medical conditions. Those with chronic pain endure frequent or constant discomfort in their daily lives, sometimes severely limiting their physical capacities. With the advent of affordable consumer-grade equipment, clinicians have access to a promising and engaging intervention for pediatric pain, both acute and chronic. In addition to providing relief from acute and procedural pain, virtual reality (VR) may also help to provide a corrective psychological and physiological environment to facilitate rehabilitation for pediatric patients suffering from chronic pain. The special qualities of VR such as presence, interactivity, customization, social interaction, and embodiment allow it to be accepted by children and adolescents and incorporated successfully into their existing medical therapies. However, the powerful and transformative nature of many VR experiences may also pose some risks and should be utilized with caution. In this paper, we review recent literature in pediatric virtual reality for procedural pain and anxiety, acute and chronic pain, and some rehabilitation applications. We also discuss the practical considerations of using VR in pediatric care, and offer specific suggestions and information for clinicians wishing to adopt these engaging therapies into their daily clinical practice.

Keywords: Virtual reality; pediatric pain; procedural pain; nonpharmacological; rehabilitation

---

1. Introduction

Children have always enjoyed games of "pretend." While immersed in a game, they often become deeply absorbed and able to ignore aversive stimuli. Immersive virtual reality (VR) is a promising and engaging intervention that may help to decrease pain and anxiety for children undergoing painful procedures and suffering from acute pain. In the context of their medical care, children may also endure chronic pain and discomfort. Because VR makes it possible to transform how patients perceive their bodies, it allows other, novel interventions that are possible in no other medium. Beyond providing distraction and enjoyment, virtual reality may provide a corrective psychological and physiological environment, and can facilitate rehabilitation for pediatric patients suffering from chronic pain, as well as neurorehabilitation for children suffering from stroke and cerebral palsy. With the advent of inexpensive consumer VR systems, the opportunities to research and deploy VR in the clinic have expanded. However, the powerful and transformative nature of many VR experiences may also pose some risks and should be utilized with caution in developing therapeutic VR interventions [1].

In this paper, we will review recent literature in pediatric virtual reality for procedural pain and anxiety, acute and chronic pain, and some rehabilitation applications. We will also discuss clinically relevant characteristics of VR experiences, such as the aspects of presence, interactivity, customization, social interaction, and embodiment. We will review how each of these requires special consideration, and in some cases adaptation of the hardware or software, for a child population. Finally, we will discuss the practical considerations of some currently available consumer VR systems, and offer specific suggestions and information for clinicians wishing to adopt these engaging therapies.

2. Review of Virtual Reality in Pediatrics

We conducted a review evaluating articles that describe the use of VR in pediatric procedural, acute and chronic pain. (see Table 1) We included articles detailing case studies or randomized trials of the use of VR. Where such studies were not available, we referred to adult studies that may offer insights into the potential use in pediatric populations, which are specifically described as pertaining to adult populations. We will discuss the selected articles and themes as they are relevant to the improved care of pediatric patients through VR. These articles can be roughly divided into two main areas of clinical relevance: acute and procedural pain and anxiety, and chronic pain and neurorehabilitation.

Table 1. The following terms were searched on PubMed (www.ncbi.nlm.nih.gov/pubmed/) between 2000 and 2017.

Key Word Search	Number of Articles Obtained	Number of Articles Deemed Relevant and Utilized in Review
Virtual Reality and Pediatric Procedures	94	13
Virtual Reality and Pediatric Anxiety	14	7
Virtual Reality and Procedural Anxiety	13	8
Virtual Reality and Pediatric Procedural Anxiety	5	5
Virtual Reality and Pediatric Chronic Pain	4	4
Virtual Reality and Pediatric Acute Pain	5	5
Virtual Reality and Pain	312	31
Virtual Reality and Acute pain	35	16
Virtual Reality and Chronic Pain	63	27

2.1. Acute and Procedural Pain

Acute pain is pain directly related to a temporary injury and typically lasts a short period of time (<6 weeks). Procedural pain and anxiety refers to distress derived from medical procedures, including intravenous (IV) injections, vaccinations, anesthesia administration, and other needle-related procedures, as well as other procedures required as part of routine care, such as burn wound dressing changes.

Virtual reality was first used to manage acute pain during painful repetitive dressing changes in patients with burn wounds [2]. Schmitt et al. demonstrated a reduction in pain of 27–44% in pediatric patients who participated in the virtual environment featuring a wintery scenario, called "SnowWorld", while undergoing dressing changes [3,4]. Jeffs et al. corroborated the efficacy of VR in burn wound pain management in adolescents [5]. In a randomized three-armed trial, 30 adolescents were assigned to standard care, watching a movie, and VR engagement with the "SnowWorld" virtual environment. The VR treatment group reported a decrease in pain compared to the passive distraction (movie) group, (difference 23.7 points decrease in pain score out of 100 total), 95% confidence interval (CI): 2.4–45.0, $p = 0.029$). In comparison to standard care, the VR group showed decreased pain as well, though the difference was not statistically significant. Of note, the VR group was the only one in which the patients' pain during the actual dressing change procedure was reported to be less than the pre-procedure pain [5].

Brown et al. performed a randomized controlled trial of an interactive VR intervention entitled "Ditto" and showed not only a decrease in self-reported pain and anxiety in pediatric patients undergoing dressing changes, but also an increased rate of epithelialization and faster wound healing in those patients undergoing VR intervention for their procedures (−2.14 days (wounds healed 2.14 days faster), CI: −4.38 to 0.1, $p = 0.061$), which was significantly faster when adjusted for mean burn depth (−2.26 days, CI −4.48 to −0.04, $p = 0.046$) [6]. Lastly, Miller et al. showed that not only was pain reduced during dressing changes, but when a multimodal intervention was utilized, the procedure required less time to complete ($p < 0.05$) [7]. Additional notable studies investigating the efficacy of VR distraction on pain and anxiety in children and adults undergoing severe burn wound care are referenced below [8,9].

Virtual reality has also proven successful at lessening procedural pain and distress related to IV placement and other needle-related procedures. In a 2006 study, Gold et al. performed a randomized control trial on 20 pediatric patients requiring IV placement [10]. The VR group received a multisensory VR experience including visual stimulation from a HMD device, tactile feedback, and music, for 5 min prior to IV placement until 5 min after placement. The control group received local anesthetic spray, but no VR intervention for the procedure. They were permitted to utilize the VR equipment for 3 min following IV placement. While children in the control group experienced a four-fold increase in pain as measured by the Wong-Baker FACES scale [11], the VR group showed no increase in affective pain following IV placement [10]. Nilsson et al. performed a similar study ($N = 42$) using a screen-based three-dimensional (3D) program [12]. Pediatric and adolescent patients undergoing venous punctures or subcutaneous venous port device insertion were randomized either to this non-immersive VR and standard care, or standard care alone. Patients did not report a significant decrease in self-reported pain for either condition; however, they did report that the VR distraction was a pleasant experience that succeeded at distraction. (We note that this intervention was not immersive).

Beyond VR's use in acute pain, it can potentially be used to make patients more familiar and comfortable with procedures. Most hospital procedures are accompanied by some stress or anxiety on the part of pediatric patients. He et al. looked at the effect of therapeutic play on perioperative anxiety, negative emotional manifestation, and postoperative pain [13]. Ninety-five children were assigned randomly to receive one hour of face-to-face therapeutic play involving objects to be used in the operation, or no intervention. Those children that participated in therapeutic play exhibited significantly lower levels of anxiety and negative emotion manifestation associated with their upcoming operation, and even showed lower levels of post-operative pain [13]. Virtual reality has the potential to familiarize children with the operation environment in a safe, controlled and playful way, and potentially decrease their pain and anxiety.

2.2. Chronic Pain

Unlike procedural or acute pain, chronic pain is persistent for a period greater than six weeks, often for months or years. It may include chronic headache, abdominal, limb, joint or back pain, neuropathic or sympathetically maintained pain such as complex regional pain syndrome (CRPS), and pain related to other medical conditions. In addition to symptom control, interventions often strive to maintain or improve function and minimize disability. While there is little research on using VR for the treatment of chronic pain in children [14], promising results in adults indicate that further research in this area is advisable. Below, we describe the use of virtual reality in neuromodulation, in physical therapy, and in biofeedback. We describe the limited research in children, and attempt to extend relevant research in adults to pediatric patients.

Virtual reality may have the potential to amplify the neuromodulatory effects of traditional mirror visual feedback (MVF), which can modify patients' pathological cortical representations in the group of chronic pain syndromes that includes phantom limb pain, complex regional pain syndrome and fibromyalgia. Mirror visual feedback was first applied to adult patients suffering from phantom limb pain (PLP) by Ramachandran and Rogers-Ramachandran [15]. This technique may exert some of its benefits by encouraging the remapping of motor and somatosensory cortices, allowing a return to a homeostatic processing mechanism and facilitating the improvement or resolution of the painful experience. Mirror visual feedback was also found to be of benefit for CRPS in a randomized controlled trial with adult patients [16]. Virtual reality has also been used in an open-label case study of five adults with CRPS, four of whom reported reduced pain intensity over five to eight sessions [17].

Besides providing a new medium for mirror therapy, VR also allows other avatar configurations to be altered. For example, patients can also experience augmented motion such that a small motion in the physical world maps to a large motion in the virtual one, or vice versa. Thus, a small movement of the arm made in real life could be rewarded by a larger, more apparent arm movement in VR. Conversely, for patients prone to guarding, movements made by patients in real life could be depicted as more restrained in the virtual world [18], which might encourage such patients to move more freely. Two studies demonstrated that adult patients with neck pain moved further and reported less pain as a result of movement when VR was used to reduce their apparent movement [18,19]. In the pediatric population, there is currently one feasibility study exploring the neuromodulatory effects of VR. Won et al. showed that a VR experience with MVF and movement augmentation properties was well tolerated by pediatric patients with CRPS during physical therapy sessions [20].

The hypothesis supporting the efficacy of neuromodulatory chronic pain therapies is founded in the association between brain connectivity changes and improvement in chronic pain symptoms. A study conducted by Lebel and colleagues found significant changes in the somatosensory processing of symptomatic pediatric CRPS when compared to post-treatment CRPS patients and control patients [21]. Because this processing resumes normality after months of traditional physical therapy, it is possible that directly altering somatosensory processing (i.e., via mirror therapy), might itself be helpful in resolving pain. Becerra et al. and Simons et al. [22,23] both showed changes in connectivity in various intrinsic brain networks after therapies that reduced pain and improved function. It is still under debate whether the association of successful recovery from CRPS symptoms is directly related to changes in brain connectivity or brain plasticity, and further research is required to determine what other factors may be involved in remapping somatosensory processing [24]. However, another piece of evidence supporting this hypothesis comes from graded motor imagery, a therapy that involves the imaginary mental rotation of one's limbs. Adult studies have shown that this therapy is associated with both changes in connectivity in the central nervous system as well as reduction in pain [25], and pediatric patients may also benefit from such therapy.

As discussed above, VR offers an engaging opportunity for children to practice motions that would be impossible or unsafe in the real world [26]. Especially in diseases like cerebral palsy, where motion is difficult, the opportunity to engage in active/repetitive motor and sensory practice can increase neuroplasticity and allow for learning to overcome some limitations of the disease [27]. In a study by Biffi et al., 12 children with Acquired Brain Injury (ABI) participated in 10 sessions using an interactive VR system called GRAIL (Gait Real-time Analysis Interactive Lab); treatment sessions led to improvement in walking abilities and enhanced engagement during training, suggesting that VR may play a role in the field of rehabilitation [28]. Although not discussing efficacy, Meyns et al. demonstrated the feasibility of using VR training to improve balance in children with cerebral palsy after lower limb surgery [29]. For a more in-depth review on neurorehabilitation applications of VR, please refer to the following excellent review by Wang et al. [26].

In addition to alterations in neuronal representation, patients with chronic pain often exhibit a debilitating fear of inducing more pain through movement. This fear not only seriously affects patients' ability to function; it can also inhibit physical therapy efforts. Trost et al. discusses the use of VR interventions to provide graded exposure treatment for pain-related fear and disability in adults with chronic low back pain [30]. Collado-Mateo et al. also found that a combined program of physical exercise and non-immersive VR improved adult patients' mobility, balance, and fear of falling in adult fibromyalgia patients [31]. Senkowski et al. cite significant promise in the use of VR-assisted therapy to aid in the decrease of fear-avoidance behavior and improvement in distorted body images [32]. Fear-avoidance is noted to be an issue in the pediatric population with chronic pain [33]; however, no VR interventions have yet been specifically designed to address this phenomenon.

2.3. Other Applications

Another possible application is the use of a virtual pain coach. A VR experience could reinforce therapeutic movements and exercises in an out-of-clinic environment. This is especially useful for long-distance patients or patients who are unable to be physically present for other reasons [34]. The variety of VR therapy options makes it an effective intervention to integrate into existing interdisciplinary programs, combining medical treatment, physical therapy and psychological interventions [35].

Finally, the effects of VR may potentially be augmented by other techniques such as biofeedback or hypnosis. Biofeedback is the process of providing the patient with information on his or her own neurological data such as heart rate variability, temperature, or muscle tension. In a recent pilot study, non-immersive VR mirror visual feedback was used successfully in combination with biofeedback to treat pediatric patients with chronic headaches [36]. Virtual reality was also used in conjunction with hypnosis in an adult case report [37].

3. Qualities of Virtual Reality

In the next section, we will discuss five qualities of VR that are of interest in considering clinical applications for children: presence, interactivity, social interactions, customization, and embodiment. We will then summarize current research on how these qualities may be useful for treating children, and note some potential areas of caution (see Table 2).

Table 2. Possible benefits and side effects of VR.

Benefits	• Provides distraction from pain • Promotes movement • Promotes imagination • Fosters sense of internal health locus of control • Promotes cortical repatterning (potentially)
Side Effects	• Visually-induced motion sickness (dizziness, nausea) • Collisions with nearby objects • As with other media, risks social isolation • In younger children, possible potential for "false memories"

3.1. Presence

Presence is the subjective feeling that the user is experiencing the environment and interactions in the virtual world are [38]. It is often measured by self-report, has been linked to physiological processes such as changes in hear rate and skin resistance [39] and behavioral measures such as not responding to stimuli in the real world [40]. Feelings of presence can be evoked by even a simple VR system, such as a 360° video viewed through a smartphone in a cardboard housing. However, a recent meta-analysis indicates that features such as improved tracking, stereoscopy, and wide field of view can make VR experiences feel more real [1]. VR is particularly promising as a distractor for procedural and acute pain because of the deep sense of presence created by virtual worlds. The immersive features of virtual reality technology immerse the patient with rich sensory stimuli, creating a realistic experience and effectively directing attention away from adverse stimuli [41,42].

Age may influence how virtual environments are experienced. For example, during burn wound care treatment with VR, pediatric patients reported higher levels of presence compared to adults receiving the same treatment [43]. Experiencing virtual environments as extremely real has important implications for how children behave and understand the world after the VR treatment. Baumgartner et al. showed that children's brains process virtual experiences differently than adults and young children may require different types of immersive experiences [44]. During early childhood (e.g., three to five-years-old) children's sense of fantasy and reality is rapidly developing [45,46]. Virtual reality can create realistic environments that may seem extremely real, particularly to young children.

Given that children may be more vulnerable to believing virtual experiences as real, virtual environments may need to be carefully selected and contextualized so that children are able to interpret their memories of the experience as derived from media rather than real life. In addition, for some age groups, debriefing post-VR experience may be necessary.

3.2. Interactivity

Virtual reality therapies incorporating tracked body movements allow for greater interactivity. In a study examining cold pressor-induced pain in 40 children of age 5–13, greater interactivity led to greater pain tolerance [47]. Children with disorders requiring intensive physical therapy, such as those with CRPS [20] or cerebral palsy [48], may benefit especially from interactive VR scenarios. Such scenarios can encourage them to engage in physical therapy while simultaneously increasing their pain tolerance.

High levels of interactivity, while effective in reducing pain, can be accompanied by a sense of nausea and increased potential for collisions with objects in the real world. Clinicians using VR as therapy should be aware of these minor risks and take appropriate precautions for pediatric patients. The more immersed users are in a virtual environment, the more the sensory input from the real world is occluded, and active users risk painful collisions.

Even adults can be at risk of falling or colliding with objects; during set-up, consumer VR systems require users to define a safe "play space", and displays are equipped with safety warnings and reminders to be careful when users approach the edge of this area. As children move around a virtual space, they may come dangerously close to objects in the real world. Even if children are seated, they should be monitored. Careful spotting is necessary to prevent them from injuring themselves or bystanders by accidentally colliding with real-world objects.

In addition, although both children and adults can be prone to "cybersickness" or feeling nausea or dizziness, children may be less able to anticipate and articulate their discomfort. Caretakers and clinicians will need to be aware of the possible signs of sickness and develop ways to measure children's discomfort in non-verbal and unobtrusive ways such as how children are moving their bodies. Another alternative is to set pre-determined timers to take short breaks.

3.3. Social Interactions in Virtual Reality

Many factors affect children's and adolescents' attraction to video games, one being their ability to share the experience with friends [49]. The use of social interactions may be particularly effective during adolescence, a time in which children are particularly sensitive to social environments [50]. Children as young as five years old respond to digital others in social ways, such as using information from a virtual character and a live person at equal rates to solve a decision-making task [51].

Children with chronic pain may have particular deficiencies in their abilities to develop and maintain peer relationships due to increased school absences, decreased physical ability to engage in sports or social activities, and decreased mood and motivation [52]. Virtual environments may offer an alternative platform for children to build these relationships by giving them access to near-real experiences that they can share with others. Children with high medical acuity, such as those in post-transplant oncology, who may be confined to a single room or unit, may benefit from access to virtual interactions if they are not able to engage with peers due to their ongoing medical condition. Since older children are already actively involved in virtual environments [53], the presence of virtual others offers new opportunities. For example, physical therapists might incorporate their own behavior into the environment via an avatar, which could help patients visualize or mimic the correct movements.

However, as in real life, children need age-appropriate environments. Social virtual environments where children can interact with others such as High Fidelity (highfidelity.io) or AltspaceVR (altVR.com) may require additional permissions so that outsiders cannot interact with patients. In addition, the risks and benefits of social media are also applicable when social media platforms provide opportunities for patients to engage virtually. While Facebook's current beta application, Spaces (oculus.com/experiences/rift/), and other environments linked with social media platforms may make it easy for children to engage with Facebook friends in immersive virtual reality, such interactions should not allow children to isolate themselves from face-to-face interactions.

3.4. *Customization*

Clinicians or patients themselves can select different virtual scenarios, and as commercial VR experiences become more common, there will be more entertainment options from which to choose. Allowing children to contribute towards selecting their virtual experience allows them agency and the ability to tailor content to their interests, as in a study by Ni et al. [54] in which pediatric patients and therapists evaluated games for degree of engagement and therapeutic usefulness together. For example, children undergoing chemotherapy who selected from a variety of virtual scenarios demonstrated reduced symptom distress [55].

Another area in which customization can be advantageous is in avatar representation. Children can select and customize their own avatar, providing them with a sense of control in a clinical setting that can significantly reduce patient stress [56]. When embodying stock avatars, children may need guidance in selecting age-appropriate material, as research suggests that users may conform their behavior to their preconceptions about the avatars they embody [57,58].

3.5. *Embodiment*

When body trackers, such as hand trackers, are used in virtual reality, participants can move their tracked limbs in real life and see their movements represented by the movements of their avatars in virtual reality. Thus, when patients are embodied in an avatar, they gain the sense that their avatar body has replaced their real body. This allows interventions that are possible in no other medium.

The tracking capabilities inherent in embodied VR experiences also offer clinicians the ability to monitor their patients' physical movements and quantify rehabilitative effort without relying on self-report data. As wearable monitors for tracking physiological data such as gait and posture become increasingly used, clinicians may observe their patients on multiple levels and tailor their treatment accordingly. As with all patient data, movement data in children must be carefully protected.

Movement is not the only aspect of patient activity that can be visualized. Biofeedback is one arena that would lend itself well to the flexibility of virtual reality, allowing the visualization of pain-linked physiological signals. This could be particularly useful for children who may not be as adept as adults at verbally describing sensory information, or translating verbal instruction into action. An example is described in a recent pilot study mentioned above, where non-immersive VR mirror visual feedback was used in combination with biofeedback to treat pediatric patients with chronic headaches [56].

In VR, patients can also be embodied in novel avatars, or avatars that do not conform to the limitations of their physical bodies [57,58]. As discussed above, Jäncke et al. propose that children may be more susceptible than adults to developing a feeling of presence in virtual environments, even in novel avatar bodies [59]. Thus, as with virtual environments, the experience of embodiment in an avatar, especially an avatar that is dissimilar to a child's real body must be contextualized. Debriefing post-VR may be necessary.

4. Practical Aspects of Virtual Reality: Hardware and Software

Clinicians looking to integrate virtual reality into their practice may benefit from the following information about the strengths and limitations of current consumer VR set-ups.

At a minimum, virtual reality requires a display in which the user sees the virtual environment. In the most common consumer systems, this is done through a head-mounted display (HMD). An HMD is a type of VR headset that displays digital images on two screens in front of the user's eyes. In phone-based VR systems such as Gear VR, Google Cardboard or Google Daydream, the HMD consists of a smartphone wrapped in an inexpensive case with lenses, such that the phone provides both the computing power and display. In more powerful VR systems, such as the Oculus Rift or HTC Vive, the content displayed on the headset is generated by a desktop or laptop computer certified as "VR ready" by the manufacturer, or, in the case of PlayStation, by a video game console. In all of these systems, the user's movements are tracked, and the system updates the content that is displayed to the user based on these tracked movements. Thus, as a child turns her head when looking around a virtual environment through an HMD, the content updates on the screens in front of her eyes, just as it would in the physical world if she turned her head to look at a different part of the room. Brief descriptions of some currently available consumer systems are found in Table 3.

4.1. Tracking Movement

Tracking users' movements while they experience VR is a key factor in creating realistic and compelling scenarios [1]. Two kinds of tracking are used in VR: orientation and position. Orientation, shown in Figure 1, tracks the user's head movements and allows her to gaze around her virtual environment.

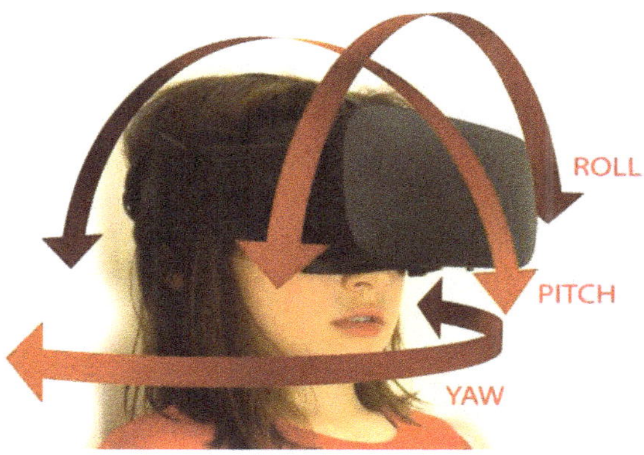

Figure 1. The child may move her head in pitch orientation, as in nodding her head, in yaw orientation, as in moving her head from side to side to look around the environment, or in roll orientation, as in touching her ear to her shoulder.

In VR systems that only have orientation, users are unable to move through scenes using their own body movement (i.e., walking). Instead, users might navigate through virtual environments using gaze, touchpad input or other less-embodied navigation techniques. Currently, smartphone-based devices tend to track only head orientation. While these systems are more limited in some respects, they are generally portable and self-contained, and require very little set-up time or space to use. They are also lighter, cheaper and potentially easier to clean and/or have disposable components, all of which may provide significant advantages when using them for pediatric patients.

In addition to orientation tracking, systems can also have positional tracking (e.g., moving forwards or backwards in VR). Position, shown in Figure 2, tracks the user's body and allows him to relocate within his environment. If the user holds hand trackers, his or her hands will also be tracked. This allows the user to interact with objects in the environment using his or her hands, and optionally see his or her hands represented by an avatar's hands. Positional tracking typically uses external sensors placed around a room that capture the position of the headset and/or additional tracked objects. Such systems allow users to walk around in the virtual space.

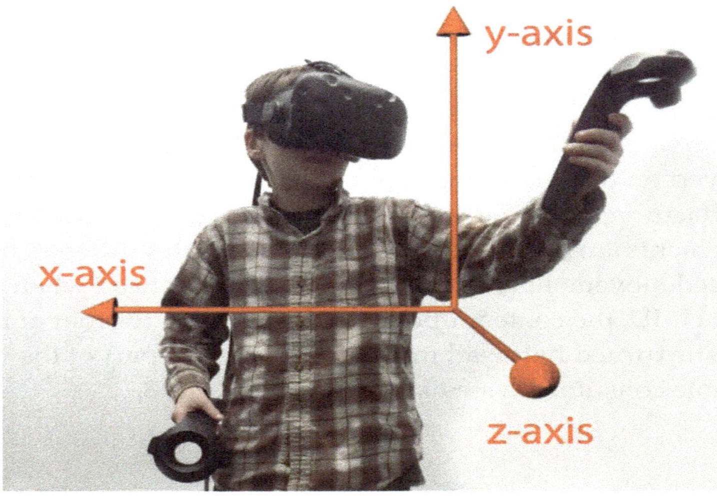

Figure 2. Virtual Reality (VR) coordinate system. In this picture, movement in the *y*-axis corresponds to moving up and down, movement in the *x*-axis corresponds to moving left and right, and movement in the *z*-axis corresponds to moving forward and backward. While global positional coordinates may vary according to set up, *y* is the up–down direction and the *z*-axis will often reflect movement towards the monitor of the desktop computer.

While they increase the level of interaction available, systems with sophisticated tracking capabilities that include hand trackers tend to be more expensive than those that only capture orientation. While still portable to an extent, more complex systems also require sufficient space for patients to safely move around, and the headsets may be heavier. They will also require more set-up time.

4.2. Hardware Issues to Consider for Children

Although consumer headsets are designed to be adjustable, they can be too heavy or too large to be easily used by smaller children, as Dahlquist, et al. speculate in their 2009 study [41]. An additional issue for hospital use is that headsets, along with hand-tracking devices, which come into close contact with users' bodies, will need to be cleaned.

These issues and more can be easily addressed through modular additions and adaptations to the basic VR unit, which would allow the technology to be effective in a wide range of clinical situations. Some consumer systems have washable covers to protect the parts of the headset that come into contact with patients' skin. Cleansing wipes can also be used on both trackers and sensors. In a 2014 study on a patient who had burn wounds on his head, a consumer HMD was mounted to an articulated arm so that the patient did not actually need to wear the device [9]. Very young children may also need the unfamiliar equipment to be decorated or disguised to be more appealing. As one of the authors has found, by introducing an HMD as a mask with a soft cover designed with a friendly face, children were more open to wearing the virtual reality equipment [60]. If trends in lightness, portability, and decreased price continue, VR systems are likely to become increasingly better adapted for pediatric patients.

Table 3. Virtual Reality (VR) head-mounted display (HMD) hardware. This table provides a non-exhaustive list of hardware

Product Name	Pricing for Headset at Time of Publication	Product Information	Description	Appropriate Ages	Limitations	Tracking
Head and Hand Tracking						
HTC Vive	$799	https://www.vive.com/us/	HMD & hand trackers, whole-room VR	(minimum 7+)	Requires "VR ready" personal computer (PC)	Positional and rotational
Oculus Rift &Touch Controllers	$599.98	https://www.oculus.com/rift/	HMD & hand trackers, can be set up on a desktop	13+	Requires "VR ready" PC	Positional and rotational
PlayStation VR	$499	https://www.playstation.com/en-us/explore/playstation-vr/	Video game console HMD and hand trackers	12+	Requires Sony PS4, compatible only with PlayStation games	Positional and rotational
Head Tracking						
Google Cardboard	$5 and up	https://vr.google.com/cardboard/	Phone-based	Unspecified; with adult supervision (single use <5–10 min)	No hand tracking, limited interactivity; requires VR-compatible phone	Rotational
Google Daydream	$79	https://vr.google.com/daydream/	Phone-based; lightweight; includes controller	13+	Currently limited software library; requires VR-compatible phone	Rotational with one controller
Gear VR	$129.99	https://www.oculus.com/gear-vr/	Phone-based, adjustable headset with hand controller	13+	Limited features compared to PC-based VR; requires VR-compatible phone	Rotational

4.3. Virtual Content

Researchers seeking virtual content have three options. They may use existing free or inexpensive consumer content. They may develop their own content. Finally, they may work with industry partners focused on the clinical use of virtual reality. The following section lists some resources available at press time.

Free or pre-existing games designed for virtual reality are becoming increasingly available and may be an appropriate option, particularly for procedural pain. Such games can be purchased and downloaded; for example, through the Steam and Oculus libraries. Another type of frequently free virtual content is 360° videos, which can be downloaded directly to the device. Some main content libraries are currently YouTube360, Within, Jaunt, NYTVR, Condition One, WSJ, and LifeVR [61]. Most content in these libraries consists of 360° videos, which allow for orientation tracking without much interaction. Finally, social interactions in a virtual space can be facilitated using social platforms such as Facebook Spaces, High Fidelity, AltSpaceVR, etc.

Virtual content can be also created for specific clinical purposes using development platforms such as Unity3D (unity3d.com), Unreal (unreal.com) and Vizard (vizard.com). Researchers seeking to create customized content, which might include those investigating rehabilitation or neurorehabilitation, may require specialized tracking and rendering or customization. Such researchers might consider collaborating with university departments, for example computer science, information science, or communication departments, or work with existing software companies. Recording one's own immersive video is also an option. Cameras ranging in complexity and price from the hundreds to thousands of dollars allow researchers to record their own video content and prepare it for viewing through a phone-based HMD.

Finally, there is increasing commercial interest in supplying clinicians with virtual reality applications. While it is outside the scope of this paper to recommend specific companies, searching for "virtual reality therapy" online will provide a list of suppliers. In addition, it is possible to make some recommendations for clinicians to take into consideration when working with a supplier. If patient data is collected as part of treatment, it may raise confidentiality issues. Developers should have experience working in a clinical setting. Compatibility with hardware should also be considered, as some application developers use proprietary hardware, while others allow the use of consumer systems. A brief list of currently available free games can be found in Table 4, below.

Table 4. Suggestions for VR games and their applications.

Game Title	Hardware Compatibility	Where to Find It	Potential Applications	Qualities
Google Earth VR	-HTC Vive -Oculus Rift	https://vr.google.com/earth/	-Anxiety -Distraction therapy -Procedural pain	-Hands-free -Cinematic -Engaging
Minecraft	-HTC Vive -Oculus Rift -Samsung -GearVR -Google -Cardboard	1. Install PC version of Minecraft 2. Install Vivecraft (http://www.vivecraft.org/) for VR compatibility	-Anxiety -Distraction therapy	-Controller required -Well-known by kids -Engaging
Guided Meditation VR	-HTC Vive -Oculus Rift -Samsung -GearVR	https://guidedmeditationvr.com/download/	-Anxiety -Distraction therapy -Procedural pain	-Hands Free -Calming
The Lab	-HTC Vive -Oculus Rift	http://store.steampowered.com/app/450390/The_Lab/	-Anxiety -Distraction therapy	-Exploration -Specific movements (archery + slingshot) -Scenic
The Blu	-HTC Vive -Oculus Rift	http://store.steampowered.com/app/451520/theBlu/	-Anxiety -Distraction therapy	-Hands-free -Cinematic -Exploration

While more research is necessary to determine the more complex aspects of VR in pediatric care, VR can be used immediately to improve the quality of life for pediatric patients. A clinician may order one of the above-mentioned devices to be kept in the clinic and made available to patients who require one of the procedures described earlier in this review. For example, a child might be given a headset and immersed in a relaxing forest scene while they are receiving an immunization or IV placement. Alternatively, a child requiring frequent dressing changes, or other painful procedures may choose to purchase a unit for home use to assist with pain management. A patient with chronic pain may find it beneficial to use VR interventions to temporarily alleviate symptoms, or to assist in performing challenging tasks while in physical or occupational therapy. The number of applications is unlimited, and can be adapted to the individual child's interests and the clinical therapeutic need.

5. Conclusions

In summary, VR is a promising new technology that offers unique opportunities to modulate the experience of pain. These opportunities include the management of acute and procedural pain and familiarizing children with future procedures via simulation. In addition, extrapolating from current evidence in adults, we propose that virtual reality may assist in the treatment of pediatric chronic pain via neuromodulation, as well as physical therapy.

Given the reduction in cost and increased ease of access, we hope that clinicians will be encouraged to explore the potential of this new modality. While the immediate adoption of VR can already engage and entertain children in a clinical setting with potential therapeutic benefits, continued study of the applications and efficacy of virtual reality in the treatment of pediatric pain is needed to better understand the impact upon quality of life for pediatric patients.

Acknowledgments: Andrea Stevenson Won's research was supported by a gift from the MAYDAY Fund through Program Officer Christina M. Spellman. Jakki O. Bailey was funded by the Sesame Workshop Dissertation Award.

References

1. Cummings, J.J.; Bailenson, J.N. How immersive is enough? A meta-analysis of the effect of immersive technology on user presence. *Media Psychol.* **2016**, *19*, 272–309. [CrossRef]
2. Hoffman, H.G.; Doctor, J.N.; Patterson, D.R.; Carrougher, G.J.; Furness, T.A., III. Virtual reality as an adjunctive pain control during burn wound care in adolescent patients. *Pain* **2000**, *85*, 305–309. [CrossRef]
3. Human Photonics Laboratory. Available online: www.Vrpain.com (accessed on 7 March 2017).
4. Schmitt, Y.S.; Hoffman, H.G.; Blough, D.K.; Patterson, D.R.; Jensen, M.P.; Soltani, M.; Carrougher, G.J.; Nakamura, D.; Sharar, S.R. A randomized, controlled trial of immersive virtual reality analgesia, during physical therapy for pediatric burns. *Burns* **2011**, *37*, 61–68. [CrossRef] [PubMed]
5. Jeffs, D.; Dorman, D.; Brown, S.; Files, A.; Graves, T.; Kirk, E.; Meredith-Neve, S.; Sanders, J.; White, B.; Swearingen, C.J. Effect of virtual reality on adolescent pain during burn wound care. *J. Burn Care Res.* **2014**, *35*, 395–408. [CrossRef] [PubMed]
6. Brown, N.J.; Kimble, R.M.; Rodger, S.; Ware, R.S.; Cuttle, L. Play and heal: Randomized controlled trial of Ditto™ intervention efficacy on improving re-epithelialization in pediatric burns. *Burns* **2014**, *40*, 204–213. [CrossRef] [PubMed]
7. Miller, K.; Rodger, S.; Bucolo, S.; Greer, R.; Kimble, R.M. Multi-modal distraction. Using technology to combat pain in young children with burn injuries. *Burns* **2010**, *36*, 647–658. [CrossRef] [PubMed]
8. Pardesi, O.; Fuzaylov, G. Pain management in pediatric burn patients: Review of recent literature and future directions. *J. Burn Care Res.* **2017**. [CrossRef] [PubMed]
9. Hoffman, H.G.; Meyer, W.J., III; Ramirez, M.; Roberts, L.; Seibel, E.J.; Atzori, B.; Sharar, S.R.; Patterson, D.R. Feasibility of articulated arm mounted Oculus Rift Virtual Reality goggles for adjunctive pain control during occupational therapy in pediatric burn patients. *Cyberpsychol. Behav. Soc. Netw.* **2014**, *17*, 397–401. [CrossRef] [PubMed]
10. Gold, J.I.; Kim, S.H.; Kant, A.J.; Joseph, M.H.; Rizzo, A.S. Effectiveness of virtual reality for pediatric pain distraction during IV placement. *CyberPsychol. Behav.* **2006**, *9*, 207–212. [CrossRef] [PubMed]
11. Wong, D.L.; Baker, C.M. Pain in children: comparison of assessment scales. *Pediatr. Nurs.* **1988**, *14*, 9–17. [PubMed]

12. Nilsson, S.; Finnström, B.; Kokinsky, E.; Enskär, K. The use of virtual reality for needle-related procedural pain and distress in children and adolescents in a paediatric oncology unit. *Eur. J. Oncol. Nurs.* **2009**, *13*, 102–109. [CrossRef] [PubMed]
13. He, H.G.; Zhu, L.; Chan, S.W.C.; Liam, J.L.W.; Li, H.C.W.; Ko, S.S.; Klainin-Yobas, P.; Wang, W. Therapeutic play intervention on children's perioperative anxiety, negative emotional manifestation and postoperative pain: A randomized controlled trial. *J. Adv. Nurs.* **2015**, *71*, 1032–1043. [CrossRef] [PubMed]
14. Shahrbanian, S.; Ma, X.; Aghaei, N.; Korner-Bitensky, N.; Moshiri, K.; Simmonds, M.J. Use of virtual reality (immersive vs. non immersive) for pain management in children and adults: A systematic review of evidence from randomized controlled trials. *Eur. J. Exp. Biol.* **2012**, *2*, 1408–1422.
15. Ramachandran, V.S.; Rogers-Ramachandran, D. Synaesthesia in phantom limbs induced with mirrors. *Proc. Biol. Sci.* **1996**, *263*, 377–386. [CrossRef] [PubMed]
16. McCabe, C.; Haigh, R.; Ring, E.; Halligan, P.; Wall, P.; Blake, D. A controlled pilot study of the utility of mirror visual feedback in the treatment of complex regional pain syndrome (type 1). *Rheumatology* **2003**, *42*, 97–101. [CrossRef] [PubMed]
17. Sato, K.; Fukumori, S.; Matsusaki, T.; Maruo, T.; Ishikawa, S.; Nishie, H.; Takata, K.; Mizuhara, H.; Mizobuchi, S.; Nakatsuka, H. Nonimmersive virtual reality mirror visual feedback therapy and its application for the treatment of complex regional pain syndrome: An open-label pilot study. *Pain Med.* **2010**, *11*, 622–629. [CrossRef] [PubMed]
18. Harvie, D.S.; Broecker, M.; Smith, R.T.; Meulders, A.; Madden, V.J.; Moseley, G.L. Bogus visual feedback alters onset of movement-evoked pain in people with neck pain. *Psychol. Sci.* **2015**, *26*, 385–392. [CrossRef] [PubMed]
19. Chen, K.B.; Sesto, M.E.; Ponto, K.; Leonard, J.; Mason, A.; Vanderheiden, G.; Williams, J.; Radwin, R.G. Use of virtual reality feedback for patients with chronic neck pain and kinesiophobia. *IEEE Trans. Neural Syst. Rehabil. Eng.* **2016**. [CrossRef] [PubMed]
20. Won, A.S.; Tataru, C.A.; Cojocaru, C.M.; Krane, E.J.; Bailenson, J.N.; Niswonger, S.; Golianu, B. Two virtual reality pilot studies for the treatment of pediatric CRPS. *Pain Med.* **2015**, *16*, 1644–1647. [CrossRef] [PubMed]
21. Lebel, A.; Becerra, L.; Wallin, D.; Moulton, E.; Morris, S.; Pendse, G.; Jasciewicz, J.; Stein, M.; Aiello-Lammens, M.; Grant, E. fMRI reveals distinct CNS processing during symptomatic and recovered complex regional pain syndrome in children. *Brain* **2008**, *131*, 1854–1879. [CrossRef] [PubMed]
22. Becerra, L.; Sava, S.; Simons, L.E.; Drosos, A.M.; Sethna, N.; Berde, C.; Lebel, A.A.; Borsook, D. Intrinsic brain networks normalize with treatment in pediatric complex regional pain syndrome. *NeuroImage Clin.* **2014**, *6*, 347–369. [CrossRef] [PubMed]
23. Simons, L.; Pielech, M.; Erpelding, N.; Linnman, C.; Moulton, E.; Sava, S.; Lebel, A.; Serrano, P.; Sethna, N.; Berde, C. The responsive amygdala: Treatment-induced alterations in functional connectivity in pediatric complex regional pain syndrome. *Pain* **2014**, *155*, 1727–1742. [CrossRef] [PubMed]
24. Makin, T.R.; Scholz, J.; Henderson Slater, D.; Johansen-Berg, H.; Tracey, I. Reassessing cortical reorganization in the primary sensorimotor cortex following arm amputation. *Brain* **2015**, *138*, 2140–2146. [CrossRef] [PubMed]
25. Walz, A.D.; Usichenko, T.; Moseley, G.L.; Lotze, M. Graded motor imagery and the impact on pain processing in a case of CRPS. *Clin. J. Pain* **2013**, *29*, 276–279. [CrossRef] [PubMed]
26. Wang, M.; Reid, D. Virtual reality in pediatric neurorehabilitation: Attention deficit hyperactivity disorder, autism and cerebral palsy. *Neuroepidemiology* **2011**, *36*, 2–18. [CrossRef] [PubMed]
27. Weiss, P.L.; Tirosh, E.; Fehlings, D. Role of virtual reality for cerebral palsy management. *J. Child Neurol.* **2014**, *29*, 1119–1124. [CrossRef] [PubMed]
28. Biffi, E.; Beretta, E.; Cesareo, A.; Maghini, C.; Turconi, A.C.; Reni, G.; Strazzer, S. An immersive virtual reality platform to enhance walking ability of children with acquired brain injuries. *Methods Inf. Med.* **2017**, *56*, 119–126. [CrossRef] [PubMed]
29. Meyns, P.; Pans, L.; Plasmans, K.; Heyrman, L.; Desloovere, K.; Molenaers, G. The Effect of additional virtual reality training on balance in children with cerebral palsy after lower limb surgery: A feasibility study. *Games Health J.* **2017**, *6*, 39–48. [CrossRef] [PubMed]
30. Trost, Z.; Zielke, M.; Guck, A.; Nowlin, L.; Zakhidov, D.; France, C.R.; Keefe, F. The promise and challenge of virtual gaming technologies for chronic pain: The case of graded exposure for low back pain. *Pain Manag.* **2015**, *5*, 197–206. [CrossRef] [PubMed]

31. Collado-Mateo, D.; Dominguez-Muñoz, F.J.; Adsuar, J.C.; Merellano-Navarro, E.; Gusi, N. Exergames for women with fibromyalgia: A randomised controlled trial to evaluate the effects on mobility skills, balance and fear of falling. *PeerJ* **2017**, *5*, e3211. [CrossRef] [PubMed]
32. Senkowski, D.; Heinz, A. Chronic pain and distorted body image: Implications for multisensory feedback interventions. *Neurosci. Biobehav. Rev.* **2016**, *69*, 252–259. [CrossRef] [PubMed]
33. Simons, L.E.; Kaczynski, K.J. The Fear Avoidance model of chronic pain: Examination for pediatric application. *J. Pain* **2012**, *13*, 827–835. [CrossRef] [PubMed]
34. Pekyavas, N.O.; Ergun, N. Comparison of virtual reality exergaming and home exercise programs in patients with subacromial impingement syndrome and scapular dyskinesis: Short term effect. *Acta Orthop. Traumatol. Turc.* **2017**, in press. [CrossRef] [PubMed]
35. Odell, S.; Logan, D.E. Pediatric pain management: The multidisciplinary approach. *J. Pain Res.* **2013**, *6*, 785–790. [CrossRef] [PubMed]
36. Shiri, S.; Feintuch, U.; Weiss, N.; Pustilnik, A.; Geffen, T.; Kay, B.; Meiner, Z.; Berger, I. A virtual reality system combined with biofeedback for treating pediatric chronic headache—A pilot study. *Pain Med.* **2013**, *14*, 621–627. [CrossRef] [PubMed]
37. Soltani, M.; Teeley, A.M.; Wiechman, S.A.; JENSEN, M.P.; SHARAR, S.R.; Patterson, D.R. Virtual reality hypnosis for pain control in a patient with gluteal hidradenitis: A case report. *Contemp. Hypn. Integr. Ther.* **2011**, *28*, 142–147.
38. Lombard, M.; Ditton, T. At the heart of it all: The concept of presence. *J. Comput. Med. Commun.* **1997**, *3*. [CrossRef]
39. Wiederhold, B.K.; Jang, D.; Kaneda, M.; Cabral, I.; Lurie, Y.; May, T.; Kim, I.; Wiederhold, M.D.; Kim, S. An investigation into physiological responses in virtual environments: an objective measurement of presence. In *Towards Cyberpsychology: Mind, Cognitions and Society in the Internet Age*; Riva, G., Galimberti, C., Eds.; IOS Press: Amsterdam, 2001; pp. 176–182.
40. Sanchez-Vives, M.V.; Slater, M. From presence to consciousness through virtual reality. *Nat. Rev. Neurosci.* **2005**, *6*, 332–339. [CrossRef] [PubMed]
41. Dahlquist, L.M.; Weiss, K.E.; Clendaniel, L.D.; Law, E.F.; Ackerman, C.S.; McKenna, K.D. Effects of videogame distraction using a virtual reality type head-mounted display helmet on cold pressor pain in children. *J. Pediatr. Psychol.* **2009**, *34*, 574–584. [CrossRef] [PubMed]
42. Law, E.F.; Dahlquist, L.M.; Sil, S.; Weiss, K.E.; Herbert, L.J.; Wohlheiter, K.; Horn, S.B. Videogame distraction using virtual reality technology for children experiencing cold pressor pain: The role of cognitive processing. *J. Pediatr. Psychol.* **2011**, *36*, 84–94. [CrossRef] [PubMed]
43. Sharar, S.R.; Carrougher, G.J.; Nakamura, D.; Hoffman, H.G.; Blough, D.K.; Patterson, D.R. Factors influencing the efficacy of virtual reality distraction analgesia during postburn physical therapy: Preliminary results from 3 ongoing studies. *Arch. Phys. Med. Rehabil.* **2007**, *88*, S43–S49. [CrossRef] [PubMed]
44. Baumgartner, T.; Speck, D.; Wettstein, D.; Masnari, O.; Beeli, G.; Jäncke, L. Feeling present in arousing virtual reality worlds: Prefrontal brain regions differentially orchestrate presence experience in adults and children. *Front. Hum. Neurosci.* **2008**, *2*, 8. [CrossRef] [PubMed]
45. Flavell, J.H.; Flavell, E.R.; Green, F.L.; Korfmacher, J.E. Do young children think of television images as pictures or real objects? *J. Broadcast. Electron. Media* **1990**, *34*, 399–419. [CrossRef]
46. Richert, R.A.; Robb, M.B.; Smith, E.I. Media as social partners: The social nature of young children's learning from screen media. *Child Dev.* **2011**, *82*, 82–95. [CrossRef] [PubMed]
47. Dahlquist, L.M.; McKenna, K.D.; Jones, K.K.; Dillinger, L.; Weiss, K.E.; Ackerman, C.S. Active and passive distraction using a head-mounted display helmet: Effects on cold pressor pain in children. *Health Psychol.* **2007**, *26*, 794–801. [CrossRef] [PubMed]
48. Bryanton, C.; Bosse, J.; Brien, M.; Mclean, J.; McCormick, A.; Sveistrup, H. Feasibility, motivation, and selective motor control: Virtual reality compared to conventional home exercise in children with cerebral palsy. *Cyberpsychol. Behav.* **2006**, *9*, 123–128. [CrossRef] [PubMed]
49. Olson, C.K. Children's motivations for video game play in the context of normal development. *Rev. Gener. Psychol.* **2010**, *14*, 180. [CrossRef]
50. Blakemore, S.-J.; Mills, K.L. Is adolescence a sensitive period for sociocultural processing? *Annu. Rev. Psychol.* **2014**, *65*, 187–207. [CrossRef] [PubMed]

51. Claxton, L.J.; Ponto, K.C. Understanding the properties of interactive televised characters. *J. Appl. Dev. Psychol.* **2013**, *34*, 57–62. [CrossRef]
52. Forgeron, P.A.; King, S.; Stinson, J.N.; McGrath, P.J.; MacDonald, A.J.; Chambers, C.T. Social functioning and peer relationships in children and adolescents with chronic pain: A systematic review. *Pain Res. Manag.* **2010**, *15*, 27–41. [CrossRef] [PubMed]
53. Beals, L.; Bers, M.U. A developmental lens for designing virtual worlds for children and youth. *Int. J. Learn. Media* **2009**, 51–65. [CrossRef]
54. Ni, L.T.; Fehlings, D.; Biddiss, E. Design and evaluation of virtual reality-based therapy games with dual focus on therapeutic relevance and user experience for children with cerebral palsy. *Games Health J.* **2014**, *3*, 162–171. [CrossRef] [PubMed]
55. Schneider, S.M.; Workman, M. Effects of virtual reality on symptom distress in children receiving chemotherapy. *CyberPsychol. Behav.* **1999**, *2*, 125–134. [CrossRef] [PubMed]
56. Li, H.C.W.; Lopez, V.; Lee, T.L.I. Effects of preoperative therapeutic play on outcomes of school-age children undergoing day surgery. *Res. Nurs. Health* **2007**, *30*, 320–332.
57. Fox, J.; Bailenson, J.N.; Tricase, L. The embodiment of sexualized virtual selves: The Proteus effect and experiences of self-objectification via avatars. *Comput. Hum. Behav.* **2013**, *29*, 930–938. [CrossRef]
58. Yee, N.; Bailenson, J. The Proteus effect: The effect of transformed self-representation on behavior. *Hum. Commun. Res.* **2007**, *33*, 271–290. [CrossRef]
59. Jäncke, L.; Cheetham, M.; Baumgartner, T. Virtual reality and the role of the prefrontal cortex in adults and children. *Front. Neurosci.* **2009**, *3*, 6. [CrossRef] [PubMed]
60. Bailey, J.O.; Bailenson, J.N.; Obradović, J.; Aguiar, N.R. The influence of Immersive virtual reality on children's inhibitory control and social behavior. Presented at the International Communication's 67th Annual Conference, San Diego, CA, USA, 25–29 May 2017.
61. Rasmussen, N.B. Top 10 Most Viewed 360° Videos of 2016. *Time*, 26 July 2016.

5

Pediatric Integrative Medicine in Residency Program: Relationship between Lifestyle Behaviors and Burnout and Wellbeing Measures in First-Year Residents

Hilary McClafferty [1,*], Audrey J. Brooks [1,*], Mei-Kuang Chen [1], Michelle Brenner [2], Melanie Brown [3], Anna Esparham [4], Dana Gerstbacher [5], Brenda Golianu [6], John Mark [5], Joy Weydert [4], Ann Ming Yeh [5] and Victoria Maizes [1]

1 Department of Medicine, Arizona Center for Integrative Medicine, University of Arizona, Tucson, AZ 85724, USA; kuang@email.arizona.edu (M.-K.C.); vmaizes@email.arizona.edu (V.M.)

2 Department of Pediatrics, Eastern Virginia Medical School/Children's Hospital of the King's Daughters, Norfolk, VA 23507, USA; michelle.brenner@chkd.org

3 Department of Pediatrics, University of Chicago Comer Children's Hospital, Chicago, IL 60637, USA; Melanie.Brown@childrensmn.org

4 Department of Pediatrics, University of Kansas School of Medicine, Kansas City, KS 66160, USA; aeesparham@cmh.edu (A.E.); jweydert@kumc.edu (J.W.)

5 Department of Pediatrics, Stanford University School of Medicine, Palo Alto, CA 94304, USA; gerst1@stanford.edu (D.G.); jmark@stanford.edu (J.M.); annming@stanford.edu (A.M.Y.)

6 Department of Anesthesiology and Pain Management, Stanford University School of Medicine, Palo Alto, CA 94304, USA; bgolianu@stanford.edu

* Correspondence: hmcclafferty@email.arizona.edu (H.M.); brooksaj@email.arizona.edu (A.J.B.)

Abstract: It is widely recognized that burnout is prevalent in medical culture and begins early in training. Studies show pediatricians and pediatric trainees experience burnout rates comparable to other specialties. Newly developed Accreditation Council for Graduate Medical Education (ACGME) core competencies in professionalism and personal development recognize the unacceptably high resident burnout rates and present an important opportunity for programs to improve residents experience throughout training. These competencies encourage healthy lifestyle practices and cultivation of self-awareness, self-regulation, empathy, mindfulness, and compassion—a paradigm shift from traditional medical training underpinned by a culture of unrealistic endurance and self-sacrifice. To date, few successful and sustainable programs in resident burnout prevention and wellness promotion have been described. The University of Arizona Center for Integrative Medicine Pediatric Integrative Medicine in Residency (PIMR) curriculum, developed in 2011, was designed in part to help pediatric programs meet new resident wellbeing requirements. The purpose of this paper is to detail levels of lifestyle behaviors, burnout, and wellbeing for the PIMR program's first-year residents (N = 203), and to examine the impact of lifestyle behaviors on burnout and wellbeing. The potential of the PIMR to provide interventions addressing gaps in lifestyle behaviors with recognized association to burnout is discussed.

Keywords: burnout; pediatrics; residents; preventive lifestyle behaviors; resilience

---

1. Introduction

Medical school and residency training are known for their scientific rigor and daunting hours of service [1,2]. Compounding burnout experienced in medical school, the life of a resident is dominated by exposure to significant human suffering, high levels of responsibility, lack of day-to-day control, steep learning curves, limited regeneration time, and chronic sleep deprivation. These realities, in conjunction with patient and family demands, subordinate ranking in the medical hierarchy, and other stressors predispose residents to high burnout prevalence [1,2].

Studies show that pediatricians and pediatric trainees experience burnout at rates comparable to other specialties, with higher prevalence in some high acuity pediatric subspecialties such as neonatology, intensive care, and hematology-oncology [3–6]. Across medical specialties and training levels, burnout has been associated with an increase in medical errors, lower adherence to best practices, substance abuse, self-medication, and poorer patient outcomes (for example, longer hospital stay), in addition to increased rates of clinician's depression, suicidal ideation, and completed suicide [7]. It has been widely reported that effective approaches must include changes at organizational, institutional, and individual levels to address the outdated culture of unrealistic endurance still pervasive in medicine [8].

Newly developed Accreditation Council for Graduate Medical Education (ACGME) core competencies in professionalism and personal development recognize the unacceptably high burnout rates in residents and present an important opportunity for programs to improve the experience of residents at all stages of training [9].

In addition to encouraging healthy lifestyle practices, the core competencies encourage cultivation of self-awareness, self-regulation skills, empathy, mindfulness, and compassion. They also highlight the need for innovation in clinical training and generate questions about how to best teach and measure success in these new areas. This endeavor provides important opportunities to introduce proactive approaches to burnout through a multidimensional model and development of educational curricula that emphasize and measure wellbeing at all phases of medical training.

To date, along with development of the new core competencies, purposeful steps taken by the ACGME include national symposia led by expert national faculty to identify actionable issues, new emphasis on education on physician wellbeing, and recommendations for annual measurement of resident burnout through its Clinical Learning Environmental Review (CLER) program which evaluates the quality of the program learning environment [10].

Despite these significant initiatives, few successful, sustainable programs in resident burnout prevention and wellness promotion have been described. Pediatricians are uniquely positioned to develop national initiatives for solution-based approaches to burnout, in part due to the timely initiation of the 2010 Pediatric Milestone Project, a collaboration between the ACGME and the American Board of Pediatrics (ABP) dedicated to development of revised core competencies. The University of Arizona Center for Integrative Medicine Pediatric Integrative Medicine in Residency (PIMR) curriculum was developed in 2011 and refined in 2012 to include a robust Self-Care unit, partly in response to the new priorities in the revised national pediatric training competencies targeting resident wellbeing outlined by the ACGME.

The 100-h curriculum is an interactive hybrid online-onsite program and has been described in detail in an earlier publication [11]. The program has been piloted since 2012 at the University of Arizona, Stanford University, the University of Kansas, the University of Chicago, and Eastern Virginia Medical School/Children's Hospital of the King's Daughters. The topics covered include: Self-; nutrition and physical activity; mind-body therapies; dietary supplements; whole systems of medicine; and clinical applications.

The curriculum was developed with the two-fold purpose of embedding foundational education in pediatric integrative medicine into residency training and introducing a 'train the trainer' model in teaching healthy lifestyle habits. In anticipation of high levels of burnout in incoming residents, the Self-Care unit was designed to provide an evidence-based 'blueprint' for learning about factors associated with lower burnout prevalence in medical trainees including: physical activity, sleep, stress management, mindfulness, and nutrition, thereby increasing resident knowledge about self-care and also providing a useful educational tool for residency programs to address new ACGME resident wellness competency requirements. An integrated evaluation arm measures resident burnout and lifestyle behaviors, and gathers feedback on perceived quality and relevance of the curriculum at four points (beginning, end Post Graduate Year (PGY) 1, end PGY2, end PGY3) of residency training.

We readily acknowledge that change is urgently needed on multiple levels to address the serious issues of preventing burnout and promoting wellbeing in medical trainees, ideally starting in pre-medical and medical students. We believe our study findings detailing the incoming resident levels of burnout, wellbeing, and lifestyle behaviors and examining the relationship between resident lifestyle habits and burnout and wellbeing measures reinforce this point and begin to explore areas of potential progress. The overarching purpose of this paper is to document the concerning state of burnout in early pediatric trainees and to examine the potential of the PIMR curriculum to provide interventions that address gaps in lifestyle behaviors with recognized association to burnout, and how they might be introduced into residency training.

2. Methods

Approval for the study was granted by the University of Arizona Institutional Review Board (Approval #12049200). First-year pediatric residents from five residencies participating in the PIMR program completed standardized wellbeing measures at the start of residency. The PIMR sites include academic and community-based programs led by pediatric faculty with fellowship training in integrative medicine, a field that blends conventional and evidence-based complementary medicine and prioritizes preventive health. Information about existing onsite physician wellness activities was collected and is presented. Data is being collected as part of a longitudinal study on resident wellbeing, burnout and lifestyle behaviors and the longitudinal impact of the PIMR curriculum.

2.1. Measures

Residents completed eight widely used, established scales assessing dimensions of well-being: perceived stress, depression symptoms, burnout (emotional exhaustion, depersonalization), life satisfaction, affect, mindfulness, emotional intelligence, and physician empathy (Table 1). A measure of lifestyle behaviors, the Arizona Lifestyle Inventory (ALI) [12], was also administered. The ALI was developed to assess changes in lifestyle behaviors in residents. The domains and items were identified from literature on evidence-based preventive services as well as other areas emphasized by integrative medicine practitioners. The items were reviewed by an expert panel of integrative medicine physicians and were revised based on their comments. The ALI primarily assesses the frequency of behaviors in the past seven days in the areas of diet/nutrition, exercise, mind-body/spiritual practices, social support activities, sleep, and work stress (see Table 2 for items by domain); areas known to mediate the relationships between stress reactivity and physical and mental health. The ALI also includes demographic variables, including hours worked, alcohol use, and health status questions, having a chronic medical condition, taking medication for a chronic medical condition, body mass index (BMI), taking prescription medication for stress or anxiety, days with pain in the past week, and days engaged in hobbies in the past week.

Site leaders completed a survey of onsite physician wellness activities in 2014 and 2016. Physician wellness activities included retreats, nutrition (healthy food options), empathy skills training, conflict resolution/communication skills training, stress management, physical activity options (e.g., exercise rooms), self-regulation skills training (e.g., mind-body skills training), and burnout prevention.

Table 1. Wellbeing measures.

Dimension	Measure	Description
Perceived stress	Perceived Stress Scale (PSS) [13]	10 items; scores 0–40
Depression symptoms	Center for Epidemiologic Studies—Depression Scale (CES-D) [14]	20 items; scores range from 0–60; score of 16 or higher indicates clinical syndrome
Burnout	Maslach Burnout Inventory (MBI) [15,16]	22 items; 3 subscales emotional exhaustion (EE), depersonalization (DEP), personal accomplishment (PA)
Life satisfaction	Satisfaction with Life Scale (SWLS) [17,18]	5 items; higher total scores indicate greater life satisfaction
Affect	Positive and Negative Affect Scale (PANAS) [19]	20 items; 2 subscales positive affect (POS), negative affect (NEG); higher score more positive, more negative affect
Mindfulness	Freiberg Mindfulness Inventory (FMI) [20]	14 items, higher score more mindful
Emotional Intelligence	Interpersonal Reactivity Index (IRI) [21]	21 items; 3 subscales perspective taking (PT), empathic concern (EC), personal distress (PD); higher scores greater perspective taking, empathic concern, personal distress
Empathy [a]	Jefferson Empathy Scale (JES) [22]	20 items, higher score greater empathy
Lifestyle Behaviors	Arizona Lifestyle Inventory [12]	35 items measuring frequency of diet/nutrition, exercise, mind-body/spiritual practices, social support activities, sleep, hobbies, alcohol consumption behaviors

[a] JES not collected in 2012 class.

2.2. Data Collection and Statistical Analysis

Data were collected directly from the residents online using an individualized link to an internet-based survey website (Survey Monkey, San Mateo, CA, USA) in the first trimester of the first year of residency. Prior to accessing the assessments, residents voluntarily completed an online informed consent form. Statistical analyses were conducted using SPSS v. 24.0 (IBM Corp. Released 2016. IBM SPSS Statistics for Windows, Version 24.0. Armonk, NY, USA).

Descriptive statistics are presented for the wellbeing measures and lifestyle behaviors. A burnout risk group variable was created utilizing medicine norms [15] as follows: high burnout consists of individuals scoring in the high range on both emotional exhaustion and depersonalization; low burnout group includes individuals scoring in the low range on both scales; remaining individuals were categorized as moderate burnout. One-way analysis of variance (ANOVA) with post hoc Tukey tests were conducted to compare wellbeing measures and lifestyle behaviors among burnout groups.

A series of multiple regression analyses were performed to examine the relationship between the lifestyle behavior domains and each of the wellbeing measures. For the lifestyle behaviors, due to variation in response format for some items, scale total scores were calculated utilizing two procedures. For scales where all items were rated on a 0–7 scale (number of days of carrying out the specific lifestyle behavior in the past seven days) the scale scores were formed using mean scores of the items in the same domain. For items where there was variation in response format, such as exercise, social support activities, and alcohol use, items were standardized first and then the means of the z-scores were used as the scale scores. Items were reverse-scored where indicated. With the exception of the work stress scale, higher scores indicate engaging in more of the behaviors in that domain. Higher scores on the work stress scale indicate a greater level of work stress. The correlation between the wellbeing measures and gender and marital status were examined. If the correlation was statistically significant, gender and/or marital status was included in the model. The initial regression models included all lifestyle variables and demographic variables, as indicated. A final regression analysis was performed dropping non-significant predictors ($p > 0.05$).

3. Results

3.1. Sample

The sample consisted of 203 first-year residents from four incoming classes (2012, $n = 15$; 2013, $n = 88$; 2014, $n = 59$; 2015, $n = 41$) at five pediatric residency programs participating in the PIMR program: (1) University of Arizona ($n = 41$); (2) University of Chicago ($n = 56$); (3) Eastern Virginia Medical School/Children's Hospital of the King's Daughters ($n = 55$); (4) University of Kansas Medical Center ($n = 26$); and (5) Stanford University ($n = 25$). The survey response rate across the cohorts was 63% and ranged between 45–88% across the residency programs. The sample was predominantly female (76%), white (71%) or Asian (13%), and non-Hispanic (94%) with an average age of 28 years old (range 24–39 years old). Half of the sample was married or cohabitating (50%) and 12% had children. The majority of residents were US Doctors of Medicine (76%), followed by foreign medical graduates (13%) and US Doctors of Osteopathic Medicine (11%). Residents completed the online surveys at the beginning of PGY1. In terms of health status, 25% ($n = 50$) reported a chronic medical condition and 19% ($n = 38$) reported taking medication for a chronic medical condition. The most common medical conditions reported were psychological (depression, anxiety, and/or attention deficit hyperactivity disorder; $n = 15$), asthma ($n = 12$) and allergies ($n = 9$). More than two-thirds (68.2%; $n = 135/198$) had a normal BMI, while 23% ($n = 46$) fell in the overweight range and 5% were in the obese range ($n = 10$). Residents reported experiencing pain an average of 1.3 days in the past seven days (range 0–7). Almost half of the residents (47%; $n = 95$) reported experiencing at least one day of pain. Few residents reported taking prescription medication for stress or anxiety ($n = 16$; 8%). Alcohol consumption averaged 2.8 drinks in the past 7 days, with a maximum of 15 drinks in the past week. Three residents reported smoking cigarettes (2%). In terms of hours worked in the past week, 92% ($n = 186$) reported working 80 h or less with 59% ($n = 119$) working 61–80 h.

3.2. Wellbeing Measures

Descriptive statistics for the wellbeing measures are presented in Table 2. The average perceived stress score (16) for this resident sample was slightly higher than normed sample data for the general public (11.9–14.7), but was consistent with ranges for healthcare students (15.5–16.7) [23]. The average depression score (12.9) was within the non-depressed range, with 70% of the sample scoring in this range. However, 30% scored over 16, the cut-off score indicating a risk for clinical depression [14,24]. Over half the sample (55%) scored in the low emotional exhaustion range. Less than half (42%) scored in the low depersonalization range. Twenty percent of residents scored in the high emotional exhaustion range and 32% scored in the high depersonalization range. Fifteen percent scored in the high burnout range on both the emotional exhaustion and depersonalization scales. The average score on personal accomplishment (29.5) was in the low range (high risk for burnout) [15]. The average life satisfaction score was 26.4 (in the satisfied range) with 68.9% scoring in the satisfied to extremely satisfied range [17,18]. The mean positive affect (35.2) and negative affect scores (20.6) were slightly better than the mid-point (30) on the Positive and Negative Affect Schedule (PANAS) scale and consistent with what was observed in incoming family medicine residents in the Integrative Medicine in Residency (IMR) program [25].

The average mindfulness score (35.4) was slightly higher than a general sample [20]. Residents in the current sample scored lower on perspective taking and empathic concern and higher on personal distress than a study of incoming internal medicine residents [26]. The average empathy score in this resident sample (110.75) is lower than means obtained in the Jefferson Empathy Scale (JES) validation study with both resident and medical student samples (118) [22].

Table 2. Measures of wellbeing—descriptive statistics.

Wellbeing Measures	*N*	*n*	Mean (SD)/% Yes	Range	Norm Data
Perceived stress	190		16.0 (5.9)	2–31	11.9–14.7 [1]
CES-D depression	190		12.9 (9.2)	0–42	
Non-depressed		132	69.5%		<16 non-depressed
Clinical depression risk		58	30.5%		≥16
MBI—Emotional exhaustion	203		18.1 (9.0)	0–54	19–26 average
Low emotional exhaustion		112	55.2%		
Moderate emotional exhaustion		50	24.6%		
High emotional exhaustion		41	20.2%		
MBI—Depersonalization	203		7.4 (4.9)	0–30	6–9 average
Low depersonalization		85	41.9%		
Moderate depersonalization		54	26.6%		
High depersonalization		64	31.5%		
MBI—Burnout risk group					
Low risk		70	34.5%		
Moderate risk		102	50.2%		
High risk		31	15.3%		
MBI—Personal accomplishment	203		29.5 (6.3)	12–48	39–34 average
Satisfaction with life	203		26.4 (5.8)	5–35	26–30 satisfied
PANAS Positive	174		35.2 (6.4)	10–50	35.3 [2]
PANAS Negative	174		20.6 (6.0)	10–42	19.6 [3]
Mindfulness	191		35.4 (7.1)	16–54	34.52 [3], 31.17 [4]
IRI Empathic concern	190		21.5 (4.0)	11–28	22.2 [5]
IRI Personal distress	190		10.4 (4.9)	0–25	8.9 [5]
IRI Perspective taking	189		18.3 (4.3)	2–28	20.6 [5]
Jefferson empathy	174		110.7 (14.2)	79–140	118 [6]

[1] General public validation sample; [2] Post Graduate Year (PGY1) Family medicine residents; [3] General sample; [4] Clinical sample; [5] PGY1 Internal medicine residents; [6] Resident and medical student mean, SD: standard deviation.

3.3. Lifestyle Behaviors

Descriptive statistics for the lifestyle behavior items by domain are presented in Table 3. Eating breakfast was the most frequent behavior (mean = 5.7 days), while eating 5 servings of fruits and vegetables was the least frequent (mean = 3.3 days). Most did not drink sugary beverages (60%). Residents reported an average of 2 days of at least 10 min moderate exercise and 1.6 days of 10 min of vigorous exercise. More than half of residents reported either 1–2 days (42%) or 3–4 days (28%) of 30 min of moderate exercise. Most residents (83%) reported sedentary behavior less than 70% on an average day. Residents reported engaging in an activity to manage stress an average of 3.3 days. The most frequent practice was prayer (mean 2.3 days). The least frequent practice was progressive muscle relaxation (mean = 0.2 days). While residents reported spending time in nurturing relationships with family or friends most days (mean = 4.8 days), much less time was spent socializing with friends (mean = 2.1 days). Most residents (74%) reported feeling a sense of belonging to a group. While getting 7–9 h of sleep (mean = 3.4 days) or waking feeling rested (mean = 3 days) averages were somewhat low, trouble staying asleep was not a frequent issue (mean = 1.4 days). Residents reported enjoying work an average of 4.6 days and feeling overwhelmed 2.6 days per week.

Table 3. Lifestyle behaviors—descriptive statistics.

Domain/Items	*N*	*n*	Mean/%	SD	Range
Diet/Nutrition					
5 Servings fruits & vegetables	203		3.3	2.2	0–7
Eat calcium rich foods	203		4.9	2.0	0–7
Eat breakfast	200		5.7	1.9	0–7
Eat home cooked dinner	203		4.2	2.0	0–7
Drank caffeinated beverages *	203		5.6	2.2	0–7
Sugary fluid drinks average day *	202		0.6	0.9	0–5
0		122	60.4%		
1		61	30.2%		
2		8	3.9%		
3		9	4.5%		
4		1	0.5%		
5 or more		1	0.5%		
Servings high fiber average day	203		2.1	1.3	0–5
0		15	7.4%		
1		51	25.1%		
2		67	33.0%		
3		43	21.2%		
4		14	6.9%		
5 or more		13	6.4%		
Vegetarian	188		0.07	0.25	0–1
Yes		13	6.9%		
Exercise					
Vigorous physical activity ≥ 10 min	202		1.6	1.8	0–7
Moderate physical activity ≥ 10 min	202		2.0	2.0	0–7
Moderate physical activity ≥ 30 min	187				
None		28	15.0%		
1–2 days		78	41.7%		
3–4 days		53	28.3%		
5–6 days		21	11.2%		
Everyday		7	3.7%		
Percent sedentary average day *	198				
Less than 5%		4	2.0%		
6–10%		8	4.0%		
11–20%		12	6.1%		
21–30%		19	9.6%		
31–40%		25	12.6%		
41–50%		36	18.2%		
51–60%		29	14.6%		
61–70%		31	15.7%		
71–80%		25	12.6%		
81–90%		9	4.5%		
91–100%		0	0%		
Mind-Body/Spiritual Practices					
Activity to relax or manage stress	202		3.3	2.4	0–7
Prayer	202		2.3	2.8	0–7
Spiritual ritual non-prayer	202		0.6	1.7	0–7
Personal reflection	201		1.5	2.2	0–7
Breathing for stress reduction	202		0.5	1.3	0–7
Progressive muscle relaxation	191		0.2	0.8	0–7
Social Support Activities					
Spend time family/friends	203		4.8	2.3	0–7
Receive healthy touch	203		4.4	2.6	0–7
Socialize with friends	202		2.1	1.6	0–7
Sense of belonging groups	203				
Yes		150	73.9%		
Not sure		20	9.9%		
No		33	16.3%		
Number groups belong	203		1.9	1.2	0–6
Sleep					
Get 7–9 h of sleep	203		3.4	2.2	0–7
Wake feeling rested	201		3.0	2.1	0–7
Trouble staying asleep *	201		1.4	2.0	0–7

Table 3. *Cont.*

Domain/Items	*N*	*n*	Mean/%	SD	Range
Hobbies	202		2.1	2.3	0–7
Number of Alcohol Drinks	200		2.8	3.0	0–15
Work					
Enjoy work *	203		4.6	1.9	0–7
Feel overwhelmed by work	203		2.6	2.2	0–7

* Items reverse-scored when creating scales.

3.4. Differences between Burnout Risk Groups on Wellbeing and Lifestyle Behaviors

In the analyses examining the impact of burnout risk level on wellbeing, all of the models were statistically significant ($p < 0.006$; Table 4). In comparing the burnout risk groups, the low burnout risk group experienced significantly greater wellbeing than the high-risk group ($p < 0.05$) in all of the models. Specifically, the low burnout risk group experienced less perceived stress, depression, negative affect, and personal distress and greater satisfaction with life, positive affect, mindfulness, empathic concern, perspective taking, and empathy than the high-risk burnout group ($p < 0.05$). Differences between the moderate burnout risk group and the high burnout risk group were also observed for perceived stress, depression, negative affect, satisfaction with life, positive affect, mindfulness, perspective taking and empathy ($p < 0.05$), with the moderate risk group experiencing greater wellbeing than the high-risk group. The low burnout risk group was significantly different from the moderate burnout risk group, experiencing less perceived stress, depression, and negative affect and greater positive affect, empathic concern, and empathy ($p < 0.05$). All post hoc group comparisons were statistically significant in the perceived stress, depression, negative affect, positive affect, and empathy analyses, indicating that wellbeing decreased significantly as burnout risk increased.

Table 4. Results of one-way variance analysis (ANOVA) for Burnout Group and wellbeing—means and standard deviations.

Wellbeing Measures	Total *N* *	Low Risk *n* = 70		Moderate Risk *n* = 102		High Risk *n* = 31		*p*-Value
		Mean	SD	Mean	SD	Mean	SD	
Perceived Stress	190	12.6 [a,c]	5.1	16.4 [b]	4.9	22.7	4.4	<0.001
CES-D Total	190	8.1 [a,c]	5.7	12.6 [b]	8.0	25.2	8.3	<0.001
Satisfaction with Life	203	27.9 [a]	4.3	27.0 [b]	5.3	21.1	7.4	<0.001
PANAS Positive	174	38.0 [a,c]	4.5	35.4 [b]	6.4	28.6	4.6	<0.001
PANAS Negative	174	17.5 [a,c]	4.6	20.5 [b]	5.2	27.8	4.9	<0.001
FMI Mindfulness	191	37.6 [a]	6.9	35.1 [b]	7.1	31.6	6.4	0.001
IRI Empathic Concern	190	22.8 [a,c]	3.7	21.2	3.9	19.7	3.9	0.001
IRI Perspective Taking	189	19.5 [a]	4.1	18.2 [b]	3.8	15.5	5.2	<0.001
IRI Personal Distress	190	9.3 [a]	4.7	10.4	4.8	12.7	4.7	0.006
Jefferson Empathy	174	115.8 [a,c]	13.0	110.6 [b]	13.2	99.2	14.1	<0.001
Lifestyle Behaviors								
Diet/Nutrition	203	0.084	0.51	0.043 [b]	0.40	−0.20	0.62	0.048
Exercise [d]	203	0.045	0.7	0.053	0.7	−0.25	0.6	0.095
Mind-body/Spiritual Practices	203	1.6	1.2	1.4	1.0	1.1	1.1	0.13
Social Support Activities [d]	203	0.018 [a]	0.7	0.075 [b]	0.6	−0.30	0.7	0.012
Sleep	203	4.4 [a]	1.5	4.1 [b]	1.4	2.9	1.3	<0.001
Hobbies	202	2.3	2.6	2.0	2.1	1.8	2.1	0.56
Alcohol drinks	200	2.5	2.7	3.2	2.9	2.5	3.6	0.32
Work Stress	203	1.7 [a,c]	1.1	2.6 [b]	1.5	4.2	1.6	<0.001

* *N* varied by measure. Post hoc Tukey tests: [a] low-risk vs. high-risk group, $p < 0.05$; [b] moderate-risk vs. high-risk group, $p < 0.05$; [c] low-risk vs. moderate-risk group, $p < 0.05$; [d] means for exercise and social relationships are *z*-scores, therefore the group mean is zero. Means greater than 0 indicate higher frequency than the group mean, while negative means indicate a frequency lower than the group mean.

For the lifestyle behaviors, the diet/nutrition, social relationships, sleep and work stress models were statistically significant ($p < 0.05$; Table 4). The post hoc group comparisons between the low-risk and high-risk groups or moderate-risk and high-risk groups, were statistically significant ($p < 0.05$) in these models. The low-risk and moderate-risk groups reported engaging in a greater frequency of social behaviors and quality sleep than the high-risk group. For diet/nutrition, the high-risk group reported a lower frequency of healthy eating behaviors than the moderate risk group. In the work stress model, the post hoc comparisons were significantly different between all burnout groups, indicating an increase in work stress as burnout risk increased ($p < 0.05$). There was no difference between the burnout risk groups for exercise, mind-body/spiritual practices, hobbies or alcohol use.

3.5. Relationship between Lifestyle Behaviors and Wellbeing Measures

Gender was significantly correlated with empathic concern and empathy and, therefore, included in those regression models. Marital status was correlated with life satisfaction and included in that regression model. The various combinations of lifestyle behaviors contributed 6% to 49% of the variance in the tested models (R^2), depending on the wellbeing measure examined (see Tables 5 and 6). Work stress was a statistically significant predictor in all but one regression model, empathic concern. Greater work stress was associated with increased perceived stress, depression, emotional exhaustion, depersonalization, negative affect, personal distress, and lower personal accomplishment, life satisfaction, positive affect, mindfulness, perspective taking, and empathy. The second-strongest predictor across the wellbeing models was exercise. A higher frequency of engaging in exercise was associated with less perceived stress, depression, negative affect, and personal distress, and higher levels of personal accomplishment, positive affect, mindfulness, perspective taking, and empathy. A higher frequency of engaging in social support activities was associated with higher life satisfaction, mindfulness, and empathic concern and less depression. More quality sleep was associated with less perceived stress, depression, emotional exhaustion, and negative affect. A greater frequency of healthy eating behaviors was associated with lower levels of depersonalization and higher life satisfaction. While a higher frequency of engaging in hobbies was associated with decreased personal distress, it was also associated with less mindfulness. Mind-body/spiritual practices were associated with increased mindfulness only. Alcohol use was non-significant in all the models. Gender was associated with empathic concern and empathy, with females having greater empathic concern and empathy, while marital status was non-significant.

Table 5. Lifestyle behavior predictors, R^2 and betas on measures of wellbeing [a].

Wellbeing Measure	Model Adjusted R^2	Model p-Value	β	t	p-Value
Perceived stress	0.39	<0.001			
Work stress			0.50	7.95	<0.001
Exercise			−0.19	−3.35	0.001
Sleep			−0.16	−2.45	0.015
CES-D Total	0.49	<0.001			
Work			0.47	7.80	<0.001
Sleep			−0.23	−3.93	<0.001
Social			−0.18	−3.14	0.002
Exercise			−0.13	−2.38	0.018
MBI emotional exhaustion	0.40	<0.001			
Work stress			0.56	9.52	<0.001
Sleep			−0.17	−2.94	0.004
MBI Depersonalization	0.16	<0.001			
Work stress			0.34	5.21	<0.001
Diet			−0.20	−3.09	0.002
MBI personal accomplishment	0.18	<0.001			
Work Stress			−0.34	−5.32	<0.001
Exercise			0.23	3.64	<0.001
Satisfaction with life [b]	0.26	<0.001			
Work stress			−0.36	−5.65	<0.001
Social			0.21	3.29	0.001
Diet			0.16	2.60	0.010

Table 5. *Cont.*

Wellbeing Measure	Model Adjusted R^2	Model p-Value	β	t	p-Value
PANAS positive	0.31	<0.001			
Work stress			−0.46	−7.29	<0.001
Exercise			0.27	4.25	<0.001
PANAS negative	0.26	<0.001			
Work stress			0.37	5.05	<0.001
Exercise			−0.17	−2.64	0.009
Sleep			−0.17	−2.34	0.021
Mindfulness	0.20	<0.001			
Work stress			−0.27	−3.95	<0.001
Exercise			0.25	3.66	<0.001
Social			0.15	2.18	0.031
Hobbies			−0.16	−2.27	0.024
Mind-body			0.14	2.01	0.046
IRI empathic concern [c]	0.06	0.001			
Gender			0.20	2.77	0.006
Social			0.17	2.41	0.017
IRI perspective taking	0.064	0.001			
Work stress			−0.20	−2.76	0.006
Exercise			0.18	2.47	0.014
IRI Personal distress	0.078	<0.001			
Exercise			−0.21	−2.94	0.004
Work stress			0.20	2.78	0.006
Hobbies			−0.15	−1.97	0.050
Jefferson empathy [c]	0.17	<0.001			
Gender			0.29	4.11	<0.001
Exercise			0.26	3.72	<0.001
Work stress			−0.17	−2.47	0.009

[a] Only statistically significant ($p < 0.05$) predictors in final model are presented. b Due to the correlation with marital status, marital status was included in the initial model. However, it was non-significant and was dropped from the final model. Married/cohabitating is coded as 1, single as 0. [c] Due to the correlation with gender, gender was included in the model. Gender is coded 1 for male, 2 for female.

Table 6. Lifestyle behavior predictors and relationship to wellbeing measures.

Lifestyle Behavior	PSS	CES-D	MBI-EE	MBI-DEP	MBI-PA	SWLS	PANAS Positive	PANAS Negative	FMI	IRI EC	IRI PT	IRI PD	JES
Work Stress	↑	↑	↑	↑	↓	↓	↓	↑	↓		↓	↑	↓
Exercise	↓	↓			↑		↑	↓	↑		↑	↓	↑
Social Support		↓				↑			↑	↑			
Sleep	↓	↓	↓					↓					
Diet/Nutrition				↓		↑							
Hobbies									↓			↓	
Gender										↑			↑
Mind-body/Spiritual									↓				
Alcohol drinks													

↑ Positive relationship between wellness behavior and wellbeing measure; ↓ Negative relationship between wellness behavior and wellbeing measure.

3.6. On-Site Physician Wellness Activities

Wellness retreats were the most frequent type of wellness activity offered, with all sites hosting wellness-focused retreats over the three-year period (see Figure 1). These retreats varied in content-based on-site faculty preferences and available resources. Most were held off-site in a private setting and provided opportunity for small group discussions and peer support, informational seminars, and experiential learning. The next-most frequently reported activity was increased nutrition options for residents, available initially at four sites, and at all sites by 2016. Physical activity options (mainly access to gyms) increased from two sites in 2014 to four sites by 2016. Burnout prevention activities increased from one site in 2014 to four sites; and by 2016, other wellness activities (empathy skills training, self-regulation skills, conflict resolution/communication, and stress management) were offered at three of the five sites.

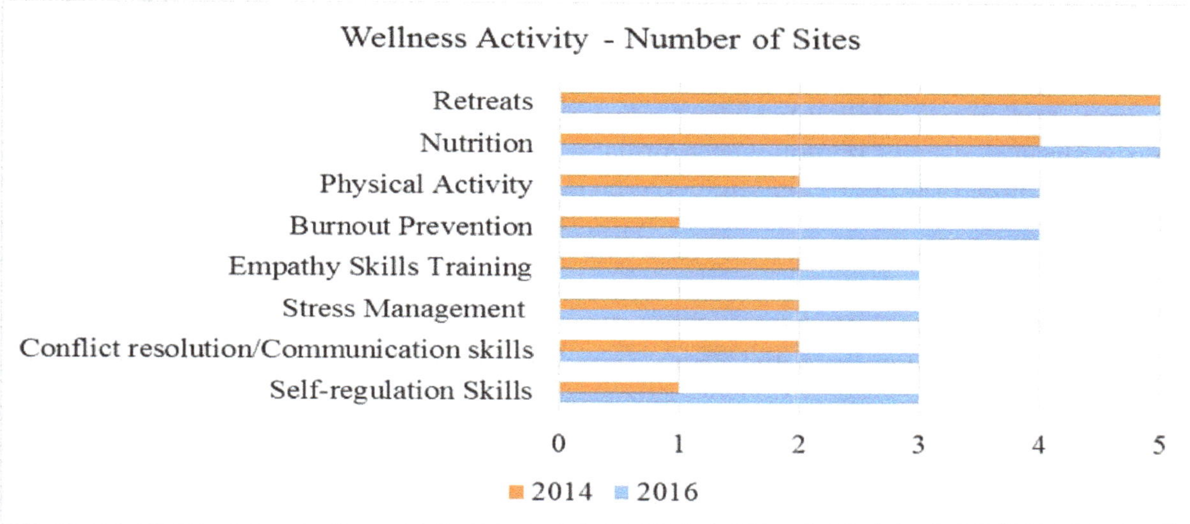

Figure 1. On-site physician wellness activities—number of sites by year.

4. Discussion

It is well established that burnout is prevalent in medical trainees and takes a steep toll on mental and physical health [2]. This highlights the need for reform of the current medical education model, and the paradox of recruiting medical students for both their academic strength and empathic qualities. A combination that may predispose talented trainees to distress during the rigors of conventional medical training. Addressing and preventing burnout from the very earliest stages of medical school training is necessary, because burnout impacts patient care, quality of patient counseling, and prevalence of medical errors [7]. The etiology of burnout is complex, involving a variety of factors at the organizational, institutional, and individual levels, requiring coordinated, systems-level solutions [8]. Surveys show that burnout rates in pediatric trainees mirror national prevalence, emphasizing the urgent need for change at the earliest stages of pediatric training in addition to preventive steps and education during medical school to avoid the recurring pitfall of receiving first-year residents already in serious stages of burnout [4,6].

To highlight this point, our study findings demonstrate that a substantial proportion of first-year pediatric residents in the PIMR pilot study began residency with higher levels of burnout and depression and poorer emotional intelligence and empathy than comparison samples, mirroring national trends [6]. Fifteen percent of residents in the study were high risk (high on both emotional exhaustion and depersonalization), 50% were in the moderate risk (high or moderate in either emotional exhaustion or depersonalization), and 35% were at low risk. In addition, with respect to depression, 30% scored in the clinical depression risk range. This is considerably higher than a study of residents and medical students that found 11% of first year residents were in the clinical depression risk range [27].

In the cohort, as burnout risk increases, overall wellbeing, empathy and emotional intelligence decreases. Residents with high burnout risk also reported more days of experiencing work stress, and had lower wellbeing, social support, stress management behaviors, emotional intelligence, and empathy than residents in the low and moderate risk groups. Overall, work stress was the strongest predictor of burnout, wellbeing, and emotional intelligence in our sample, significant in all models except empathic concern. The sense of feeling overwhelmed and lack of work enjoyment appears to permeate all areas of the resident's life, increasing burnout and decreasing wellbeing, emotional intelligence, mindfulness, and empathy.

Residents in the high-risk burnout group reported lower frequencies of healthy eating, social support activities, and quality sleep than their peers. One in four residents were living with a chronic illness, and 28% of residents entering the PIMR program were either overweight (23%) or obese (5%), highlighting the links between chronic stress and upregulation of inflammatory cytokines, depression, and other related comorbidities [28–30].

Exercise was a strong predictor of wellbeing and emotional intelligence, associated with less stress and depression, greater personal accomplishment, affect, mindfulness, emotional intelligence and empathy, although not distinguishing between burnout groups. Inadequate sleep was associated with emotional exhaustion, as well as stress, depression, and negative affect, similar to the burnout risk models. Social support activities were associated with less depression and greater life satisfaction, mindfulness, and empathic concern, although contrary to the burnout models, they were not associated with the burnout measures. Higher quality diet/nutrition behaviors were associated with less depersonalization and greater life satisfaction. Female gender was associated with greater empathic concern and empathy.

In our study, mind-body spiritual practices were not associated with any of the burnout, wellbeing, or emotional intelligence measures. One reason for these findings may be due to the low frequency of engagement in these behaviors in this sample. The narrow range may have limited the ability to detect an association to the burnout, wellbeing, and emotional intelligence variables. Fortunately, some residency programs are beginning to teach these behaviors, and future studies will be able to examine the role of mind-body practices in prevention of burnout.

In summary, a majority of residents in the study were at either moderate or high risk of burnout, not meeting basic recommendations for healthy lifestyle habits, and stood a 1 in 4 chance of being overweight or obese. Our findings are consistent with other surveys that document high levels of burnout in graduating US medical students [31], and mirror studies demonstrating lack of regular physical activity in residents [32,33], and published reports of lower levels of stress and burnout in medical students who exercised regularly [34–36]. While the percentage of overweight residents was lower in our sample (23%) when compared to a study of first year residents from multiple specialties (34%) [37], the rate of obese residents in our sample of pediatric residents was higher (5% vs. 0%). In addition to the protective lifestyle behaviors mentioned, the remaining wellness activities (empathy skills training, self-regulation skills, conflict resolution/communication, stress management) were offered at 3 of the 5 sites. Ideally, these would serve to help moderate perceived work stress and help build connections at work, cultivating social resilience, which has been shown to be protective against burnout in medical training [38].

National surveys have shown that organizational and institutional measures to reduce and prevent burnout are effective [39,40], and a prudent financial investment [41]. Despite these findings, and widespread recognition of burnout's mental and physical toll, few programs offer approaches to promote self-care activities associated with lower burnout prevalence [34,42–44].

The PIMR program addresses these gaps in two important ways. First, by embedding a curriculum on protective lifestyle behaviors into residency training, the concept of self-care is acknowledged and normalized. Second, engagement of a critical mass of residents and faculty instructors participating in and teaching these activities drives broader culture change within individual organizations. In our study, this is borne out by the increase in program wellness activities over time. Perhaps most notable is the increase from only 1 site offering burnout prevention activities in 2014 to 4 sites with burnout prevention activities in 2016. Newly revised ACGME competencies mandating specific attention to resident wellbeing will hopefully provide critical leverage to move this initiative forward [9].

Furthermore, promotion of healthy lifestyle behaviors in residents aligns with developing themes in the medical literature suggesting that trainees with healthier lifestyle habits are more likely to counsel patients on healthy lifestyle habits, and to do so more effectively than their less healthy colleagues [45–47]. This point has special relevance in pediatric trainees, who have the potential to encourage a lifetime of healthy habits in their young patients.

Limitations

One of the main limitations of this study is the limited generalizability of the findings. The five participating residencies were not randomly selected but volunteered to participate to pilot a new integrative medicine curriculum. Given that there are nearly 200 pediatric residencies nationwide, it is not possible to determine the representativeness of these 5 sites. In addition, the response rate was 63% across the sites, with variation in the response rate between the sites, also limiting our ability to generalize our findings. Data was collected during the first trimester of residency and does not reflect the full measure of residency stressors that accumulate throughout residency.

A second limitation is our primary emphasis on lifestyle behaviors as potential mediators/moderators in the relationship between stress and burnout and its consequent effects. Individual factors that can mediate the impact of stress, such as cognitive appraisals, coping styles and strategies, self-efficacy expectations, grit, optimism, resiliency, hardiness, and social competence were not assessed. System level factors were also not assessed. These include current rotations, prior experience, and levels of faculty support and burnout and how this influences resident burnout, all areas of active study. The newly developed lifestyle behavior instrument used in this study may not have fully captured the lifestyle behaviors most critical to wellbeing. Further, the lifestyle behaviors were captured retrospectively, thus it was not possible to confirm the accuracy of the self-reported lifestyle behaviors with other methods, such as daily recording of the behavior. Lastly, the study utilized online self-report surveys which may be subject to recall bias and social desirability influences.

Future directions could address efforts to increase the reach of the PIMR program by increasing the number of enrolled sites and residents, thereby increasing reach and diversity. Another strategy might include a more tailored rollout of self-care curriculum modules designed to educate leaders and encourage a culture of wellness and engagement within the top levels of organizations [48].

5. Conclusions

Accruing research suggests that first-year residents enter training with high levels of burnout, emphasizing the need for effective solutions to address burnout in medical education. Burnout prevalence in our study supported these findings. Furthermore, high burnout risk was associated with a decrease in overall wellbeing, increased work stress, inadequate sleep, fewer social support activities, and poorer diet quality. New mandates from the ACGME to promote resident wellbeing are encouraging, yet few educational programs currently exist to meet these requirements. National surveys show that organizational measures designed to reduce burnout have proven effective. The PIMR program offers an innovative curriculum that residency programs can use to target protective lifestyle behaviors correlated with decreased burnout measures. These include physical activity, sleep, nutrition, and stress management/coping skills. Within the PIMR program, education about these behaviors is delivered in a train the trainer educational model that will ideally equip residents to become more effective role models and counselors to their young patients.

Author Contributions: H.M. and A.J.B. conceived and designed the study; H.M., A.J.B., M.-K.C., M.B., M.B., A.E., D.G., B.G., J.M., J.W., and A.M.Y. participated in study design and data collection; H.M., A.J.B. and M.-K.C. analyzed and interpreted the data; H.M. and A.J.B. wrote the body of the paper, and all authors contributed substantially to individual sections and editing of drafts.

Acknowledgments: Sincere thanks to all the residents and faculty participating in the PIMR pilot program, as well as to all faculty involved in the early adopter phase including: Maria Mascarenhas and Miriam Stewart, Children's Hospital of Philadelphia; Carmen Herrera, University of New Mexico; Alexandra Russell, Vanderbilt University; Rukmani Vasan, University of Southern California; Marian Eckert, Kinderkrankenhaus St. Marien; Elena Ladas, Columbia University; Hillary Franke, University of Arizona; J. Paige Frazer, Eastern Virginia Medical School, Children's Hospital of the King's Daughters. Thanks also go to Paula Cook, Research Specialist, and Rhonda Hallquist, Instructional Web Developer, for their many contributions. And a special thanks to Emily Sherbrooke, IMR/PIMR Program Coordinator Sr.; and to Janice Curtis, Administrative Associate, for their administrative support and expert help in manuscript preparation. Funding was received from the David and Lura Lovell Foundation, the Weil Foundation, the Gerald J. and Rosalie E. Kahn Family Foundation, Inc., the John F. Long Foundation, the Resnick Foundation, and the Sampson Foundation.

References

1. Dyrbye, L.N.; West, C.P.; Satele, D.; Boone, S.; Tan, L.; Sloan, J.; Shanafelt, T.D. Burnout among US medical students, residents, and early career physicians relative to the general US population. *Acad. Med.* **2014**, *89*, 443–451. [CrossRef] [PubMed]
2. Dyrbye, L.; Shanafelt, T. A narrative review on burnout experienced by medical students and residents. *Med. Educ.* **2016**, *50*, 132–149. [CrossRef] [PubMed]
3. McClafferty, H.; Brown, O.W. Physician health and wellness. *Pediatrics* **2014**, *134*, 830–835. [CrossRef] [PubMed]
4. Pantaleoni, J.L.; Augustine, E.M.; Sourkes, B.M.; Bachrach, L.K. Burnout in pediatric residents over a 2-year period: A longitudinal study. *Acad. Pediatr.* **2014**, *14*, 167–172. [CrossRef] [PubMed]
5. Mahan, J.D. Burnout in pediatric residents and physicians: A call to action. *Pediatrics* **2017**, *139*, e20164233. [CrossRef] [PubMed]
6. Baer, T.E.; Feraco, A.M.; Sagalowsky, S.T.; Williams, D.; Litman, H.J.; Vinci, R.J. Pediatric resident burnout and attitudes toward patients. *Pediatrics* **2017**, *139*, e20162163. [CrossRef] [PubMed]
7. Jennings, M.L.; Slavin, S.J. Resident wellness matters: Optimizing resident education and wellness through the learning environment. *Acad. Med.* **2015**, *90*, 1246–1250. [CrossRef] [PubMed]
8. Shanafelt, T.D.; Dyrbye, L.N.; West, C.P. Addressing physician burnout: The way forward. *JAMA* **2017**, *317*, 901–902. [CrossRef] [PubMed]
9. Accreditation Council for Graduate Medical Education (ACGME). Revised Common Program Requirements, Section VI, The Learning and Working Environment. Available online: https://www.acgmecommon.org/press_release (accessed on 2 March 2017).
10. Accreditation Council for Graduate Medical Education (ACGME). Physician Wellbeing. Available online: http://www.acgme.org/What-We-Do/Initiatives/Physician-Well-Being (accessed on 3 February 2017).
11. McClafferty, H.; Dodds, S.; Brooks, A.J.; Brenner, M.; Brown, M.; Frazer, P.; Mark, J.; Weydert, J.; Wilcox, G.; Lebensohn, P.; Maizes, V. Pediatric integrative medicine in residency (PIMR): Description of a new online educational curriculum. *Children* **2015**, *2*, 98–107. [CrossRef] [PubMed]
12. Lebensohn, P.; Brooks, A.J.; Chen, M.K. A multi-dimensional integrative health measure to assess wellness behaviors—The Arizona lifestyle inventory. In Proceedings of the International Conference to Promote Resilience, Empathy and Well-Being in Health Care Professions (CENTILE 2017), Washington, DC, USA, 22–25 October 2017.
13. Cohen, S.; Kamarck, T.; Mermelstein, R. A global measure of perceived stress. *J. Health Soc. Behav.* **1983**, *24*, 385–396. [CrossRef] [PubMed]
14. Radloff, L.S. The CES-D scale: A self-report depression scale for research in the general population. *Appl. Psychol. Meas.* **1977**, *1*, 385–401. [CrossRef]
15. Maslach, C.; Jackson, S.E.; Leiter, M.P. *Maslach Burnout Inventory*, 3rd ed.; Consulting Psychologists Press: Palo Alto, CA, USA, 1996.
16. Maslach, C.; Jackson, S.E.; Leiter, M. *Maslach Burnout Inventory Manual*, 4th ed.; Mind Garden Inc.: Menlo Park, CA, USA, 2016.
17. Diener, E.; Emmons, R.A.; Larsen, R.J.; Griffin, S. The satisfaction with life scale. *J. Pers. Assess.* **1985**, *49*, 71–75. [CrossRef] [PubMed]
18. Pavot, W.; Diener, E. Review of the satisfaction with life scale. *Psychol. Assess.* **1993**, *5*, 164–172. [CrossRef]
19. Watson, D.; Clark, L.A.; Tellegen, A. Development and validation of brief measures of positive and negative affect: The PANAS scales. *J. Pers. Soc. Psychol.* **1988**, *54*, 1063–1070. [CrossRef] [PubMed]
20. Walach, H.; Buchheld, N.; Buttenmüller, V.; Kleinknecht, N.; Schmidt, S. Measuring mindfulness—The Freiburg mindfulness inventory (FMI). *Pers. Individ. Dif.* **2006**, *40*, 1543–1555. [CrossRef]
21. Davis, M.H. Measuring individual differences in empathy: Evidence for a multidimensional approach. *J. Pers. Soc. Psychol.* **1983**, *44*, 113–126. [CrossRef]
22. Hojat, M.; Mangione, S.; Nasca, T.J.; Cohen, M.J.M.; Gonnella, J.S.; Erdmann, J.B.; Veloski, J.; Magee, M. The Jefferson scale of physician empathy: Development and preliminary psychometric data. *Educ. Psychol. Meas.* **2001**, *61*, 349–365. [CrossRef]

23. Birks, Y.; McKendree, J.; Watt, I. Emotional intelligence and perceived stress in healthcare students: A multi-institutional, multi-professional survey. *BMC Med. Educ.* **2009**, *9*, 61. [CrossRef] [PubMed]
24. Weissman, M.M.; Sholomskas, D.; Pottenger, M.; Prusoff, B.A.; Locke, B.Z. Assessing depressive symptoms in five psychiatric populations: A validation study. *Am. J. Epidemiol.* **1977**, *106*, 203–214. [CrossRef] [PubMed]
25. Lebensohn, P.; Dodds, S.; Brooks, A.J.; Cook, P.; Schneider, C.D.; Woytowicz, J.; Maizes, V. A longitudinal study of well-being, burnout and emotional intelligence in family medicine residents. In Proceedings of the International Research Congress on Integrative Medicine and Health, Miami, FL, USA, 13–16 May 2014.
26. Bellini, L.M.; Shea, J.A. Mood change and empathy decline persist during three years of internal medicine training. *Acad. Med.* **2005**, *80*, 164–167. [CrossRef] [PubMed]
27. Goebert, D.; Thompson, D.; Takeshita, J.; Beach, C.; Bryson, P.; Ephgrave, K.; Kent, A.; Kunkel, M.; Schechter, J.; Tate, J. Depressive symptoms in medical students and residents: A multischool study. *Acad. Med.* **2009**, *84*, 236–241. [CrossRef] [PubMed]
28. Park, Y.-M.; Zhang, J.; Steck, S.E.; Cohen, M.J.M.; Gonnella, J.S.; Erdmann, J.B.; Veloski, J.; Magee, M. Obesity mediates the association between Mediterranean diet consumption and insulin resistance and inflammation in US Adults. *J. Nutr.* **2017**, *147*, 563–571. [CrossRef] [PubMed]
29. Chao, A.M.; Jastreboff, A.M.; White, M.A.; Grilo, C.M.; Sinha, R. Stress, cortisol, and other appetite-related hormones: Prospective prediction of 6-month changes in food cravings and weight. *Obesity* **2017**, *25*, 713–720. [CrossRef] [PubMed]
30. Razzoli, M.; Pearson, C.; Crow, S.; Bartolomucci, A. Stress, overeating, and obesity: Insights from human studies and preclinical models. *Neurosci. Biobehav. Rev.* **2017**, *76*, 154–162. [CrossRef] [PubMed]
31. Dyrbye, L.N.; Moutier, C.; Durning, S.J.; Massie, F.S., Jr.; Power, D.V.; Eacker, A.; Harper, W.; Thomas, M.R.; Satele, D.; Sloan, J.A.; Shanafelt, T.D. The problems program directors inherit: Medical student distress at the time of graduation. *Med. Teach.* **2011**, *33*, 756–758. [CrossRef] [PubMed]
32. Daneshvar, F.; Weinreich, M.; Daneshvar, D.; Sperling, M.; Salmane, C.; Yacoub, H.; Gabriels, J.; McGinn, T.; Smith, M.C. Cardiorespiratory fitness in internal medicine residents: Are future physicians becoming deconditioned? *J. Grad. Med. Educ.* **2017**, *9*, 97–101. [CrossRef] [PubMed]
33. Williams, A.S.; Williams, C.D.; Cronk, N.J.; Kruse, R.L.; Ringdahl, E.N.; Koopman, R.J. Understanding the exercise habits of residents and attending physicians: A mixed methodology study. *Fam. Med.* **2015**, *47*, 118–123. [PubMed]
34. Dyrbye, L.N.; Satele, D.; Shanafelt, T.D. Healthy exercise habits are associated with lower risk of burnout and higher quality of life among US medical students. *Acad. Med.* **2017**, *92*, 1006–1011. [CrossRef] [PubMed]
35. Olson, S.M.; Odo, N.U.; Duran, A.M.; Pereira, A.G.; Mandel, J.H. Burnout and physical activity in Minnesota internal medicine resident physicians. *J. Grad. Med. Educ.* **2014**, *6*, 669–674. [CrossRef] [PubMed]
36. Frank, E.; Tong, E.; Lobelo, F.; Carrera, J.; Duperly, J. Physical activity levels and counseling practices of US medical students. *Med. Sci. Sports Exerc.* **2008**, *40*, 413–421. [CrossRef] [PubMed]
37. Leventer-Roberts, M.; Zonfrillo, M.R.; Yu, S.; Dziura, J.D.; Spiro, D.M. Overweight physicians during residency: A cross-sectional and longitudinal study. *J. Grad. Med. Educ.* **2013**, *5*, 405–411. [CrossRef] [PubMed]
38. McKenna, K.M.; Hashimoto, D.A.; Maguire, M.S.; Bynum, W.E. The missing link: Connection is the key to resilience in medical education. *Acad. Med.* **2016**, *91*, 1197–1199. [CrossRef] [PubMed]
39. West, C.P.; Dyrbye, L.N.; Erwin, P.J.; Shanafelt, T.D. Interventions to prevent and reduce physician burnout: A systematic review and meta-analysis. *Lancet* **2016**, *388*, 2272–2281. [CrossRef]
40. Panagioti, M.; Panagopoulou, E.; Bower, P. Controlled interventions to reduce burnout in physicians: A systematic review and meta-analysis. *JAMA Intern. Med.* **2017**, *177*, 195–205. [CrossRef] [PubMed]
41. Shanafelt, T.; Goh, J.; Sinsky, C. The business case for investing in physician well-being. *JAMA Intern. Med.* **2017**, *177*, 1826–1832. [CrossRef] [PubMed]
42. Heinen, I.; Bullinger, M.; Kocalevent, R.D. Perceived stress in first year medical students—Associations with personal resources and emotional distress. *BMC Med. Educ.* **2017**, *17*, 4. [CrossRef] [PubMed]
43. Thompson, G.; McBride, R.B.; Hosford, C.C.; Halaas, G. Resilience among medical students: The role of coping style and social support. *Teach. Learn. Med.* **2016**, *28*, 174–182. [CrossRef] [PubMed]
44. Ward, S.; Outram, S. Medicine: In need of culture change. *Intern. Med. J.* **2016**, *46*, 112–116. [CrossRef] [PubMed]
45. Howe, A.; Smajdor, A.; Stockl, A. Towards an understanding of resilience and its relevance to medical training. *Med. Educ.* **2012**, *46*, 349–356. [CrossRef] [PubMed]

46. Frank, E.; Rothenberg, R.; Lewis, C.; Belodoff, B.F. Correlates of physicians' prevention-related practices. Findings from the Women Physicians' Health Study. *Arch. Fam. Med.* **2000**, *9*, 359–367. [CrossRef] [PubMed]
47. Frank, E.; Breyan, J.; Elon, L. Physician disclosure of healthy personal behaviors improves credibility and ability to motivate. *Arch. Fam. Med.* **2000**, *9*, 287–290. [CrossRef] [PubMed]
48. McClafferty, H.; Ricker, M.; Brooks, A.J.; Lebensohn, P. Cracking the nut: Wellbeing in training, increasing resilience in both individuals & across healthcare organizations. In Proceedings of the International Conference to Promote Resilience, Empathy and Well-Being in Health Care Professions (CENTILE 2017), Washington, DC, USA, 22–25 October 2017.

6

Mind–Body Therapy for Children with Attention-Deficit/Hyperactivity Disorder

Anne Herbert [1] and Anna Esparham [2,*]

1 Gottlieb Memorial Hospital, Loyola University Health System, 701 North Ave, Melrose Park, IL 60160, USA; anne.herbert@luhs.org
2 Division of Integrative Medicine, University of Kansas Medical Center, 3901 Rainbow Blvd, Mailstop 1017, Kansas City, KS 66160, USA
* Correspondence: aesparham@kumc.edu

Abstract: Attention-deficit/hyperactivity disorder (ADHD) is pervasive among the pediatric population and new treatments with minimal adverse effects are necessary to be studied. The purpose of this article is to review current research studying mind–body therapies for treatment of children diagnosed with ADHD. Literature was reviewed pertaining to the effectiveness of movement-based therapies and mindfulness/meditation-based therapies for ADHD. Many positive effects of yoga, Tai Chi, physical activity, and meditation may significantly improve symptoms of ADHD among children.

Keywords: attention-deficit/hyperactivity disorder (ADHD); mind–body; pediatric; children; mindfulness; meditation; yoga; integrative medicine; alternative; complementary

---

1. Introduction

Attention-deficit/hyperactivity disorder (ADHD) is a widespread chronic disorder affecting children's well-being and success in life. The historical understanding of ADHD has changed over the years [1]. ADHD was defined in the Diagnostic and Statistical Manual of Mental Disorders (DSM)-III-R in 1987 as a disorder with a specific diagnostic checklist and three subtypes: primarily inattentive, primarily hyperactive, and combined. According to the American Psychiatric Association in the DSM-V, to be considered ADHD, a child must have symptoms before the age of 12, for at least six months, and affecting two domains of life. The prevalence of the three subtypes of ADHD are: primarily inattentive (20–30% of diagnosed population), primarily hyperactive-impulsive (less than 15%), and combined subtype (50–75%) [2]. The prevalence of ADHD in the US among children is estimated at 11% [3]. ADHD is very common among children and adolescents, consisting of about 50% of child psychiatric diagnoses [1].

2. Attention-Deficit/Hyperactivity Disorder

2.1. Etiology

A landmark theory about the primary dysfunction of ADHD was developed by Russel Barkley called the Hybrid Neuropsychological Model of Executive (Self-Regulatory) Function [4]. This theory explains ADHD as primarily a disorder of maladaptive behavioral inhibition and impairment of four executive functions. According to Barkley, behavioral inhibition has three functions: inhibiting a prepotent response, stopping an ongoing response, and controlling interference. Behavioral inhibition creates an opportunity for the executive functions to take place leading to a response. The four executive functions Barkley identified are (a) working memory, (b) self-regulation of affect, motivation and arousal, (c) internalization of speech, and (d) reconstitution. In individuals with ADHD, behavioral inhibition is dysfunctional, thereby impairing the four executive functions. In turn, motor response in the forms of motor control, fluency and syntax are affected because these actions are controlled directly by the four executive functions. Therefore, individuals with ADHD have a cascade of dysfunction, beginning with a deficit in behavioral inhibition, leading to an impairment of the four executive functions, resulting in altered motor responses [4]. Barkley's theory must be considered in the present literature review regarding how mind–body therapy has the potential to affect executive functioning in ADHD.

ADHD has been correlated with many different genetic and environmental influences. It has been identified that genetic factors, environment, brain structure, neural pathways, and neurotransmitter levels influence ADHD and its symptoms [2,5,6]. In-utero influences such as alcohol and tobacco exposure during pregnancy, low birth weight, toxemia, eclampsia, poor maternal health, maternal age, and certain complications during labor can predispose a child to ADHD. Furthermore, psychosocial adversity in a child's life such as marital discord, low socioeconomic level, paternal criminality, maternal mental disorders, large family size, or foster care placement have been correlated with an increased risk for ADHD [5]. Further areas of study may be necessary to include the mechanism of action on how these predisposing risks affect executive function in children with ADHD.

ADHD has been identified as a *complex trait* disorder meaning that it is affected by many susceptibility genes. Each gene affects the risk of developing the disorder on a small scale (p. 51) [6]. Research on genetic associations with ADHD exhibit significant amounts of inconsistent results most likely due to its complexity. Twin and adoption studies show that genetic factors may account for over 70% of the of ADHD symptom variance. Mean heritability for ADHD has been shown to be 77% in twin studies [5]. An extensive meta-analysis by Gizer et al. reviewed the candidate genes associated with ADHD. Their analysis showed significant associations for several genes that influence neurotransmitter function including serotonin, dopamine and norepinephrine regulation. These were found to include *DAT1*, *DRD4*, *DRD5*, *5HTT*, *HTR1B*, and *SNAP25* [6]. One of the most extensively studied was the candidate gene *DAT1*, which codes for a carrier protein that allows for the reuptake of dopamine into the presynaptic neuron [6]. Studies also show genetic differences for the norepinephrine transporter (*NET*) that affects ADHD functioning [7,8]. Dysregulation of dopamine and norepinephrine is thought to play a role in ADHD symptoms [5,7]. The genetic variations associated with ADHD decrease norepinephrine and dopamine activity in the synapses. Stimulant medications, such as methylphenidate and amphetamine, may help overcome this by increasing the availability of norepinephrine and dopamine by inhibiting transporter functions [7].

A longitudinal study among children showed that children homozygous for the major A allele for *NET* were more likely to have a lifetime diagnosis of ADHD [7]. The major A allele may also be associated with higher ADHD symptoms scores. Sigurdardottir et al. found that individuals with the major A allele showed higher *NET* binding potential than controls. Higher *NET* availability was found to be associated with higher symptom scores on the Conners' Adult ADHD Rating Scale: The Self-Report Screening Version (CAARS-S:SV) and Observer-Screen Version (CAARS-O:SV) [8]. Specific brain regions and neurotransmitters have been identified as playing a role in ADHD symptoms. Previous theories explain that the prefrontal cortex of the brain has the overall function of forming "cross-temporal structures of behavior that have a unifying purpose or goal" (p. 71) [4]. The prefrontal cortex is hypothesized to have a role in self-regulation of drive and motivational states that precede goal-directed actions. Because of this, the prefrontal cortex and its executive functions have an influence over motor control in the form of response, anticipatory setting to respond, or inhibition of response. Persons with damage to the prefrontal cortex present with similar symptoms to those with ADHD, having deficient inhibition and executive functioning [4]. Decreased volume of total cerebral brain matter in the frontal cortex, cerebellum and subcortical structures are also associated with ADHD. Hypofunction of anterior cingulate cortex may be associated with disinhibition in ADHD. Furthermore, frontosubcortical pathways that operate with catecholamines are affected in

ADHD. Stimulant medications act on these pathways to increase inhibition of frontal cortical activity on subcortical regions. In addition, the corpus callosum and cerebellum play a role in cognitive functioning. Communication between the two regions may be degraded in ADHD [2].

Certain brain wave activity and patterns have been found among individuals with ADHD that set them apart from their counterparts. Electroencephalography (EEG) is used to analyze brain activity in individuals with ADHD. EEG studies can be analyzed both quantitatively and qualitatively. Certain studies investigate waveform amplitude, absolute and relative power, dominant and subordinate frequency analysis, wave percentage time, and coherence between regions. EEG provides a measure of the "background state" of the brain. Since the 1930s, EEG studies have identified that a subgroup of children with ADHD tend to have an increase in theta and delta slow wave activity, mostly in the frontal region [1]. During inattentive or unfocused states, the slow theta waves (3.5–8.0 Hz) dominate the prefrontal and frontal cortices, as well as other midline loci of the brain. During relaxed, wakeful states, alpha waves (9.0–11 Hz) take over these areas of the brain. Increasing awareness, planning, and purposeful actions cause the sensorimotor rhythm (12–15 Hz) to appear in the motor cortex [9]. Training the sensorimotor rhythm through neurofeedback has been hypothesized to improve inhibitory responses and control of attention in children with ADHD [10,11]. Focused attention or sustained mental effort causes beta-1 (13–21 Hz) and beta-2 activity (22–30 Hz) to be active in the prefrontal, frontal and central midline areas (p. 434) [9]. As the brain moves from a sleeping to attentive state, the wave frequency in central, midline and frontal regions increases and the amplitude decreases. Many individuals with ADHD have been shown to exhibit increased theta/beta wave ratios. Individuals with ADHD also exhibit differences in Event-Related Potential (ERP) tests. The ERP tests evaluate the brain's electrical response to stimuli directly after the stimulus. It is conducted by presenting two types of stimuli, "Go" and "No-Go." When presented with the "Go" stimulus, the participant must respond, while when the "No-Go" stimulus is presented, the participant is supposed to inhibit a response. According to the review by Monastra et al., participants with ADHD perform significantly poorer on "Go," "No-Go" tests. Slow Cortical Potentials (SCPs) are event-related current shifts in the brain that originate from the upper cortical layer and last 300 msec to a few seconds. Negative electrical shifts have been linked to reduced activation of regions related to orientation and attention, which is of interest to ADHD research. SCP biofeedback training is currently being studied where participants in this treatment receive "feedback" related to their regulation of positive or negative current shifts. Reduced ADHD symptoms were reported in two studies of SCP biofeedback training, but there is not enough controlled research to be able to consider it as an effective treatment at this time [9]. However, it is not yet universal that EEG-neurofeedback can diagnose ADHD based on brainwaves as it may only differentiate a relatively small group of these children.

Lazzaro et al. investigated brain wave activity of adolescents with ADHD compared to age- and sex-matched counterparts [12]. The study recruited 54 male adolescents 11–17 years of age, 34 were unmedicated, and the rest were taken off of medication two weeks prior to the study. They were age-matched with 54 male adolescents without ADHD as a control group. The participants underwent a baseline resting, open-eye EEG and then the experimental EEG where they were asked to focus their sight on a black dot 60 cm away to limit eye movement. Brain activity was then measured for two minutes. There was significantly increased theta and alpha-1 activity across anterior, midline, posterior, left and right hemisphere brain regions among ADHD participants. Delta and alpha-2 activity was not significantly increased among ADHD participants compared to control [12]. In summary, the majority of individuals with ADHD presented with excess theta activity and decreased beta in the frontal and central midline regions, also known as cortical hypoarousal. However, there is a minority of individuals with ADHD who exhibit cortical hyperarousal or no changes in quantitative electroencephalography (QEEG) compared to healthy controls. As far as diagnostic value of QEEG, the reported sensitivity and specificity of the theta/beta power ratio has been shown to be comparably accurate in differentiating ADHD from healthy counterparts when compared with behavioral rating scale measures [9].

Heart rate variability (HRV) may be a useful marker for therapeutic changes in ADHD and illustrates the relationship between ADHD and the autonomic nervous system. Abnormal catecholaminergic function has been linked to ADHD, resulting in "underarousal of the sympathetic system in children with ADHD" (p. 1366) [13]. Stimulants increase the dopamine and norepinephrine activity. In turn, studies have shown increases in blood pressure and heart rate due to these medications. One study consisting of 37 children with ADHD, ages 6–12 years, showed a significant change in HRV from baseline to endpoint. Prior to the study, children were either medication naive or taken off medication for at least two months. Square root of the mean squared difference of successive normal-to-normal intervals (RMSSD) and high frequency (HF) were calculated as indicators of parasympathetic vagal tone. Both of these measures were significantly decreased after introduction of methylphenidate treatment from baseline to endpoint. Average heart rate significantly increased from baseline to endpoint. These results may indicate that the children with ADHD may exhibit decreased parasympathetic activity as indicated by increased HRV following pharmacological intervention [13]. Another study by Rukmani et al. exhibited similar results, finding that medication-naive children with ADHD had reduced overall heart rate variability compared to age and gender-matched controls. They hypothesized that these results indicate catecholamine dysregulation and parasympathetic dominance in ADHD [14]. However, this needs to be further studied due to the heterogeneity of ADHD, as catecholamine and the autonomic nervous system imbalance may be different in subgroups of individuals with ADHD. Mind–body therapies may offer an effect on functioning of the autonomic nervous system. Future research should investigate effects of mind–body therapy on measures of heart rate variability in order to compare its effects to that of pharmacological treatment.

2.2. Current Treatments

ADHD presents with a complex etiology and has multiple treatment options. Stimulant medication is the most often used medication for the disorder in younger children, and more recently, non-stimulant medications are used for children and adolescent populations. Other treatments include behavior modification, which includes therapy from clinicians, family or parent training and therapy, and school-based interventions in the classroom [15].

A recent study of 152 children with ADHD revealed that initial treatment behavior modification was less costly than initial treatment with a low dose of stimulant medication. This experimental study found that, on average, children who underwent successful behavior modification training had a cost of $392 versus $1448 for pharmacological treatment over a 10-month school year [16]. In addition, the Multimodal Treatment Study demonstrated that medication did have any long-term benefits in reducing ADHD symptom severity [17]. Adverse effects that are most common of stimulant medications are appetite loss, abdominal pain, headaches, and sleep disturbance [15]. Common effects of non-stimulant medications, such as atomoxetine, include initial somnolence, gastrointestinal disturbances, and decreased appetite. Other non-stimulant medications, such as clonidine or guanfacine, may cause somnolence and dry mouth [15].

Behavioral interventions and pharmaceutical regimens have been shown to be effective at reducing ADHD symptoms significantly, especially when used in combination [18]. It deserves to be explored if the integration of mind–body therapy, with these already accepted treatments would further decrease ADHD symptoms and improve functioning. Mind–body therapies offer a wide range of effects on psychosocial, emotional, and neurobiological functioning, making it a promising addition to current therapy regimens.

3. Mind–Body Therapies

3.1. Current Treatments

Integrative medicine offers an alternative or addition to pharmacological or cognitive-behavioral therapies for treatment of ADHD. There are limited well-designed studies of integrative therapies, making it difficult to generalize results. Current therapies to improve ADHD symptoms identified through evidence-based medicine include diet, nutrient supplementation, gut health, environmental health, and neurofeedback [19].

Mind–body therapy includes but is not limited to mindfulness, biofeedback, deep breathing, guided imagery, progressive relaxation, hypnotherapy, and yoga [20]. A reason for incorporating more integrative therapies is motivated by consumer interest and the need to improve treatment outcomes. Mind–body medicine encompasses various therapies that are non-invasive techniques with the aim of "harnessing positive thought and emotion for the purpose of enhancing health" (p. 102) [20]. The practice of mindfulness and meditation is a conscious exercise that builds attention control and inhibitory skills [21].

3.2. Yoga

One field of mind–body medicine is the practice of yoga. Yoga is an ancient physical practice, derived from Sanskrit word "yuj" meaning "to yoke," and refers to uniting the body, mind and spirit. Yoga teaches individuals to master certain poses and breathing techniques which may promote self-control, attention, awareness and adaptive skills. Yoga has been used as a form of exercise and meditation. It has been currently studied as therapy for the treatment of stress, chronic pain, asthma, irritable bowel syndrome, and ADHD [20].

Yoga has various components to unite the body, mind and spirit. It is comprised of the asanas (physical postures), pranayamas (breathing techniques), and dharana/dhyana (meditation practices) [22]. The goal of these components is to connect the breathing, thoughts, emotions, and body into awareness of the present moment. The conditions affected by yoga explored by Rosen et al. included emotional, mental and behavioral health. The studies reviewed showed significant decreases among children practicing yoga in a variety of measures such as: negative stress response behaviors, total mood disturbance, negative affect, anger, resilience, and fatigue/inertia [22]. There are few studies that may suggest that yoga influences HRV and autonomic function, but more rigorous studies are needed to report any firm conclusions [23].

One study by Hariprasad et al. investigated the effects of yoga as a complementary therapy for children with ADHD who were admitted in a child psychiatry unit [24]. The sample was made of nine children, ages 5–16 years. Eight of the nine children were on medications. The children underwent eight yoga sessions over the course of their inpatient stay. The children were rated on Conners' abbreviated rating scale (CARS), ADHD-rating scale IV (ADHD-RS IV), and clinical global impression (CGI)-Severity. They were rated at the beginning of the study, discharge, and at one month, two months and three months following the study. It was found that CARS, and ADHD-RS IV, and CGI-S were significantly improved among the patients upon discharge. Confounding variables are that this study lacked a control group and the group represents a more severely impaired population of ADHD individuals as evidenced by their need for inpatient treatment. Additionally, the children were taking medication and influenced by other inpatient interventions besides yoga. While yoga may offer some benefit as a complementary therapy in an inpatient setting, this study lacks controls and a large enough sample needed to recommend yoga as an add-on intervention [24].

Sahaja yoga practice as family therapy may have a positive effect on ADHD symptoms and could possibly reduce dosage of medication in some cases. Another study investigated effects of Sahaja yoga meditation as a family treatment for children with ADHD [25]. There were 48 participants in the study, 31 receiving medication, 14 not on medication, and 3 unknown. The participants went through a six-week program of 90-minute clinic sessions twice a week and regular meditation at home.

Effects of the yoga were measured by pre- and post-assessment of child self-ratings and parent's rating of ADHD symptoms, self-esteem and child–parent relationship quality. The results of the study indicated that parents reported significant improvements in ADHD symptoms, with an average decrease calculated at 35%. The researchers also compared scores of the six non-medicated versus the medicated children and found that there were no significant differences in symptoms, indicating that the changes were likely not due to pharmacologic treatment. In addition, 11 of the 20 children who were medicated could reduce their dose of medication throughout the yoga program. In addition to improvement in symptoms, parents also reported improved self-esteem and relationships, feeling less stressed and had a better ability to handle their children's behavior. Children self-reported better sleep patterns, less anxiety, more ability to focus at school, and less conflicts. However, this study relies on unblended ratings of parents and lacked a control group, which makes it difficult to infer that Sahaja yoga may be an effective adjunctive therapy for ADHD. Sahaja yoga has also been reported to increase gray volume matter associated with sustained attention, self-control, compassion, and interoceptive perception in older adults [26]. Additionally, the yoga as a form of stress reduction for parents of children with ADHD is a valid topic to be explored by future research.

Yoga may also help increase time on task for students with ADHD in the educational setting. One study investigated the effect of a yoga practice intervention on children's time on task in school [27]. The participants were 10 children, ages 6–10, with attention problems. The children completed three weeks of two sessions per week for 30 min in each session. The time to task was measured by observation during morning class work in school. The observers used the Behavioral Observation Form where time on task was defined as the percentage of intervals when students had eye contact with the teacher or assigned task and performed assignments. Cohen's effect size was calculated, with small effect being 0.20 or greater, moderate 0.50 or greater and, large effect 0.80 or greater. Effect size for each grade was calculated by taking the difference between the mean of the baseline and intervention phases divided by the standard deviation of the baseline phase. The effect sizes regarding behavioral observation scores were found to be from 1.51 to 2.72 for the three grade groups, showing a large effect. At follow-up, the effect sizes were decreased, but still showing a moderate to great effect at 0.77 and 1.95. Observation as a measurement of student behavior has both strengths and limitations. A limitation is that observation may include rater bias, especially when the observer is not blinded to the purpose of the study as was the case in the present study. On the other hand, teacher-ratings are often used in ADHD research such as the Conner's parent/teacher rating scale. Another positive result of this study was that children reported enjoying the yoga videos and that video format is an inexpensive and easy method of presenting the therapy. Yoga may have the potential to increase time on task in class and be an enjoyable and cost-effective treatment for children with attention problems [27].

There are few experimental studies exploring the effects yoga on attention mechanisms. One study investigated how 20 yoga sessions for boys with ADHD would help attention versus a control of cooperative game activities [28]. The experimental group consisted of 11 participants and control of eight boys. The two groups were assessed pre-and post-intervention using the Conners' Parent and Teacher Rating scale and scores were compared by one-way ANOVA. Qualitative data was also taken from parents. The scores in five subscales of the measurement were improved for the yoga group post-intervention. Parents also reported that the relaxation and breathing techniques were beneficial when their children were restless, needed sleep, and affected their behavior in the immediate period after class. The participants in both groups were receiving medication throughout the study. This experiment shows that yoga can be an effective complementary therapy for children with ADHD that are receiving medication [28]. The breathing and relaxation techniques that are learned through yoga practice may be used by children to focus attention and decrease hyperactivity.

In reference to the theory of executive dysfunction being the hallmark of ADHD, yoga practice must be evaluated in regards of its effect on these functions. Chou and Huang found that an eight-week yoga program significantly improved sustained attention and discrimination function in children with

ADHD compared with a control group [29]. The researchers created two groups of children 8–12 years old from the same suburban area: yoga (n = 24) and control (n = 25). The two groups were matched, so there were no significant differences in extraneous variables. They measured children at baseline and after intervention on the Visual Pursuit Test and Determination Test. These types of measurements may limit the application of this study because these two tests have not been used among ADHD populations. However, the Visual Pursuit Test is used in psychological diagnostics for selective and sustained attention and was used because attention deficits are symptoms of ADHD. Additionally, the Determination Test assesses for reaction speed, attention deficits, and reactive stress tolerance in the presence of external sensory stimuli. Findings revealed that the group who underwent yoga intervention had significantly better reaction time and response accuracy at the two measurements [29].

Another recent study investigated yoga and physical activity on measures of executive functioning [30]. They examined 30 female undergraduate students' scores on the Flanker task, a measure relating to inhibitory control, and the N-back task, a measure relating to working memory, under three different conditions: baseline, aerobic exercise and yoga. It was found that response accuracy to the Flanker task was significantly increased under the yoga condition compared to aerobic exercise. The researchers believe that the positive effects exhibited under the yoga condition on the two measures may be due to improvements in mood and its focus on body awareness and breathing. By these mechanisms, it is hypothesized that yoga would have positive effects on attentional ability [30].

3.3. *Tai Chi*

Tai Chi is an ancient Chinese martial art consisting of slow movements coordinated with balancing body weight and breathing deeply. There may be potential benefit for improving ADHD symptoms of anxiety and hyperactivity with regular Tai Chi practice. A sample of 13 adolescents with ADHD was studied to find the effect of a five-week Tai Chi intervention on symptoms according to the Conners' Scale rated by teachers. The participants were rated at baseline, at the end of the five weeks and two weeks after intervention. During the five weeks, participants completed two 30-minute sessions per week. It was found that the adolescents exhibited significantly decreased anxiety, decreased daydreaming, decreased inappropriate emotions, decreased hyperactivity, and increased conduct after the Tai Chi intervention. The scores persisted to be significantly affected even at the two-week post-intervention post-test [31]. Researchers hypothesized that these effects may be due to lower levels of stress and cortisol release, which has been shown as an effect of Tai Chi in previous research studies [32]. According to the theory that executive functions are impaired in ADHD, Tai Chi may help improve executive functioning because it requires a combination of focused attention on movement and breath as guided by the teacher. This study shows that Tai Chi may have some beneficial effects on adolescents with ADHD as an adjunctive therapy [31].

3.4. *Physical Activity*

In human studies, physical activity and fitness has shown to affect brain structure and increase brain activity that is associated with conflict and attentional control. Though ADHD is a disorder with a complex etiology, there are a few factors contributing to the likelihood of ADHD that may be affected by physical activity. Exercise has also been shown to improve dopamine function, known to be dysregulated in ADHD [33]. Brain derived neurotrophic factor (BDNF) has also been found to play a role in ADHD symptoms through recent research [34]. This factor helps development of neurons in the dopaminergic pathways in the brain, which may be of importance to impulse control and attention. According to animal studies, BDNF expression is increased with stimulant medications [35]. The prefrontal and frontal regions contribute to regulation of catecholaminergic pathways involved in ADHD. According to Madras et al., there may be a decreased ability for people with ADHD to reload these catecholamines effectively [36]. Physical activity may affect these same neurological factors and brain regions. It has been shown that physical activity increases cerebral blood flow, thereby potentially helping where ADHD exhibits a deficit in blood flow to the prefrontal and frontal regions. Hunter et al.

demonstrated that physical activity may increase the amount of dopamine and norepinephrine in synaptic clefts which activate catecholaminergic pathways [37]. High impact running significantly increased measurements of dopamine, epinephrine and BDNF activity. Additionally, these increases were correlated with significant improvements in memory and learning ability tasks among the study participants [37].

A recent meta-analysis demonstrated that physical activity increases executive function and cognitive functioning with an effect size of 0.535 [38]. In another meta-analysis, pre-adolescent children were found to have increased executive function after one aerobic exercise session (effect size 0.540) [39]. One study investigating karate and its impact on motor and cognitive development showed that this particular martial arts form resulted in improved attention through the Tower of London test (effect size 0.88, $p < 0.05$) [40]. Martial arts teach children to practice self-control, concentration and meditation that may ultimately result in improvements of executive function. A study by Medina et al. showed that boys with ADHD had significantly improved attention after high-intensity treadmill exercise lasting for 30 min with or without medication [33]. The impact on cognitive function and academic performance needs to be further studied, as a recent systematic review found that the evidence for the effect of exercise on ADHD is equivocal and limited in quantity and quality [41]. While the preliminary evidence supports physical activity as an adjunctive treatment for ADHD, the data is insufficient to support it as a stand-alone treatment. A literature review by Gapin et al. suggests that future research should investigate physical activity as a stand-alone therapy for individuals that prefer alternative treatments as this topic has not been extensively tested in research [42].

4. Mindfulness-Based Therapies

Mindfulness and meditation have been found to "change brain activation patterns, contribute to enhanced mood, reduce anxiety, improve stress management, reduce pain and enhance immune function" [43] (p. 510). These effects imply that mind–body therapies could be well-suited for symptoms of ADHD in children. Mindfulness is "defined as a process of bringing one's complete attention to the present experience on a moment-to-moment basis" (p. 64) [44]. In other descriptions, it has been known as bringing awareness to the present experience without a judgmental attitude, but rather attentive and curious [45]. Mindfulness was developed from ancient cultural meditation practices and has now been adopted by Western psychology and medicine as treatment for stress reduction therapy [44]. Additionally, mindfulness therapy has been found to be satisfying and without unwanted side effects for persons with ADHD [45,46]. Meditation has been defined as a mental training technique that can enhance an altered state of consciousness, resembling its similarity to mindfulness [47]. Mindfulness and meditation have also been found to increase connectivity amongst brain regions associated with executive function [48].

Meditation/Mindfulness

The effect of an eight-week mindfulness training program for adults and adolescents with ADHD was considered [46]. The group consisted of 24 adults and eight adolescents who completed the intervention of eight weeks with 2.5 hours of training per day and additional "homework" meditation of 5 to 15 min. Measurements for pre- and post-intervention included the ADHD Rating Scale IV and SNAP-IV scale (for ADHD symptoms), the Attention Network Test (ANT) (for alerting, orienting and conflict attention), and the Stroop task (for attentional conflict), the Trail Making Test (for set-shifting and inhibition), the Digit Span (for working memory) in addition to other measurements. Substantial effects of the meditation were exhibited. In addition, 78% of participants reported a significant reduction in their ADHD symptoms with 30% reporting at least a 30% reduction. Significant improvement in attentional conflict and set-shifting was also found from pre- to post-intervention. Participant satisfaction was rated at a 9/10 on the visual analog scale and no adverse side effects were reported from the therapy. This study supports the hypothesis that mindfulness training may reduce self-reported ADHD symptoms and improved performance on certain attentional and cognitive tests [46].

This study by Crescentini et al. examined the effects of mindfulness training on 16 healthy primary school children ages seven to eight years old. The training consisted of three sessions per week for eight weeks [45]. A pre-test and post-test were taken by the main teacher of the students measuring behavior, social, emotion, and attention regulation skills. The children also self-reported mood and depression symptoms. There was a positive effect of the intervention on reduction of attention and internalizing issues. Children did not report any change in depressive symptoms after the intervention. This study shows support that mindfulness training has beneficial effects on attention and ADHD symptoms [45]. Mindfulness training can be incorporated into classroom activities or at home easily. Unlike medications, there are no harmful side effects and the training can be virtually at no cost to parents or teachers if they are educated on how to carry out the sessions for children

The effects of meditation on attention were studied by Jha et al. [44]. Two experimental conditions were created to study mindfulness and its effect on attention. Three realms of attention were studied: alerting, orienting and conflict-monitoring. These areas of attention were measured by scores on the Attention Network Test (ANS) at Time 1 before treatment and Time 2 after treatment. Group 1 underwent an eight-week long, three-hour daily course. Group 2 underwent an intensive retreat for one month where they completed 10–12 h of mindfulness practice. Group 3 was a control group of persons with no previous mindfulness experience. Group 1 also had no previous mindfulness experience, while Group 2 had previous mindfulness practice and therefore could be compared as "experienced" in mindfulness. Results showed that participants in Group 1 had significantly improved scores of orienting-type attention and endogenous orient attention in comparison with the other two groups. Group 2 exhibited improved scores in exogenous stimulus detection when compared to the other two groups [44].

Another study by Van de Weijer-Bergsma et al. incorporated parents and tutors into the mindfulness intervention [49]. Ten adolescents, 19 parents and seven academic tutors underwent mindfulness training for eight weeks for 1.5 h sessions. The training consisted of sitting meditation, body scan, and breathing space exercises along with interventions to improve awareness of one's distractability, impulsivity, and hyperactivity. Measurements were completed before the training as a pretest, at the end of the eight-week training and then again after 16 weeks. Measures consisted of scales measuring behavior problems, executive functioning, mindful awareness, parenting stress, parenting style, fatigue, happiness, and a computerized test of attention. Statistical analysis was carried out from pre-test to post-test to follow-up by paired t-tests with significant effects at $p < 0.10$ in a two-tailed t-test. At eight weeks, it was found that the adolescents had improvements in attention problems, executive functioning and performance on the computerized attention test [49]. The significance of their findings should be interpreted with caution, as the significance level is more liberal at $p < 0.10$. Further study should explore effects on mindfulness, perhaps with the same measurements but with larger sample sizes and interpreted with more strict significance scoring.

Studies show that meditative practice causes measurable changes within brain-wave activity. One experiment by Lagopoulos et al. investigated the effects of nondirective meditation on theta and alpha activity in the brain as recorded by EEG [50]. Eighteen participants who engaged in regular meditation for many years were recruited for the study. The experiment compared the theta and alpha activity between 20 minutes of non-directed meditation to non-meditative relaxation among the participants. There was a significant increase in alpha and theta activity among all three brain regions during meditation when compared to the relaxation session. Delta activity was significantly greater in the temporal central region during meditation as compared to relaxation. There was significantly greater alpha activity in the posterior region when compared to the frontal region, whereas theta activity was greater in the frontal and temporal-central regions compared to the posterior [50]. Meditation's effects on brainwaves may be an important area of study to determine what brainwave changes occur in children with ADHD practicing mind–body therapies, such as meditation.

An important factor to consider in the discussion of mindfulness or meditation for ADHD treatment is the type of meditation being used. Certain forms of mindfulness lead participants to greater awareness or attention on breathing or emotions, while others encourage free, relaxed mental states of "inattention." For example, one form of meditation, known as Yoga Nidra, is characterized by leading participants to "lose executive control" and has been shown to cause decreased blood flow to areas of the brain that regulate executive functions [51]. This study showed increased theta activity, which supports other meditation studies on brain wave activity. Because persons with ADHD already exhibit increased theta activity, it is counterintuitive that meditation could exhibit a beneficial effect on symptoms by causing a potential further increase. One potential mechanism by which meditation might affect ADHD symptoms is through the regulation of dopamine. Kjaer et al. found that dopamine release was significantly increased in the ventral striatum during Yoga Nidra meditation practice [51]. Through a C-raclopride Positron Emission Tomography (PET) scan, they found that there was as great as a 65% increase in dopamine among their participants [51]. Since medications for ADHD primarily target dopamine and norepinephrine transporters to increase synaptic levels, there may be a possibility that meditation could exhibit similar effects to these medications by the same means [7,51].

5. Conclusions

Potential benefits and mechanism of action of mind–body therapies have been evidenced through research and continue to be explored. Compared to pharmacological treatment, mind–body therapies have little to no unwanted side effects. There is little cost compared to clinical therapy since the only cost is for training or sessions that are typically conducted in groups. Activities such as yoga or Tai Chi can be practiced at home or school. Families and teachers can access videos online or purchase videos from reliable sources as resources to guide the therapy.

Mindfulness and meditation can be done anywhere and at any time. Furthermore, mindfulness is a learned skill. It is counterintuitive that meditation has positive effects on ADHD symptoms because theta to beta ratios are typically increased in ADHD, and meditation further increases theta wave activity [48]. Meditation and mindfulness may improve symptoms not because of the quantity of brainwave activity, but because of the learned skill to control attention and focus to a specific purpose or action (i.e., the breath). Further study of whether persons with ADHD can perform meditation and mindfulness more effectively because of their naturally increased theta activity is worth exploration. How mind–body therapies affect neuroanatomical and neurotransmitter function may also support its therapeutic use.

Mind–body training for parents has an added benefit to children's ADHD symptoms. Parents who practice mindfulness with parenting techniques report better outcomes in ADHD symptoms of their children [48]. It is probable that the effects of the studies involving children and parents could be not only due to the intervention itself, but the lasting actions of the child–parent interaction at home following the mind–body sessions. A parent who learns mindfulness through yoga or meditation may have improved methods of disciplining and responding to a child's behavior, and, in turn, the child may learn from the parent how to change their behavior in a positive way. Furthermore, having parents involved in the same treatment as their children helps continuation of mindful practice at home rather than limiting training to individual sessions.

Limitations of current research are primarily due to small sample sizes and lack of control groups. More research needs to be done with larger sample sizes and more controlled settings. Many of the studies reviewed also gathered data from subjective self-report or parent/teacher surveys. More objective data should be measured alongside subjective data in future research.

Acknowledgments: No grants or funds were received for this review article. The authors wish to thank their division of KU Integrative Medicine and Department of Internal Medicine for their continued support and encouragement in the advancement of the field, integrative medicine.

Author Contributions: Anne Herbert contributed to the writing and editing of the manuscript. Anna Esparham contributed to the writing and editing of the manuscript.

References

1. Barry, R.J.; Clarke, A.R.; Johnstone, S.J. A review electrophysiology in attention-deficit/hyperactivity disorder: I. Qualitative and quantitative electroencephalopathy. *Clin. Neurophysiol.* **2003**, *114*, 172–183. [CrossRef]
2. Spencer, T.J.; Biederman, J.; Mick, E. Attention-deficit/hyperactivity disorder: Diagnosis, lifespan, comorbidities, and neurobiology. *Ambul. Pediatr.* **2007**, *7*, 73–81. [CrossRef] [PubMed]
3. Centers for Disease Control and Prevention. Attention-Deficit/Hyperactivity Disorder. 2013. Available online: http:www.cdc.gov/ncbddd/adhd/data.html (accessed on 18 November 2016).
4. Barkley, R.A. Behavioral inhibition, sustained attention, and executive function: Constructing a unified theory of ADHD. *Psychol. Bull.* **1997**, *121*, 65–94. [CrossRef] [PubMed]
5. Purper-Ouakil, D.; Ramoz, N.; Lepagnol-Bestel, A.M.; Gorwood, P.; Simonneau, M. Neurobiology of attention deficit/hyperactivity disorder. *Pediatr. Res.* **2011**, *69*, 69R–76R. [CrossRef] [PubMed]
6. Gizer, I.R.; Ficks, C.; Waldman, I.D. Candidate gene studies of ADHD: A meta-analytic review. *Hum. Genet.* **2009**, *126*, 51–90. [CrossRef] [PubMed]
7. Hohmann, S.; Hohm, E.; Treutlein, J.; Blomeyer, D.; Jennen-Steinmetz, C.; Schmidt, M.H.; Esser, G.; Banaschewski, T.; Brandeis, D.; Laucht, M. Association of norepinephrine transporter (*NET, SLC6A2*) genotype with ADHD-related phenotypes: Findings of a longitudinal study from birth to adolescence. *Psychiatry Res.* **2015**, *226*, 425–433. [CrossRef] [PubMed]
8. Sigurdardottir, H.L.; Kranz, G.S.; Rami-Mark, C.; James, G.M.; Vanicek, T.; Gryglewski, G.; Kautzky, A.; Hienert, M.; Traub-Weidinger, T.; Mitterhauser, M.; et al. Effects of norepinephrine transporter gene variants on NET binding in ADHD and healthy controls investigated by PET. *Hum. Brain Mapp.* **2016**, *37*, 884–895. [CrossRef] [PubMed]
9. Monastra, V.J. Quantitative electroencephalography and attention-deficit/hyperactivity disorder: Implications for clinical practice. *Curr. Psychiatry Rep.* **2008**, *10*, 432–438. [CrossRef] [PubMed]
10. Mohammadi, M.R.; Malmir, N.; Khaleghi, A.; Aminiorani, M. Comparison of sensorimotor rhythm (SMR) and beta training on selective attention and symptoms in children with attention deficit/hyperactivity disorder (ADHD): A trend report. *Iran. J. Psychiatry* **2015**, *10*, 165–174. [PubMed]
11. Ter Huurne, N.; Lozano-Soldevilla, D.; Onnink, M.; Kan, C.; Buitelaar, J.; Jensen, O. Diminished modulation of preparatory sensorimotor mu rhythm predicts attention-deficit/hyperactivity disorder severity. *Psychol. Med.* **2017**, 1–10. [CrossRef] [PubMed]
12. Lazzaro, I.; Gordon, E.; Li, W.; Lim, C.L.; Plahn, M.; Whitmont, S.; Clarke, S.; Barry, R.J.; Dosen, A.; Meares, R. Simultaneous EEG and EDA measures in adolescent attention deficit hyperactivity disorder. *Int. J. Psychophysiol.* **1999**, *34*, 123–134. [CrossRef]
13. Kim, J.H.; Yan, J.; Lee, M. Changes of heart rate variability during methylphenidate treatment in attention-deficit hyperactivity disorder children: A 12-week prospective study. *Yonsei Med. J.* **2014**, *56*, 1365–1371. [CrossRef] [PubMed]
14. Rukmani, M.R.; Sephardi, S.P.; Thennarasu, K.; Raju, T.R.; Sathyaprabha, T.N. Heart rate variability in children with Attention Deficit/Hyperactivity Disorder: A pilot study. *Ann. Neurosciences* **2016**, *23*, 81–88. [CrossRef] [PubMed]
15. Wolraich, M.; Brown, L.; Brown, R.T.; DuPaul, G.; Earls, M.; Feldman, H.M.; Ganiats, T.G.; Kaplanek, B.; Meyer, B.; Perrin, J.; et al. ADHD: Clinical practice guideline for the diagnosis, evaluation, and treatment of attention-deficit/hyperactivity disorder in children and adolescents. *Pediatrics* **2011**, *128*, 1007–1022. [PubMed]
16. Page, T.F.; Pelham, W.E., III; Fabiano, G.A.; Greiner, A.R.; Gnagy, E.M.; Hart, K.C.; Coxe, S.; Waxmonsky, J.G.; Foster, E.M.; Pelham, W.E. Comparative cost analysis of sequential, adaptive, behavioral, pharmacological, and combined treatments for childhood ADHD. *J. Clin. Child Adolesc. Psychol.* **2016**, *45*, 416–427. [CrossRef] [PubMed]

17. Swanson, J.M.; Arnold, L.E.; Molina, B.S.G.; Sibley, M.H.; Hechtman, L.T.; Hinshaw, S.P.; Abikoff, H.B.; Stehli, A.; Owens, E.B.; Mitchell, J.T.; et al. Young adult outcomes in the follow-up of the multimodal treatment study of attention-deficit/hyperactivity disorder: Symptom persistence, source discrepancy, and height suppression. *J. Child Psychol. Psychiatry.* **2017**. [CrossRef] [PubMed]
18. Pelham, W.E.; Fabiano, G.A.; Waxmonsky, J.G.; Greiner, A.R.; Gnagy, E.M.; Pelhamm, W.E., III; Coxe, S.; Verley, J.; Bhatia, I.; Hart, K.; Karch, K.; et al. Treatment sequencing for childhood ADHD: A multiple-randomization study of adaptive medication and behavioral interventions. *J. Clin. Child Adolesc. Psychol.* **2016**, *45*, 396–415. [CrossRef] [PubMed]
19. Esparham, A.; Evans, R.G.; Wagner, L.E.; Drisko, J.A. Pediatric integrative medicine approaches to attention deficit hyperactivity disorder (ADHD). *Children* **2014**, *1*, 186–207. [CrossRef] [PubMed]
20. McClafferty, H. Complementary, holistic and integrative medicine. *Pediatrics Rev.* **2011**, *32*, 201–203. [CrossRef] [PubMed]
21. Kaunhoven, R.J.; Dorjee, D. How does mindfulness modulate self-regulation in pre-adolescent children? An integrative neurocognitive review. *Neurosci. Biobehav. Rev.* **2017**, *74*, 163–184. [CrossRef] [PubMed]
22. Rosen, L.; French, A.; Sullivan, G. Complementary, holistic, and integrative medicine: Yoga. *Pediatrics Rev.* **2015**, *36*, 468–474. [CrossRef] [PubMed]
23. Tyagi, A.; Cohen, M. Yoga and heart rate variability: A comprehensive review of the literature. *Int. J. Yoga* **2016**, *9*, 97–113. [PubMed]
24. Hariprasad, V.R.; Arasappa, R.; Varambally, S.; Srinath, S.; Gangadhar, B.N. Feasibility and efficacy of yoga as an add-on intervention in attention deficit-hyperactivity disorder: An exploratory study. *Indian J. Psychiatry* **2013**, *55*, S379–S384. [PubMed]
25. Harrison, L.J.; Manocha, R.; Rubia, K. Sahaja yoga meditation as a family treatment programme for children with attention deficits-hyperactivity disorder. *Clin. Child Psychol. Psychiatry* **2004**, *9*, 479–497. [CrossRef]
26. Hernández, S.E.; Suero, J.; Barros, A.; González-Mora, J.L.; Rubia, K. Increased grey matter associated with long-term Sahaja yoga meditation: A voxel-based morphometry study. *PLoS ONE* **2016**, *11*, 1–16. [CrossRef] [PubMed]
27. Peck, H.L.; Kehle, T.J.; Bray, M.A.; Theodore, L.A. Yoga as an intervention for children with attention problems. *Sch. Psychol. Rev.* **2005**, *34*, 415–424.
28. Jensen, P.S.; Kenny, D.T. The effects of yoga on the attention and behavior of boys with attention-deficit/hyperactivity disorder (ADHD). *J. Atten. Disorders* **2004**, *7*, 205–216. [CrossRef] [PubMed]
29. Chou, C.; Huang, C. Effects of an 8-week yoga program on sustained attention and discrimination in children with attention deficit hyperactivity disorder. *PeerJ* **2017**. [CrossRef] [PubMed]
30. Gothe, N.; Potifex, M.B.; Hillman, C.; McAuley, E. The acute effects of yoga on executive function. *J. Phys. Act. Health* **2013**, *10*, 488–495. [CrossRef] [PubMed]
31. Hernandez-Reid, M.; Field, T.M.; Thimas, E. Attention deficit hyperactivity disorder: Benefits from Tai Chi. *J. Bodyw. Mov. Ther.* **2000**, *5*, 120–123. [CrossRef]
32. Converse, A.K.; Ahlers, E.O.; Travers, B.G.; Davidson, R.J. Tai chi training reduces self-report of inattention in healthy young adults. *Front. Hum. Neurosci.* **2014**, *8*, 1–7. [CrossRef] [PubMed]
33. Medina, J.A.; Netto, T.L.; Muszkat, M.; Medina, A.C.; Botter, D.; Orbetelli, R.; Scaramuzza, L.F.; Sinnes, E.G.; Vilela, M.; Miranda, M.C. Exercise impact on sustained attention of ADHD children, methylphenidate effects. *Atten. Defic. Hyperact. Disord.* **2010**, *2*, 49–58. [CrossRef] [PubMed]
34. Chen, C.; Nakagawa, S.; An, Y.; Ito, K.; Kitaichi, Y.; Kusumi, I. The exercise-glucocorticoid paradox: How exercise is beneficial to cognition, mood, and the brain while increasing glucocorticoid levels. *Front. Neuroendocrinol.* **2017**, *44*, 83–102. [CrossRef] [PubMed]
35. Fumagalli, F.; Cattaneo, A.; Caffino, L.; Ibba, M.; Racagni, G.; Carboni, E.; Gennarelli, M.; Riva, M.A. Sub-chronic exposure to atomoxetine up-regulates BDNF expression and signalling in the brain of adolescent spontaneously hypertensive rats: Comparison with methylphenidate. *Pharmacol. Res.* **2010**, *62*, 523–529. [CrossRef] [PubMed]
36. Madras, B.K.; Miller, G.M.; Fischman, A.J. The dopamine transporter and attention-deficit/hyperactivity disorder. *Biol. Psychiatry* **2005**, *57*, 1397–1409. [CrossRef] [PubMed]
37. Winter, B.; Breitenstein, C.; Mooren, F.C.; Voelker, K.; Fobker, M.; Lechtermann, A.; Krueger, K.; Fromme, A.; Korsukewitz, C.; Floel, A.; et al. High impact running improves learning. *Neurobiol. Learn. Mem.* **2007**, *87*, 597–609. [CrossRef] [PubMed]

38. Vyniauske, R.; Verburgh, L.; Oosterlaan, J.; Molendijk, M.L. The effects of physical exercise on functional outcomes in the treatment of ADHD: A meta-analysis. *J. Atten. Disord.* **2016**. [CrossRef]
39. Ludyga, S.; Gerber, M.; Brand, S.; Holsboer-Trachsler, E.; Pühse, U. Acute effects of moderate aerobic exercise on specific aspects of executive function in different age and fitness groups: A meta-analysis. *Psychophysiology* **2016**, *53*, 1611–1626. [CrossRef] [PubMed]
40. Alesi, M.; Bianco, A.; Padulo, J.; Vella, F.P.; Petrucci, M.; Paoli, A.; Palma, A.; Pepi1, A. Motor and cognitive development: the role of karate. *Muscle Ligaments Tendons J.* **2014**, *4*, 114–120.
41. Li, J.W.; O'Connor, H.; O'Dwyer, N.; Orr, R. The effect of acute and chronic exercise on cognitive function and academic performance in adolescents: A systematic review. *J. Sci. Med. Sport* **2017**. [CrossRef] [PubMed]
42. Gapin, J.I.; Laban, J.D.; Etnier, J.L. The effects of physical activity on attention deficit hyperactivity disorder symptoms: The evidence. *Prev. Med.* **2011**, *52*, 570–574. [CrossRef] [PubMed]
43. Edwards, E.; Mischoulon, D.; Rapaport, M.; Stussman, B.; Weber, W. Building an evidence base in complementary and integrative healthcare for child and adolescent psychiatry. *Child Adolesc. Psychiatr. Clin. N. Am.* **2013**, *22*, 509–522. [CrossRef] [PubMed]
44. Jha, A.P.; Krompinger, J.; Baime, M.J. Mindfulness training modifies subsystems of attention. *Cogn. Affect. Behav. Neurosci.* **2007**, *7*, 109–119. [CrossRef] [PubMed]
45. Crescentini, C.; Capurso, V.; Furlan, S.; Fabbro, F. Mindfulness-oriented meditation for primary school children: Effects on attention and psychological well-being. *Front. Psychol.* **2016**, *7*. [CrossRef] [PubMed]
46. Zylowska, L.; Ackerman, D.L.; Yang, M.H.; Futrell, J.L.; Horton, N.L.; Hale, T.S.; Pataki, C.; Smalley, S.L. Mindfulness meditation training in adults and adolescents with ADHD. *J. Atten. Disord.* **2008**, *11*, 737–746. [CrossRef] [PubMed]
47. Nash, J.D.; Newberg, A. Toward a unifying taxonomy and definition for meditation. *Front. Psychol.* **2013**, *4*. [CrossRef] [PubMed]
48. Taren, A.A.; Gianaros, P.J.; Greco, C.M.; Lindsay, E.K.; Fairgrieve, A.; Brown, K.W.; Rosen, R.K.; Ferris, J.L.; Julson, E.; Marsland, A.L.; et al. Mindfulness meditation training and executive control network resting state functional connectivity: A randomized controlled trial. *Psychosom. Med.* **2017**. [CrossRef] [PubMed]
49. Van de Weijer-Bergsma, E.; Formsma, A.R.; de Bruin, E.I.; Bögels, S.M. The effectiveness of mindfulness training on behavioral problems and attentional functioning in adolescents with ADHD. *J. Child Fam. Stud.* **2012**, *21*, 775–787. [CrossRef] [PubMed]
50. Lagopoulos, J.; Xu, J.; Rasmussen, I.; Vik, A.; Malhi, G.S.; Eliassen, C.S.; Arnsten, I.E.; Sæther, J.G.; Hollup, S.; Holen, A.; et al. Increased theta and alpha EEG activity during nondirective meditation. *J. Altern. Complement. Med.* **2009**, *15*, 1187–1192. [CrossRef] [PubMed]
51. Kjaer, T.W.; Bertelsen, C.; Piccini, P.; Brooks, D.; Alving, J.; Lou, H.C. Increased dopamine tone during meditation-induced change of consciousness. *Cogn. Brain Res.* **2002**, *13*, 255–259. [CrossRef]

7

Implementing Integrative Nursing in a Pediatric Setting

Megan E. Voss * and Mary Jo Kreitzer

Center for Spirituality and Healing, University of Minnesota, Minneapolis, MN 55455, USA; kreit003@umn.edu
* Correspondence: vossx146@umn.edu

Abstract: Pediatric blood and marrow transplantation (BMT) is one of the most challenging allopathic treatments a patient and family can be faced with. A large Midwest academic health center, and leader in pediatric BMT, made the decision in 2013 to incorporate integrative nursing as the care delivery model. Nurses trained in advanced nursing practice and specialized in integrative health and healing performed a deep-dive needs assessment, national benchmarking, a comprehensive review of the literature, and ultimately designed a comprehensive integrative program for pediatric patients and their families undergoing BMT. Four years after implementation, this paper discusses lessons learned, strengths, challenges and next phases of the program, including a research agenda. The authors conclude that it is feasible, acceptable and sustainable to implement a nurse-led integrative program within an academic health center-based pediatric BMT program.

Keywords: pediatric integrative nursing; program development; pediatric blood and marrow transplant

---

1. Introduction

Integrative nursing has emerged as a framework for delivering sound patient care over the past five years. Principles closely aligned with the Institute for Healthcare Improvement's (IHI) Quadruple Aim can be used to help clinicians work with their patients to achieve better outcomes at lower costs, while at the same time tending to clinician well-being [1]. In the current healthcare environment, clinicians are consistently asked to do more with less. Nurses are caring for patients at much higher acuity levels than ever before, and often with higher nurse-to-patient ratios. Clinician burnout and early exit from the field are reaching alarming levels [2]. Integrative nursing as a care delivery model can be used as a strategy for mitigating the challenges faced by today's acute care nurses [3,4]. The aspirational vision of the pediatric blood and marrow transplantation (BMT) program's integrative model of care was to add an additional layer of supportive care that would palliate the patient and family on all dimensions: mind, body and spirit. The vision has remained closely aligned with the IHI Quadruple Aim. The goals of implementing integrative nursing are to improve the care experience of the patient and family, improve symptom management, and enhance the patient and family's capacity to cope. Additionally, in alignment with the IHI fourth aim, the program aspires to meet the self-care needs of staff from an organizational standpoint and to give providers and staff the tools they need to meet their individual responsibilities for self-care.

2. Methods

A team of advanced nursing practice leaders with specialty training in integrative health and healing performed a four-month long deep-dive needs assessment in order to develop a customized integrative program to complement the pediatric BMT program. Otto Scharmer's Theory U (Figure 1) served as the framework for the needs assessment. In this model of transformational change, there is a major focus on deeply listening to and understanding the needs of stakeholders in the organization;

in this case patients, families, staff and leaders, and to engage them in planning for the desired future [5]. Those five stages are outlined in Figure 1.

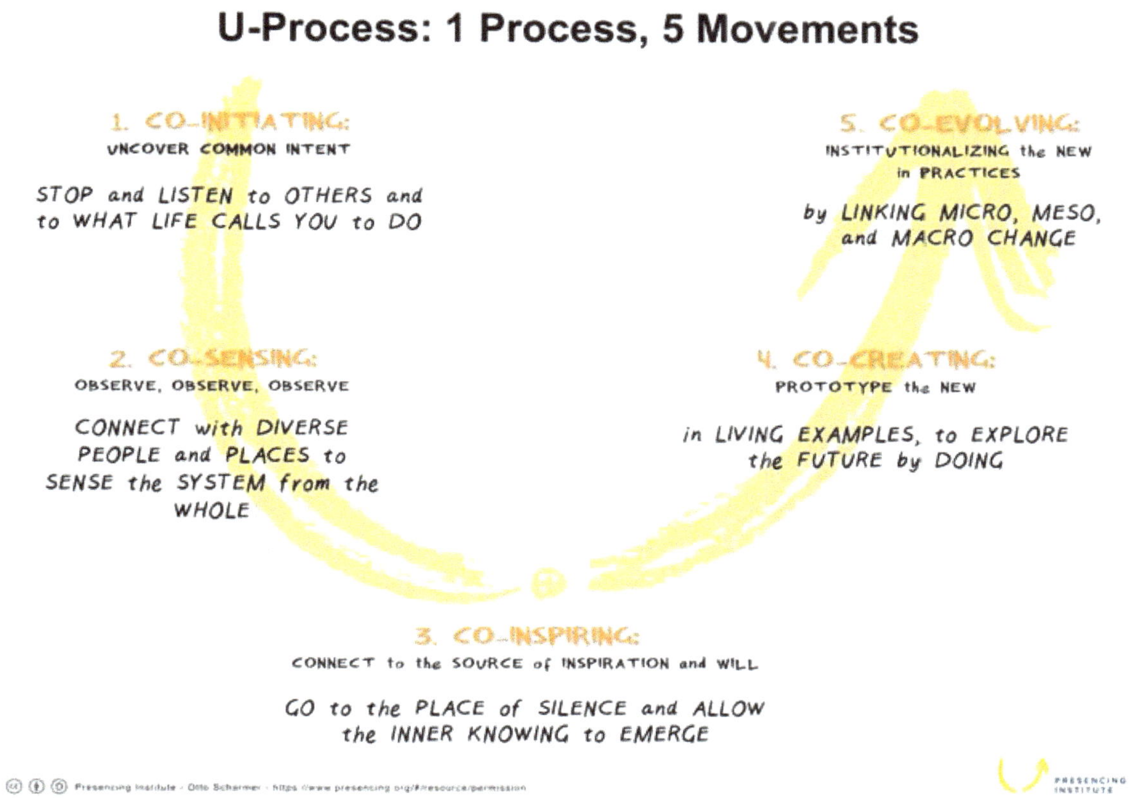

Figure 1. Theory U, reprinted with permission from [5].

2.1. Integrative Nursing as a Framework for Practice

The principles of integrative nursing (Table 1) informed the design, implementation and evaluation of the program. Integrative nursing is a whole person, whole system way of caring and healing that shapes and impacts patient care across the continuum. While the first text explicating the principles of integrative nursing was published in 2014, the concepts are timeless, are aligned with major nursing theorists, and date back to the philosophy, values and practices first introduced by Florence Nightingale in the 1800s [3,4].

Table 1. Principles of integrative nursing [3,6].

Human beings are whole systems inseparable from their environments.
Human beings have the innate capacity for health and well-being.
Nature has healing and restorative properties that contribute to health and well-being.
Integrative nursing is person-centered and relationship-based.
Integrative nursing practice is informed by evidence and uses the full range of therapeutic modalities to support/augment the healing process, moving from least intensive/invasive to more, depending on need and context.
Integrative nursing focuses on the health and well-being of caregivers as well as those they serve.

2.2. Program Design and Components

The pediatric BMT integrative therapy program was designed based on the outcomes of a four-month long needs assessment. The needs assessment included the following five components:

- Stakeholder dialogue—Interviews were conducted with clinical and administrative leadership as well as with frontline clinical staff.
- Shadowing practice—Current state of nursing and supportive care staff practice was observed to identify areas of opportunity.
- Prototyping—Experiential and educational sessions were conducted to engage staff and enhance their understanding of integrative modalities.
- Benchmarking—Other pediatric integrative therapy programs were examined through site visits, phone interviews, and extensive internet searches. These were reviewed for best practices.
- Staff survey—Nursing staff (N = 32) on the unit were surveyed to assess the knowledge, perceptions and comfort level with integrative modalities and care delivery.

Through this assessment, it was ascertained that the system overall had strong interest in and readiness for an integrative therapy program. The medical director was enthusiastically devoted to supporting this effort both clinically and financially. Many other pediatric hospitals around the nation have established integrative therapy programs; therefore, it was suddenly a market disadvantage to not offer what was becoming a standard of care in the eyes of patients and families [7]. While these strengths culminated to create a culture of momentum, there were still many challenges identified during the needs assessment.

2.2.1. Challenges

- Skepticism from staff—Due to historic start/stop efforts and initiatives that lacked structure, momentum and institutional support, staff doubted the likelihood of ever forming a sustainable, consistent and reliable integrative therapy program. There was distrust of the system and fatigue from working around system failures.
- Perceived barriers—Ranked by nursing staff in descending order: time, lack of skills, lack of knowledge, and comfort with integrative modalities.
- Inconsistencies in infrastructure—Processes, policies, procedure and methods of providing staff education had many variations across the board between the clinic and the hospital settings. These inconsistencies made it challenging to assess what existed, let alone what could be built.
- Lack of clinical expertise—The system did not employ any clinician with the level of training necessary to ensure that safe and effective integrative therapies were being utilized to the fullest potential to meet the needs of patients and families.

Ultimately, it was determined that a historic lack of cohesive institutional effort to form a comprehensive integrative therapy program led to the development of many variations in integrative therapy practices throughout the institution. While this demonstrates a high level of staff dedication to patient needs and adaptability, it also lends itself to inconsistency in standards of practice, policies, procedures and staff education. These types of efforts leave patients and families with minimal access to a consistent, reliable and safe set of services. Despite these challenges, several goals and a common vision emerged as part of the needs assessment process.

2.2.2. Vision

The vision was to create a world-class comprehensive integrative therapy program that would provide a seamless experience for pediatric BMT patients and families from the time of diagnosis through survivorship or bereavement. Additionally, the vision was to align the program with the organizational vision and mission and with national health care goals, including the Quadruple

Aim: improving the patient experience, the health of populations, reducing the cost of health care delivery, and improving care team well-being [2]. The program aimed to be viewed as a means to achieving essential health care outcomes by aligning fluidly with the challenges of today's health care environment. Integrative nursing is a key strategy in improving outcomes, enhancing patient/family satisfaction, and reducing the cost of care delivery, while at the same time improving its quality [3].

2.2.3. Goals

- Improve symptom management.
- Improve patient experience.
- Enhance patient and family resilience and capacity to cope.
- Provide patient and family with tools for incorporating integrative health practices before, during and after hospitalization.
- Improve care team well-being.
- Grow and support integrative health and healing research.
- Embed integrative approaches in every patient's care plan and every clinician's workflow.

2.2.4. Recommendations

The recommendations for achieving this vision and these goals were clear, yet extensive and arduous. To build a sustainable program, it would take years to accomplish every essential element. The following list of recommendations was developed five years ago following the initial needs assessment.

- Create an infrastructure and commit resources that are commensurate with the program vision and goals.
    - Hire or appoint an organizational lead.
    - Establish standards of care as well as policies and procedures that support those standards.
    - Create flowsheets and templates in the electronic medical record that not only allow for documentation of integrative approaches to care, but also allow for easy assessment of outcomes.
- Design a robust and comprehensive program evaluation strategy.
- Establish strong staff education and support.
- Offer access to a consistent set of therapeutic approaches that are evidenced-informed and focused on improved symptom management and quality of life.
- Expand patient and family education.
- Develop parent support resources to engage them in self-care and stress management, and to empower them to participate in comforting and caring for their child through the use of integrative approaches.
- Create an integrative health consult service for expertise, leadership and guidance to staff, patients and families.
- Establish an integrative health and healing research program focused on pediatric BMT patients' needs and clinical outcomes.

The program has three main components: care of patients and their families, staff well-being, and outcome evaluation. The components have been developed and implemented in that order. This order of evolution has been successful for several reasons. Nursing staff often does not recognize the need for self-care, does not identify burnout correctly or timely, or is reluctant to make changes. By implementing care of patients and families first, nurses and other frontline staff experienced secondary benefits of employing integrative strategies in the hospital setting. Nursing frequently received positive feedback from patients and families on the benefits they were experiencing from using integrative modalities.

2.2.5. Care Delivery Model

The framework for the nursing care delivery model comes from the integrative nursing work of Mary Jo Kreitzer and Mary Koithan [3]. The six principles of integrative nursing guide the practice of every nurse in the institution. Additionally, two doctoral prepared nurses with advanced nursing practice study in integrative health and healing lead the delivery of integrative therapy and integrative health consultation. Each new patient receives an integrative health consult with one of the integrative health doctor of nursing practice (DNP) nurses. These consults are triggered in the system to happen automatically for every patient. There is no fee associated with consultation or administration of integrative care. These services are offered to all patients regardless of insurance coverage or ability to pay. During this initial consultation, the patient and family's historical use of integrative therapies is discussed, an assessment of current or anticipated needs, symptoms and challenges is performed, as is a discussion of current skills, strengths and coping mechanisms. Safety and compatibility of integrative therapies with upcoming treatment regimen is discussed during this consult, and education is provided if a patient is currently using or desiring to use an integrative approach that might pose a safety risk during or immediately following the period of chemotherapy and radiation. Finally, a plan for integrative care during hospitalization is discussed and designed. Upon admission to the BMT unit, patients can choose to receive integrative services daily, as needed, or on a consultation basis only. The most common reasons patient engage in integrative therapies are for pain control, nausea, insomnia, anxiety and benefit of forming a therapeutic relationship with the clinician. Supplementary Materials Table S1 describes the integrative therapies that are offered consistently and reliably on the BMT unit.

2.3. Program Evaluation

Entering into the fifth year of the program, data has been gathered showing an uptick in integrative therapy utilization since year one. The authors hypothesize this could be due to several factors: (1) the first year of the program, there was only one full-time clinician dedicated to providing integrative services to patients and families. Currently, there are two-and-a-half full-time equivalent employees providing integrative services. (2) Patients and families affected by childhood cancer, and other rare diseases for which BMT is utilized as a treatment, are very well connected to one another. Patients and families now report having heard about the benefits of integrative therapies from people in their disease-specific communities before ever arriving to the facility. (3) Clinicians have indubitably become more skilled at applying integrative therapies to unique patient populations. Clinicians are skilled at assessing the root cause of a patient's symptom and applying the therapy that will modify the root cause rather than simply eliminating the symptom. For example, young children often experience nausea and/or vomiting before or after medication administration or in anticipation of chemotherapy. It is important to assess the characteristics of and the circumstances surrounding the nausea and/or vomiting. Often, it is anxiety or anticipatory anxiety that leads to sudden onset nausea and/or vomiting [8]. Mind/body techniques are more effective at mitigating the risk of emesis related to anxiety or a conditioned response to treatment than a pharmaceutical antiemetic [8]. Finally, (4) it is plausible that providers and staff recommend integrative therapies more often and demonstrate more confidence in integrative therapies now than they did four years ago. Once providers and staff began having first-hand observations and experiences with integrative therapies achieving positive results for their patients, they were more likely to recommend them.

The BMT program treats approximately 80 patients per year. Patients are engaged in treatment for a minimum of three to four months. Some patients remain in the system and seek in- and outpatient care intermittently for up to two years. Year one of the program, 51% of BMT patients engaged in integrative therapies. By year two, that number increased to 70%, and at the conclusion of year three, approximately 94% of patients participated in integrative therapies throughout their BMT experience. Patient and family engagement with the integrative therapy team ranges from a one-time consult to daily sessions of 30–60 min. The average patient is seen two or three times per week for approximately 30 min. Over the course of hundreds of integrative therapy sessions over the past four years, the program reports no adverse events. Practice guidelines and safety recommendations have been developed based on available literature, clinician experience, patient report, and occasionally "near misses".

2.4. Emerging Research Agenda

Establishing a research program was one of the eight original goals. This has been the most challenging goal to accomplish and was, by design, delayed for the first few years. Infrastructure needed to be built before clean data collection could occur. Now that a consistent set of services is offered by experienced clinicians, the program is ripe for an integrative research agenda. Several quality improvement surveys and one qualitative study have been completed and played an important role in shaping the research agenda. The first study published by the program examined themes around the usefulness of music therapy [9]. Table 2 outlines the research initiatives that are underway and projects that will be implemented over the next two years.

Table 2. Research agenda.

Study Concept	Description
Music therapy as a method to physical rehabilitation	Qualitative data has revealed that even when children are too physically ill or mentally reluctant to participate in physical rehabilitation therapies, many are still motivated to get out of bed and participate in music therapy. It is hypothesized that active participation in music therapy can help achieve physical rehabilitation goals in some patients [9].
Retrospective review of utilization and safety	Data mining will be done to assess the most common therapy used by each age group, adverse reactions in patients with safety considerations such as thrombocytopenia or impaired skin integrity, responses of pain, nausea and anxiety to integrative therapy, and average length and number of visits (inpatient and outpatient) each patient requests.
Self-assessment of change after the implementation of an integrative iherapy ilan of care	The self-assessment of change is a retrospective pre/post assessment that measures a variety of psychosocial indicators. The tool was designed specifically to capture change produced by integrative therapy.
Survivorship well-being for patients and families	Interactive online content based on the University of Minnesota's Wellbeing Model (Figure 2) will be developed and focused on teenagers and young adults. Virtual support groups will accompany content. Groups will be facilitated by a variety of healthcare professionals with an integrative lens. Data will be collected to assess the impact on overall well-being including indicators such as self-management, perceived stress, quality of life, anxiety, depression and resilience.
Microbiome	This study will examine the effects of chemotherapy and prolonged prophylactic antibiotic use on patients after engraftment and full recovery from pancytopenia. It will also look at the potential for the safe and judicial use of supplements to restore intestinal tissue integrity and the microbiome.
Staff self-care	Continuous data collection efforts have been and will continue to be underway assessing staff burnout and other components of well-being.

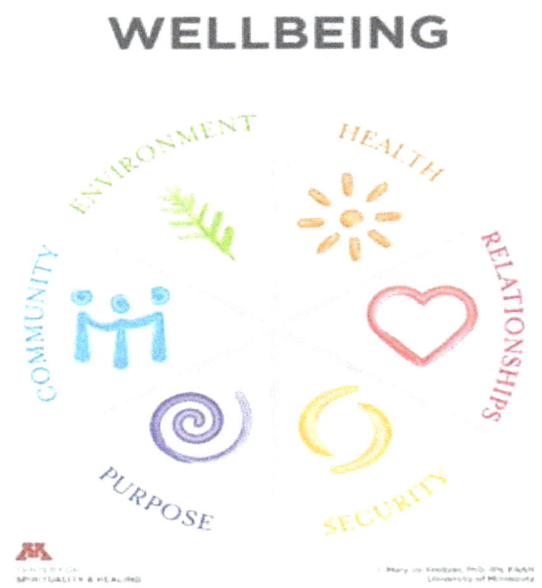

Figure 2. University of Minnesota's Wellbeing Model [6].

3. Results and Discussion

The integrative therapy program is entering into its fifth year of existence. It has grown and matured since the original design, but remains true to its initial mission, vision and goals. By all objective measures, the program has been deemed a success. Rates of patient engagement and utilization, increase in grant funding and institutional support, and provider and front-line clinician acceptance all speak to the accomplishments of the program over the past four years. The authors conclude that it is both feasible and acceptable to implement a nurse-led integrative program within an academic health center-based pediatric BMT program.

The success and sustainability of the program may be in large part due to nursing leadership. Nurses are uniquely positioned to assess and treat patients from a whole-person, whole-system framework. Nurses are by nature nurturing, caring and attuned to using their own self as a therapeutic intervention. Furthermore, by having advanced nursing practice consultation available, the model is more financially sustainable than a physician-centric integrative consult service. Patients receive competent assessment and continuity of care with nurses trained in integrative modalities accessible to them on a daily basis.

4. Conclusions

The work over the past few years has demonstrated that there is a strong clinical and business case for implementing integrative nursing within an acute-care pediatric setting. Patients and families are voicing a desire for this approach to care and there is increasing evidence that integrative approaches can improve clinical outcomes including symptom management [8]. If embedded into the ongoing delivery of care, the implementation of integrative nursing is both feasible and sustainable. It requires investment in education and leadership and perhaps most importantly a culture change that embraces a whole-person, whole-system approach to patient care.

Author Contributions: M.J.K. has been an active advisor and mentor to the growth and development of the pediatric BMT integrative program since its conceptualization in 2012. M.E.V. began work on the pediatric BMT integrative program by joining the team that conducted the initial needs assessment under the guidance of M.J.K. and John E. Wager, executive medical director for pediatric BMT in 2013. M.E.V. continues to direct the program and its research efforts.

Acknowledgments: The authors would like to acknowledge the perpetual support of John E. Wagner, the executive medical director of the pediatric BMT program. Without his vision, leadership and support, this program would not exist. Without the constant administrative support of Janet Hegland, program director pediatric BMT, this program would not have made it off the ground. Hegland's leadership and dedication are appreciated. The other members of the original needs assessment team, Janet Tomaino and Rachel Trelstad Porter, the authors appreciate the initial work that helped to pave the path and plant the seeds of inspiration for this program. The insights and contributions of that group still play a daily role in the program evolution. Finally, the authors would like to thank all of the frontline staff working with pediatric BMT patients. The faculty, hospitalists, nurses, nurse practitioners, physicians' assistants, chaplains, social workers and support staff are the true essence of healing presence in the lives of these children.

References

1. Institute for Healthcare Improvement: IHI Home Page. Available online: http://www.ihi.org:80/ (accessed on 29 June 2018).
2. Clinician Resilience and Well-Being. National Academy of Medicine. Available online: https://nam.edu/initiatives/clinician-resilience-and-well-being/ (accessed on 29 June 2018).
3. Kreitzer, M.J.; Koithan, M. *Integrative Nursing*; Oxford University Press: New York, NY, USA, 2018.
4. Koithan, M.S.; Kreitzer, M.J.; Watson, J. Linking the unitary paradigm to policy through a synthesis of caring science and integrative nursing, linking the unitary paradigm to policy through a synthesis of caring science and integrative nursing. *Nurs. Sci. Q.* **2017**, *30*, 262–268. [CrossRef] [PubMed]
5. Presencing Institute—Theory U: Leading from the Future as It Emerges. Available online: https://www.presencing.org/#/aboutus/theory-u (accessed on 29 June 2018).
6. Integrative Nursing. Available online: https://www.csh.umn.edu/education/focus-areas/integrative-nursing (accessed on 6 July 2018).
7. Jacobs, S.S. Integrative therapy use for management of side effects and toxicities experienced by pediatric oncology patients. *Children* **2014**, *1*, 424–440. [CrossRef] [PubMed]
8. Roscoe, J.A.; Morrow, G.R.; Aapro, M.S.; Molassiotis, A.; Olver, I. Anticipatory nausea and vomiting. *Support. Care Cancer* **2011**, *19*, 1533–1538. [CrossRef] [PubMed]
9. Yates, G.J.; Beckmann, N.B.; Anderson, M.R.; Voss, M.E.; Silverman, M.J. Caregiver perceptions of music therapy for children hospitalized for a blood and marrow transplant: An interpretivist investigation. *Glob. Adv. Health Med.* **2018**. [CrossRef] [PubMed]

8

A Pilot Study of Mindfulness Meditation for Pediatric Chronic Pain

Lynn C. Waelde [1,2], Amanda B. Feinstein [3], Rashmi Bhandari [3], Anya Griffin [3], Isabel A. Yoon [3] and Brenda Golianu [3,*]

1 Pacific Graduate School of Psychology, Palo Alto University, Palo Alto, CA 94304, USA; lwaelde@paloaltou.edu
2 Department of Psychiatry and Behavioral Sciences, Stanford University School of Medicine, Stanford, CA 94305, USA
3 Department of Anesthesia, Stanford University School of Medicine, Stanford, CA 94305, USA; abfein@stanford.edu (A.B.F.); rbhandar@stanford.edu (R.B.); anyag@stanford.edu (A.G.); iayoon@stanford.edu (I.A.Y.)
* Correspondence: bgolianu@stanford.edu

Abstract: Despite advances in psychological interventions for pediatric chronic pain, there has been little research examining mindfulness meditation for these conditions. This study presents data from a pilot clinical trial of a six-week manualized mindfulness meditation intervention offered to 20 adolescents aged 13–17 years. Measures of pain intensity, functional disability, depression and parent worry about their child's pain were obtained at baseline and post-treatment. Results indicated no significant changes in pain or depression, however functional disability and frequency of pain functioning complaints improved with small effect sizes. Parents' worry about child's pain significantly decreased with a large effect size. Participants rated intervention components positively and most teens suggested that the number of sessions be increased. Three case examples illustrate mindfulness meditation effects and precautions. Mindfulness meditation shows promise as a feasible and acceptable intervention for youth with chronic pain. Future research should optimize intervention components and determine treatment efficacy.

Keywords: mindfulness; meditation; pediatric; chronic pain; adolescent; group therapy

1. Introduction

Pediatric chronic pain is a significant problem in the United States, with prevalence rates across pain subtypes ranging from 11% to 38% [1]. Children with chronic pain experience impairments in emotional [2], social [3], and school functioning [4,5]. Chronic pain in childhood not only pervasively impacts quality of life [6], but also leaves youth at risk for progression of pain into adulthood [7].

Psychological approaches to pain management are known to be an important part of interdisciplinary treatment for pediatric chronic pain [8]. Such approaches typically include cognitive behavioral therapy [9,10], biofeedback [11], and hypnosis [12]. Research suggests that psychological therapies may improve pain and functioning [13].

Mindfulness, often defined as paying attention on purpose and nonjudgmentally in the present moment [14], is a strategy that has received little attention in the field of pediatric pain, despite the growing application of mindfulness-based interventions to address chronic pain in adults [15]. Mindfulness-based interventions for youth have ranged from delivering mindfulness strategies within broader cognitive behavioral packages [16] to developmentally modifying the Mindfulness-Based Stress Reduction (MBSR) program [17]. Jastrowski-Mano et al. [18] published the first small (n = 6) randomized controlled pilot study on MBSR for pediatric pain. Due to high attrition and difficulties with recruitment, they were unable to draw conclusions about the efficacy or feasibility of MBSR for this population. Ruskin and colleagues [19] reported on the development of an MBSR group for adolescents with chronic pain and cited challenges as well, including insufficient post-test data which affected their ability to draw conclusions about outcomes. Two more recent studies examining mindfulness-based programs for adolescents with chronic pain indicated that such interventions were feasible and acceptable [20,21]. Chadi et al. [20] utilized a combination of MBSR and Mindfulness-Based Cognitive Therapy adapted to adolescents and reported no improvements in psychological or pain symptoms, though they did report pre/post-reductions in salivary cortisol levels. Ali et al. [21] utilized a developmentally modified MBSR protocol in a pilot cohort study and reported significant pre/post-improvements in fibromyalgia symptoms, anxiety, and functional disability. Given that previous studies utilizing mindfulness for pediatric chronic pain have reported feasibility and some positive outcomes, more research is needed to further explore the acceptability and efficacy of therapeutic modalities that incorporate mindfulness for this challenging patient population.

The current study was designed to pilot a mindfulness meditation program using a manualized intervention entitled Inner Resources for Teens (IRT) [22], a six-week protocol developed and adapted for teenagers from a similar course utilized for adults named Inner Resources for Stress [23]. Like MBSR, the IRT program teaches mindfulness in daily life and mindfulness meditation, but also includes techniques such as breath-focused imagery and repetition of cue words that are intended to provide additional cognitive structure. Unlike MBSR, IRT does not include hatha yoga or movement-based practices. Previous randomized controlled trials (RCT) of the Inner Resources for Stress intervention for adults have demonstrated pre/post-improvements relative to control groups in diurnal cortisol slope, life satisfaction, and remission from chronic depression [24,25].

The aims of this study were to examine the feasibility, acceptability, and usefulness of the mindfulness meditation intervention, as well as the acceptability of specific treatment components of the IRT program. A secondary aim of this study was to document qualitative case descriptions from three participants to highlight benefits and challenges of using mindfulness meditation with this population.

2. Methods

2.1. Participants and Setting

Twenty patients diagnosed with chronic pain were recruited from a university-based pediatric pain management clinic. All participants had a history of chronic pain for more than 12 months. They continued to receive multidisciplinary pain management standard of care throughout the intervention. The mean age of participations was 15.1 (standard deviation (SD) = 1.36) and ages ranged from 13 to 17. Two participants (10%) were male. Types of pain included abdominal pain, headaches, fibromyalgia, musculoskeletal pain, complex regional pain syndrome, and joint pain (see Table 1). The mean duration of chronic pain was 2.8 years (range 2.2 to 7).

Table 1. Types of Pain Experienced by Participants.

Pain Type	*n* (%)
Headache	7 (35)
Abdominal pain	6 (30)
Joint pain, rheumatologic	2 (10)
Musculoskeletal pain	2 (10)
Flank pain, polycystic kidney disease	1 (5)
Complex regional pain syndrome	1 (5)
Erythromelalgia	1 (5)

2.2. Procedures

This study was conducted at a tertiary pediatric pain clinic within a children's hospital setting on the West Coast in the United States. The study was approved by the university's Institutional Review Board. Consent and assent procedures took place at the clinic visit. Participants completed baseline questionnaires on the day of the first mindfulness session, including demographics, pain intensity ratings, and domains of physical and psychological functioning. Following the final session, they also completed ratings of pain and function and responded to open-ended questions evaluating the feasibility and acceptability of the intervention.

2.3. Intervention

The mindfulness intervention consisted of a six-session group-based intervention to teach and practice skills for maintaining sustained nonjudgmental present moment awareness. Three groups were held four months apart, containing nine, three and eight participants, respectively. The intervention was led by a clinical psychologist (author L.W.) and a clinical psychology doctoral student who was trained and supervised in the intervention. The techniques were adapted specifically for adolescents and included a guided body tour, tension release, mindfulness meditation, breath-focused imagery, and repetition of cue words. The Guided Body Tour consisted of noticing and then visualizing breath flow to parts of the body. Complete Breath involved noticing every part of the breath from the inhalation through the exhalation. Repetition of secular cue words consisted of repeating the sounds "Hum Sah," meant to represent the sound of breathing in synchrony with the breath, repeating "Hum" with every inhalation and "Sah" with the exhalation. Tension Release was a breath-focused visualization exercise designed to enhance participants' ability to let go of any "tension or holding",

Sessions were 60 min in length, and began and ended with a 20-min period of therapist-led teaching and practice of mindfulness meditation. The middle 20 min of each session included therapist presentations of didactic material, including the discussion of ways to apply the practice to presenting problems. A major focus of the didactic/discussion sessions was to encourage use of mindfulness skills and techniques in daily life, particularly in response to dealing with pain. Participants were asked to practice these techniques at home for at least 15 min per day for six weeks and to practice them as much as possible in daily life. Participants were provided with a manual, entitled *Inner Resources for Teens* [22] which contained age-appropriate readings and suggestions for the daily practice of the techniques. The manual included four 15-min audio recordings of guided mindfulness meditations that participants used for home practice. The audio recordings were provided on compact disc (CD) and participants were encouraged to convert the recordings to other listening devices.

2.4. Measures

Demographic information collected from participants included age, sex, and duration of chronic pain problem. Qualitative information was obtained from written surveys.

Pain Intensity: Adolescents rated their usual pain intensity and worst pain intensity in the past seven days on the 11-point Numeric Rating Scale (NRS-11) from 0 = "No pain" to 10 = "Worst pain possible" at baseline and post-treatment [26]. The NRS-11 has evidenced validity in the assessment of pain intensity in children and adolescents [26].

Depression: The Children's Depression Inventory (CDI) is a self-report assessment of symptoms of depression that includes 27 items that are scored on a 3-point scale [27]. Total scores range from 0 to 54. Psychometric evidence supporting its use in youth are described by other authors [28,29].

Functional Disability: The 15-item Functional Disability Inventory (FDI) [30] evaluates the physical impact of chronic condition as reported by youth and their caregivers (proxy report) on activities of daily living (e.g., walking, school, sleep) on a Likert scale ranging from 0 = "No trouble" to 4 = "Impossible", where higher scores signify greater functional impairment. The measure has shown sound reliability and validity when used with youth who experience chronic medical challenges [31].

The Stanford Pediatric Pain Functioning Inventory (SPPFI): The SPPFI is a clinical tool which evaluates the frequency of pain functioning complaints during the past week. The survey consisted of 24 questions designed for teenagers (aged 13–18) and a similar version for their parents (proxy report). The item stem for the first five items states: "Due to my pain in the past week, it was hard for me to . . . ." Some of the items for this stem include "Walk more than a block," and "Do physical education (PE), sports, or exercise." The next 15 items have the stem "Because of my pain in the past week, I . . . ." Some of the items following this stem include "Spent time on my bed or couch," "Had low energy," "Had trouble paying attention," and "Worried about making my pain worse." The last four items had the stem "In the past week my pain . . . ." Some of the items for this stem included "Interrupted family activities," "Made my parents worry," and "Made my parents miss work." Parent items had the stem "This past week, my child's pain . . . " which included items such as "Caused me to worry," "Affected our family's activities," "Caused me/my spouse to miss work." Participants rated items on a 5-point response scale with 0 = "Never," 1 = "Almost never," 2 = "Sometimes," 3 = "Often," 4 = "Always",

The Project Evaluation questionnaire was administered at post-treatment and included open-ended questions assessing the feasibility and acceptability of the treatment. Participants and parents indicated the desired length and number of sessions the intervention should include. Participants also rated the components of the intervention on a scale 6-point scale, with 0 = "Not sure," 1 = "Not at all useful," 2 = "A little bit useful," 3 = "Moderately useful," 4 = "Quite a bit useful," and 5 = "Extremely useful." Ratings of 0 and 1 were reported as "Not useful," and ratings of 2–5 were reported as "Useful."

3. Results

Of the 20 participants enrolled the study, four did not meet the attendance criteria of four out of six sessions (attrition rate = 20%). Attrition was due to transportation difficulties ($n = 1$), a new medical condition that precluded group participation ($n = 1$), and participant concerns that the sessions were not adequately reducing pain ($n = 2$). Two additional participants were lost to follow-up because they were not able to attend the last session and scheduling difficulties prevented them from scheduling an in-person post-treatment assessment; therefore, follow-up assessment data were available for 14 participants.

Paired t-tests examined changes from baseline to post-treatment (see Table 2). Participant ratings of pain intensity (usual pain and worst pain) did not change from baseline to post-treatment. Likewise, participant ratings of depression were unchanged. Although improvements in ratings of functional disability frequency of pain functioning complaints were not statistically significant, there were numerical pre/post-decreases equivalent to a small Cohen's d effect size [32]. Parents' ratings of the worry caused by their child's pain significantly decreased from baseline to post-treatment, with a large effect size.

Table 2. Means, Standard Deviations, and Effects Sizes of Change from Baseline to Post-treatment.

	Baseline $n = 20$		Post-Treatment $n = 14$			
Variable	*M*	*SD*	*M*	*SD*	*t*	*d*
NRS-usual pain	5.6	1.9	5.6	2.0	−0.4	0
NRS-most severe pain	8.6	1.6	8.8	1.4	−0.8	0
CDI	38.7	7.1	38.9	6.9	−0.1	0
FDI	13.8	6.6	12.5	9.9	0.6	0.20
Teen SPPFI	31.8	14.9	27.4	17.5	0.83	0.30
Parent SPPFI-child's pain caused me to worry [a]	2.7	1.2	1.8	1.2	3.3 *	0.75

Note: NRS = Numerical Rating Scale; SPPFI = Stanford Pediatric Pain Functioning Inventory; CDI = Children's Depression Inventory; FDI = Functional Disability Inventory. [a] Parent SPPFI were available for 11 parents. * $p < 0.01$. M = Mean; SD = standard deviation; t = paired t-test; d = Cohen's d effect size

The program evaluation questionnaire assessed the acceptability of aspects of the intervention. Participants and parents also provided data on the acceptability of the number of sessions the intervention should include (see Table 3). None of the participants indicated that they thought the intervention should be shorter. Less than one-third (n = 4; 28.6%) of participants indicated that six weeks was the ideal length for the mindfulness meditation program, and the remaining participants (n = 10; 71.4%) endorsed that the intervention should include more than 8 or 10 sessions. None of the participants indicated that the intervention should be shorter than 60 min. The majority of the participants (n = 10; 71.4%) indicated that 60 min was the ideal session length and less than a third (n = 4; 28.6%) indicated that it should be longer. Only one parent thought the intervention should be shorter in terms of number and length of sessions, and around half of parents agreed that the current format of six 60 min sessions was preferred. Results indicated that the majority of participants rated the intervention components as useful (see Table 4). Practice in daily life and the group sessions were the most highly rated components, with 12 participants (85.7%) rating them as useful. Meditation and repetition of cue words, unguided by an audio recording, was rated as useful by 11 participants (78.6%). Of the four audio recordings of guided practice, Complete Breath and "Hum Sah" were the most highly rated, followed by the Guided Body Tour and Tension Release.

Table 3. Participant and Parent Recommendations for Intervention Duration from Project Evaluation.

	Teen Participants n (%)	**Parents n (%)**
Number of weekly sessions		
4	0	1 (9.1)
6 (number of pilot sessions)	4 (28.6)	5 (45.5)
8	4 (28.6)	1 (9.1)
10	6 (42.9)	4 (36.4)
Length of weekly session in minutes		
30	0	1 (9.1)
60 (length of pilot sessions)	10 (71.4)	7 (63.6)
90	4 (28.6)	3 (27.3)

Table 4. Number and Proportion of Participants Rating Intervention Components as Useful.

Intervention Component	**n (%)**
Inner Resources for Teens manual	10 (71.4)
Guided Body Tour CD	9 (64.3)
Complete Breath CD	10 (71.4)
Hum Sah CD	10 (71.4)
Tension Release CD	8 (57.1)
Meditation practice without CD	11 (78.6)
Hum Sah practice without CD	11 (78.6)
Practice in daily life	12 (85.7)
Group sessions	12 (85.7)

Note: CD = audio recording on compact disc used for guided practice.

Case Illustrations

Case #1. A 15-year-old male participant with multiple pain complaints, including headaches and myofascial pain, was able to learn and practice the meditation techniques and use them to cope with stressors associated with his medical conditions. Although his awareness of pain was slightly increased during the initial sessions, after approximately three weeks of practicing the techniques he became aware that the pain increased his distress and that he could use mindful awareness to reduce his experience of stress, feel more relaxed, and attenuate his experience of pain. He attended all six sessions. He continued to improve after the conclusion of the intervention, by self-report and clinical assessment in follow-up medical visits.

Case #2. A 14-year-old female with fibromyalgia and depression reported improvements in both physical and emotional symptoms after participating in the full six-week program. She reported that this intervention was helpful and described through the program evaluation questionnaires that she learned a new method for coping with her symptoms. Peer support seemed to be of particular benefit to this participant, as she was able to normalize the experience of chronic pain. She especially liked the practice of cue word repetition during periods of sitting meditation and in her daily life, as she reportedly found that it decreased her worry and rumination and reduced her experience of pain. At the midpoint of the intervention, she reported that mindfulness allowed her to address the emotional impact of chronic pain, particularly anxiety, resulting in self-reported reduction in usual pain level. This improvement increased her ability to begin and maintain a daily exercise program and led to full symptom resolution three months after completion of the intervention.

Case #3. A 16-year-old female participant with functional abdominal pain and a longstanding history of participation in pain management treatments (e.g., interventional blocks, multiple medication trials and psychological interventions) reported that she utilized distraction as her primary method of coping with chronic pain. Although she reported successful use of the techniques for coping with anxiety, such as when trying to fall asleep or prior to a music competition, she found the concurrent use of mindfulness and distraction to cope with pain to be confusing and ineffective, resulting in exacerbation of pain symptoms. Due to the focus on body awareness with mindfulness practice, she reported that she became more aware of pain sensations and increasingly distressed. With support of the study team, she was withdrawn from the mindfulness program after two sessions. She continued to participate in outpatient pain management, including psychological services. There were no long-term sequelae and her pain level returned to baseline upon termination of the intervention.

4. Discussion

The current study examined a novel intervention for training in mindfulness meditation, Inner Resources for Teens, which combined mindfulness in daily life, meditation practices, breath-focused cue word repetition, and visualization for adolescents with chronic pain. The intervention was reported as feasible, acceptable, and useful for the majority of participants by adolescent- and parent-report (as well as case study description). There were small quantitative improvements in functioning and reduced disability, suggesting a small effect size; however, due to the small number of patients these were not found to be statistically significant. Parent's concern and worry about their child demonstrated a statistically significant decrease with a large effect size. The adolescents in our pilot study demonstrated acceptable adherence to the intervention, with 80% attending at least four of the six sessions. The majority of participants reported satisfaction with the intervention and expressed the desire for additional sessions after the six weekly sessions were completed. The 60-min session length used in the current study was preferred by most participants and parents.

The group format of the intervention was a highly rated component, consistent with previous work indicating that social support is a valued component of mindfulness interventions for pediatric chronic pain [21]. Practice in daily life was also highly rated, similar to work with adults showing that integrating mindfulness practice in daily life was more commonly practiced than sitting meditation [25]. At the end of the six-week program, participants preferred the unguided meditation and cue word repetition over practice using audio recordings. It is possible that the guided practices were more important at an earlier stage, when participants were first learning the practices. Of the four audio recordings of guided practice, Complete Breath and "Hum Sah" were the most highly rated, followed by the Guided Body Tour and Tension Release. Both the Guided Body Tour and Tension Release may serve to focus attention on bodily sensations to a greater degree than breath-focused meditations and may be less tolerable for adolescents with chronic pain.

As illustrated in Case #3, increased body awareness may be difficult for adolescents with chronic pain, particularly if they primarily rely upon distraction as a pain coping strategy. It is notable that all of the intervention components were rated as useful by a majority of participants, suggesting that the combination of mindfulness, cue word repetition, and meditation exercises was acceptable within the scope of a single intervention. This combination of components differs from interventions such as MBSR, which do not include visualization and cue word repetition [17]. However, as illustrated in Cases #1 and #2, these practices were useful for stress and anxiety. Case #1 noted that his pain initially increased as he brought awareness to his breathing and body, but he was able to tolerate the minor exacerbation in pain intensity until he experienced reduced stress and anxiety about the pain, which in turn reduced his perception of pain. Case #2 reported that the use of breath-focused cue word repetition was helpful in redirecting her attention from worry and rumination and provided useful structure during the initial phases of learning the techniques.

There were no significant changes post-intervention in pain intensity or depression quantitative measures, which is not a surprising finding. Previous studies of mindfulness [20,21] have not reported reductions in pain as an outcome of the intervention, so it may be that these practices are more specific to the distress and dysregulation that accompany the pain experience [33]. Alternatively, it may be that the timing of teaching intervention components is the critical factor. Previous work shows that initial instructions to observe and accept experience—a defining feature of most mindfulness approaches—reduces pain tolerance relative to a control condition and may tax self-regulatory capacity [34]. Longer training may be required to use mindfulness techniques to control or down-regulate the pain experience [35]. Focused practices, such as visualization or cue word repetition, may provide useful structure for teens who are unable to tolerate increased present moment awareness during the initial phase of training.

Parents demonstrated reduced worry about their child's chronic pain over the six-week intervention period. It may be that parents had increased confidence in their child's ability to implement self-management skills, and this confidence decreased parental worry and catastrophizing. Increased parental catastrophizing has been associated with increased child disability in pediatric patients with chronic pain [36], therefore this parent outcome is a promising target for future implementations of mindfulness training.

Limitations of the study include reliance on self-report measures with only limited inclusion of parent-reported data. In addition, the measure of parent worry was based on an item from an assessment tool (i.e., SPPFI), limiting the interpretation of this construct. Although the heterogeneity of pain complaints may be a limitation that restricts recommending this intervention to specific pain populations, it is also a strength with regard to generalizability across pain conditions in terms of the usefulness of this intervention. Not providing intervention components to family members was an additional limitation that was expressly desired by families and should be addressed in future research.

Future Directions

Given that most of the teen participants indicated that the number of sessions should be increased, future implementations should consider a longer format (8 to 10 weekly sessions). The 60-min session length used in the current study seemed optimal to most participants. The impact of the intervention on parents' worry about their child's pain appears indicative of benefits that parents, themselves, may receive through their child's knowledge and implementation of pain coping skills. With additional parent-proxy report measures utilized in future studies, it may be possible to further delineate parental perspectives on functional improvements gained via mindfulness interventions, in the context of other parental self-reported outcomes. Future work is recommended to explore how parents may directly benefit from their own mindfulness training within the context of concurrent adolescent and parent groups. Given that previous research and the results of this pilot study indicate that pain experience may initially fluctuate with mindfulness training, introducing more structured practice, such as cue word repetition, during the first session of the intervention may provide the necessary support for patients as they gain skills to reduce anxiety and increase self-regulatory capacity.

Likewise, future studies should consider the coping style of individual participants as well as their developmental needs, as the focus of mindfulness practice on present moment awareness and physical sensations may seem overwhelming for some adolescents at first. It may be that initially distraction techniques may provide some much-needed relief from the painful sensations, whereas at a later stage, the use of mindfulness techniques may help to decrease anxiety and amplification of the pain experience. The gradual incorporation of mindfulness techniques into the therapy process may produce optimal results. Additional work is also needed to study the method of delivery as a group intervention compared to individual instruction. The group intervention may allow for much-needed social interaction as well as peer validation, whereas the individualized approach may allow for further personalization of the techniques. Future research may explore the relative merits of both distraction and mindfulness techniques to determine the most beneficial use of these strategies for different pain contexts and strategies. Moreover, improved clarification about the aim and rationale for mindfulness treatment may align participant expectancies with the aims of the intervention during each phase of the training. Because the current brief intervention did not demonstrate decreases in pain or increases in functioning, future studies are needed to explore dose and duration of treatment to optimize pain and symptom management.

5. Conclusions

In conclusion, a mindfulness program such as the IRT shows promise as an intervention for helping adolescents with chronic pain and appears to be a feasible tool in the armamentarium of non-pharmacological treatments. The results of this pilot study demonstrate the continued need to further develop pediatric chronic pain mindfulness interventions, exploring a variety of treatment components to determine the most feasible, acceptable and efficacious interventions for this population within the context of a multidisciplinary approach to pediatric chronic pain management.

Author Contributions: L.C.W., B.G., and R.B. conceived and designed the study. B.G., L.C.W., and R.B. recruited and tested subjects. L.C.W. analyzed data. All authors were involved in data interpretation and writing of the manuscript. Aaron Fett and Jason Thompson served as co-interventionists. David Spiegel, M.D. provided invaluable consultation regarding study design.

References

1. King, S.; Chambers, C.T.; Huguet, A.; MacNevin, R.C.; McGrath, P.J.; Parker, L.; MacDonald, A.J. The epidemiology of chronic pain in children and adolescents revisited: a systematic review. *Pain* **2011**, *152*, 2729–2738. [CrossRef] [PubMed]
2. Pinquart, M.; Shen, Y. Depressive symptoms in children and adolescents with chronic physical illness: An updated meta-analysis. *J. Pediatr. Psychol.* **2011**, *36*, 375–384. [CrossRef] [PubMed]
3. Forgeron, P.A.; King, S.; Stinson, J.N.; McGrath, P.J.; MacDonald, A.J.; Chambers, C.T. Social functioning and peer relationships in children and adolescents with chronic pain: A systematic review. *Pain Res. Manag.* **2010**, *15*, 27–41. [CrossRef] [PubMed]
4. Chan, E.; Piira, T.; Betts, G. The school functioning of children with chronic and recurrent pain. *Pediatr. Pain Lett.* **2005**, *7*, 11–16.
5. Simons, L.E.; Logan, D.E.; Chastain, L.; Stein, M. The relation of social functioning to school impairment among adolescents with chronic pain. *Clin. J. Pain* **2010**, *26*, 16–22. [CrossRef] [PubMed]
6. Gold, J.I.; Yetwin, A.K.; Mahrer, N.E.; Carson, M.C.; Griffin, A.T.; Palmer, S.N.; Joseph, M.H. Pediatric chronic pain and health-related quality of life. *J. Pediatr. Nurs.* **2009**, *24*, 141–150. [CrossRef] [PubMed]
7. Walker, L.S.; Dengler-Crish, C.M.; Rippel, S.; Bruehl, S. Functional abdominal pain in childhood and adolescence increases risk for chronic pain in adulthood. *Pain* **2010**, *150*, 568–572. [CrossRef] [PubMed]
8. Eccleston, C.; Palermo, T.M.; Williams, A.C.d.C.; Lewandowski Holley, A.; Morley, S.; Fisher, E.; Law, E. Psychological therapies for the management of chronic and recurrent pain in children and adolescents. *Cochrane Libr.* **2014**.

9. Robins, P.M.; Smith, S.M.; Glutting, J.J.; Bishop, C.T. A randomized controlled trial of a cognitive-behavioral family intervention for pediatric recurrent abdominal pain. *J. Pediatr. Psychol.* **2005**, *30*, 397–408. [CrossRef] [PubMed]
10. Kashikar-Zuck, S.; Ting, T.V.; Arnold, L.M.; Bean, J.; Powers, S.W.; Graham, T.B.; Passo, M.H.; Schikler, K.N.; Hashkes, P.J.; Spalding, S. Cognitive behavioral therapy for the treatment of juvenile fibromyalgia: A multisite, single-blind, randomized, controlled clinical trial. *Arthritis Rheumatol.* **2012**, *64*, 297–305. [CrossRef] [PubMed]
11. Labbé, É.L.; Williamson, D.A. Treatment of childhood migraine using autogenic feedback training. *J. Consult. Clin. Psychol.* **1984**, *52*, 968–976. [CrossRef] [PubMed]
12. Vlieger, A.M.; Menko–Frankenhuis, C.; Wolfkamp, S.C.; Tromp, E.; Benninga, M.A. Hypnotherapy for children with functional abdominal pain or irritable bowel syndrome: A randomized controlled trial. *Gastroenterology* **2007**, *133*, 1430–1436. [CrossRef] [PubMed]
13. Fisher, E.; Heathcote, L.; Palermo, T.M.; de C Williams, A.C.; Lau, J.; Eccleston, C. Systematic review and meta-analysis of psychological therapies for children with chronic pain. *J. Pediatr. Psychol.* **2014**, *39*, 763–782. [CrossRef] [PubMed]
14. Kabat-Zinn, J. *Full catastrophe living: The program of the stress reduction clinic at the University of Massachusetts Medical Center*; Delta: New York, NY, USA, 1990.
15. Cherkin, D.C.; Sherman, K.J.; Balderson, B.H.; Cook, A.J.; Anderson, M.L.; Hawkes, R.J.; Hansen, K.E.; Turner, J.A. Effect of mindfulness-based stress reduction vs cognitive behavioral therapy or usual care on back pain and functional limitations in adults with chronic low back pain: A randomized clinical trial. *JAMA* **2016**, *315*, 1240–1249. [CrossRef] [PubMed]
16. Pielech, M.; Vowles, K.E.; Wicksell, R. Acceptance and Commitment Therapy for Pediatric Chronic Pain: Theory and Application. *Children* **2017**, *4*, 10. [CrossRef] [PubMed]
17. Kabat-Zinn, J.; Lipworth, L.; Burney, R. The clinical use of mindfulness meditation for the self-regulation of chronic pain. *J. Behav. Med.* **1985**, *8*, 163–190. [CrossRef] [PubMed]
18. Jastrowski Mano, K.E.; Salamon, K.S.; Hainsworth, K.R.; Anderson Khan, K.J.; Ladwig, R.J.; Davies, W.H.; Weisman, S.J. A randomized, controlled pilot study of mindfulness-based stress reduction for pediatric chronic pain. *Altern. Ther. Health Med.* **2013**, *19*, 8–14. [PubMed]
19. Ruskin, D.; Kohut, S.A.; Stinson, J. The development of a mindfulness-based stress reduction group for adolescents with chronic pain. *J. Pain Manag.* **2014**, *7*, 301.
20. Chadi, N.; McMahon, A.; Vadnais, M.; Malboeuf-Hurtubise, C.; Djemli, A.; Dobkin, P.L.; Lacroix, J.; Luu, T.M.; Haley, N. Mindfulness-based Intervention for Female Adolescents with Chronic Pain: A Pilot Randomized Trial. *J. Can. Acad. Child Adolesc. Psychiatry* **2016**, *25*, 159. [PubMed]
21. Ali, A.; Weiss, T.R.; Dutton, A.; McKee, D.; Jones, K.D.; Kashikar-Zuck, S.; Silverman, W.K.; Shapiro, E.D. Mindfulness-Based Stress Reduction for Adolescents with Functional Somatic Syndromes: A Pilot Cohort Study. *J. Pediatr.* **2017**, *183*, 184–190. [CrossRef] [PubMed]
22. Waelde, L.C. *Inner Resources for Teens: Treatment Manual and Materials*; Inner Resources Center, Pacific Graduate School of Psychology, Palo Alto University: Palo Alto, CA, USA, 2011.
23. Waelde, L.C. *Inner Resources for Stress: Treatment Manual and Materials*; Inner Resources Center, Pacific Graduate School of Psychology, Palo Alto University: Palo Alto, CA, USA, 2005.
24. Butler, L.D.; Waelde, L.C.; Hastings, T.A.; Chen, X.H.; Symons, B.; Marshall, J.; Kaufman, A.; Nagy, T.F.; Blasey, C.M.; Seibert, E.O.; et al. Meditation with yoga, group therapy with hypnosis, and psychoeducation for long-term depressed mood: A randomized pilot trial. *J. Clin. Psychol.* **2008**, *64*, 806–820. [CrossRef] [PubMed]
25. Waelde, L.C.; Meyer, H.; Thompson, J.T.; Thompson, L.; Gallagher-Thompson, D. Randomized controlled trial of Inner Resources meditation for family dementia caregivers. *J. Clin. Psychol.* **2017**, (in press). [CrossRef] [PubMed]
26. Miró, J.; Castarlenas, E.; Huguet, A. Evidence for the use of a numerical rating scale to assess the intensity of pediatric pain. *Eur. J. Pain* **2009**, *13*, 1089–1095. [CrossRef] [PubMed]
27. Rush, A.J.; Beck, A.T.; Kovacs, M.; Hollon, S. Comparative efficacy of cognitive therapy and pharmacotherapy in the treatment of depressed outpatients. *Cognit. Ther. Res.* **1977**, *1*, 17–37. [CrossRef]
28. Saylor, C.F.; Finch, A.; Spirito, A.; Bennett, B. The Children's Depression Inventory: A systematic evaluation of psychometric properties. *J. Consult. Clin. Psychol.* **1984**, *52*, 955. [CrossRef] [PubMed]

29. Strauss, C.C.; Forehand, R.; Frame, C.; Smith, K. Characteristics of children with extreme scores on the Children's Depression Inventory. *J. Clin. Child Adolesc. Psychol.* **1984**, *13*, 227–231. [CrossRef]
30. Walker, L.S.; Greene, J.W. The functional disability inventory: measuring a neglected dimension of child health status. *J. Pediatr. Psychol.* **1991**, *16*, 39–58. [CrossRef] [PubMed]
31. Claar, R.L.; Walker, L.S. Functional assessment of pediatric pain patients: psychometric properties of the functional disability inventory. *Pain* **2006**, *121*, 77–84. [CrossRef] [PubMed]
32. Cohen, J. *Statistical Power Analysis for the Behavioral Sciences*, 2nd ed.; Lawrence Erlbaum Associates, Inc: Hillsdale, NJ, USA, 1988.
33. Chapman, C.R.; Tuckett, R.P.; Song, C.W. Pain and stress in a systems perspective: reciprocal neural, endocrine, and immune interactions. *J. Pain* **2008**, *9*, 122–145. [CrossRef] [PubMed]
34. Evans, D.R.; Eisenlohr-Moul, T.A.; Button, D.F.; Baer, R.A.; Segerstrom, S.C. Self-regulatory deficits associated with unpracticed mindfulness strategies for coping with acute pain. *J. Appl. Soc. Psychol.* **2014**, *44*, 23–30. [CrossRef] [PubMed]
35. Kingston, J.; Chadwick, P.; Meron, D.; Skinner, T.C. A pilot randomized control trial investigating the effect of mindfulness practice on pain tolerance, psychological well-being, and physiological activity. *J. Psychosom. Res.* **2007**, *62*, 297–300. [CrossRef] [PubMed]
36. Palermo, T.M.; Law, E.F.; Essner, B.; Jessen-Fiddick, T.; Eccleston, C. Adaptation of Problem-Solving Skills Training (PSST) for Parent Caregivers of Youth with Chronic Pain. *Clin. Pract. Pediatr. Psychol.* **2014**, *2*, 212–223. [CrossRef] [PubMed]

9

The Elephant in the Room: The Need for Increased Integrative Therapies in Conventional Medical Settings

Missy Hall [1,*], Susanne M. Bifano [1], Leigh Leibel [2], Linda S. Golding [3] and Shiu-Lin Tsai [4]

1 Child Life Department, NewYork-Presbyterian Morgan Stanley Children's Hospital Columbia University Medical Center, 3959 Broadway, New York, NY 10032, USA; sub9053@nyp.org

2 Division of Hematology/Oncology, Columbia University Medical Center, 161 Ft. Washington Ave, Suite 922, New York, NY 10032-3789, USA; LL3125@cumc.columbia.edu

3 Pastoral Care, NewYork-Presbyterian Milstein Columbia University Medical Center, 622 W. 168th St., New York, NY 10032-3789, USA; lig9048@nyp.org

4 Division of Pediatric Emergency Medicine, Department of Emergency Medicine, Columbia University College of Physicians and Surgeons, 3959 Broadway, CHN-W116, New York, NY 10032; st166@cumc.columbia.edu

* Correspondence: mmh9010@nyp.org

Abstract: Pediatric integrative therapy programs are essential to the treatment and well-being of patients. Identifying an effective integrative therapy model within conventional pediatric medical settings, however, often proves difficult. Our goal in this article is to explore varied solutions to increase access and inclusion of integrative therapies in an effort to promote best practice and holistic care. The main methods applied in this article are vignettes that illustrate how the integrative therapies in a metropolitan academic hospital successfully treat the patient by complementing conventional medicine. This leads to comprehensive care. The central finding of the article proposes viable solutions to increase interdisciplinary collaboration both internally within the institution and externally. Integrative therapists detail how they were able to increase visibility and yield best practice through increased educational initiatives and interdisciplinary collaboration.

Keywords: Integrative therapies; art therapy; music therapy; yoga therapy; acupuncture; pastoral care; creative arts therapy; pediatrics

---

1. Introduction

And so these men of Indostan, disputed loud and long,
each in his own opinion, exceeding stiff and strong,
Though each was partly in the right, and all were in the wrong!

So, oft in theologic wars, the disputants, I ween,
Rail on in utter ignorance, of what each other mean,
And prate about an Elephant
Not one of them has seen!

John Godfried Saxe [1]

The parable of the blind men and the elephant has long illustrated the importance of considering multiple viewpoints in order to see the full picture. The story tells of a group of blind men who are asked to characterize an elephant by touching a different part of its body, such as the tail, the ear, or the trunk. The result is that the elephant is universally mischaracterized because each man makes assumptions based on his partial interaction with the animal. The moral of the parable is that in order to attain a comprehensive version of the truth, we must first acknowledge our limitations and seek out other perspectives.

This parable mirrors conventional healthcare. Current medical practice routinely emphasizes treating the "diagnosis" at the expense of the patient. Doing so results in clinical "blindness" that inhibits best practice and limits comprehensive care.

For this reason, conventional medicine is increasingly trending toward interdisciplinary practice [2–4]. This practice acknowledges the patient and the person thereby targeting and treating the whole system.

One way to increase interdisciplinary practice is to promote integrative health care. This involves combining standard medical treatment with mind-body practices. This holistic approach to health care includes treating all parts of the patient, including the "mental, emotional, functional, spiritual, social and community aspects" [5].

Mind and body practices are centered around the patient-practitioner relationship and incorporate all available evidence-based therapies to treat the patient [6]. Acupuncturists, yoga therapists, and creative arts therapists engage in non-traditional mind-body practices that fall under this umbrella. Yoga therapists and creative arts therapists are mental health clinicians trained in psychotherapy and the psychology of their modality (yoga, art, music, dance, and poetry).

At NewYork-Presbyterian Morgan Stanley Children's Hospital, Columbia University Medical Center, mind-body therapies serve a variety of diverse populations. In an effort to advance integrative health care within this major metropolitan academic institution, these writers embarked upon several hospital-wide initiatives to educate the medical community on evidence-based mind-body interventions. To change culture, they organized a full day conference entitled Creative Arts Therapies Conversations in Healthcare and Therapeutic Transformations (CAT CHATTs): "*What Does Health Look Like in Healthcare Today? Sustaining Identity as an Integrative Therapist in Medicine*". They invited art, music, dance-movement and yoga therapists, chaplains, physicians, social workers, nurses, psychiatrists, and acupuncturists from major academic institutions to present and discuss numerous ways integrative therapists yield best practice, mitigate effects of invasive procedures, treat physical and emotional pain, and increase communication among staff and with family members for responsible care. This event was supported by NewYork-Presbyterian Morgan Stanley Children's Hospital (NYP MSCH) and attended by approximately 100 professionals representing all levels of health care providers across New York State. Feedback from evaluations was overwhelmingly favorable and highlighted the need to make integrative healthcare a universal practice in conventional medical settings.

The following are vignettes from five different integrative clinicians at our urban teaching hospital. They serve to illustrate how integrative therapies are effective and evidence-based disciplines that when used in conjunction with standard medical treatment can promote best practice. All patients' names and identifiers have been changed or replaced with initials to maintain anonymity and privacy.

2. Acupuncture in the Pediatric Emergency Department

"Doc, need you in room 23 stat! We have an eight-year-old boy with paraphimosis since last night and clinic just sent him to us for reduction!" It's now 1:30 p.m. and the foreskin has been in the retracted position since CJ showered last night over 15 h ago. CJ appeared anxious and tearful due to pain from a swollen and red foreskin. After placing him in a Trendelenburg position, topical 2% Lidocaine and D50W plus ice were placed on the area to decrease pain and swelling. Next, intranasal Fentanyl was administered for pain and a child life specialist was at the bedside, providing breathing coaching and an iPad for distraction. The first attempt to release the foreskin was met with such pain and crying that the procedure was aborted. Urology was in the operating room, unavailable to assist. Should I give CJ another dose of opioids? Inject local anesthetics, but risk causing further swelling and emotional trauma? In this case, I offered the family auricular acupuncture to decrease CJ's pain and anxiety.

Oftentimes, children who are in pain or waiting to undergo a painful procedure are already afraid and anxious. In order to break this tension and dispel their trepidation of acupuncture, I would often jokingly say, "The acupuncture needle is the biggest one in our whole emergency room"! and then dramatically pull out a tiny needle as everyone laughs. To introduce acupuncture to CJ and his family, I first showed them how filamentous the acupuncture needle is by bending it along my finger. Next, I mimicked the pin prick needle sensation by gently pinching the dorsum of his hand while saying, "You might feel the acupuncture needle like a little pinch". This process helped to put CJ and his family more at ease and they agreed to give acupuncture a try. To further empower CJ at this time when he may feel especially vulnerable, I said, "Let me know if the needle bothers you. We can stop anytime you like". Using the Battlefield auricular acupuncture protocol [7], CJ calmly allowed me to place five needles in his right auricle. Within minutes we were able to perform a second attempt and successfully reduced the paraphimosis manually, thus avoiding surgery. CJ, his parents, and our emergency medical team were all very happy with the outcome.

This case demonstrates how a child benefited from a collaborative effort using standard pain medications and other non-pharmacologic therapies, including breathing techniques, distraction with iPad, and acupuncture. This multimodal, integrated approach resulted in a successful outcome-something no single therapy could have accomplished.

Acupuncture has been used in China for thousands of years to treat pain [8] and is recognized by the National Institutes of Health as a safe and effective therapy for pain [9]. The mechanisms for acupuncture analgesia have been extensively studied and include the involvement of the autonomic nervous system, endogenous endorphin release, brain region modulation, connective tissue and local needling effects [10–13]. While many caretakers have heard of acupuncture, most have never heard of its use in pediatrics and are pleasantly surprised when acupuncture is offered in the Pediatric Emergency Department (PED).

Acupuncture is often offered to pediatric patients undergoing radiation and chemotherapy on the Hematology-Oncology service at NYP MSCH because it mitigates symptoms, including nausea, vomiting, pain, and anxiety [14–16]. For children with sickle cell pain crisis who present to the MSCH PED, acupuncture is sometimes used in conjunction with standard pharmaceuticals to help decrease pain and anxiety [17], and the amount of opioids needed.

Nursing and physician colleagues in the PED have witnessed first-hand the positive result of acupuncture. For this reason they frequently refer patients for acupuncture when standard of care, including pharmaceuticals, fails to achieve sufficient pain relief. In a study conducted at NYP MSCH PED, patients were treated with acupuncture for diverse painful conditions, including headaches, otitis externa, torticollis, constipation, dysmenorrhea, and knee and ankle sprains. Acupuncture was well accepted, with 96% of patients and families reporting satisfaction with acupuncture and 52% achieving complete pain resolution. Unlike pharmaceuticals, acupuncture offers the additional advantage of low adverse side effects, and avoids medication interactions. Given our nation's opioid crisis, the integrative practices at NYP MSCH PED conform to the recommendations from the Centers for Disease Control and Prevention and the U.S Food and Drug Administration that nonpharmacologic therapies, including acupuncture, be offered to treat patients with pain [18,19].

It is gratifying to be able to relieve a patient's pain and suffering; to see a child's face change from a grimace to a smile. The practice of acupuncture has afforded me opportunities to show families and colleagues that medication alone is not always the solution, nor is it the only answer. With growing evidence on its efficacy and high safety profile, acupuncture may one day become an invaluable staple in our therapeutic armament to help treat pain in pediatrics.

3. Pastoral Care as an Integrating Practice

Ravi is a two-and-a-half-year-old boy with a hyphenated Jewish and Italian last name. He has been on the Neurology Unit for one month with seizures. Ravi's skin is very dark in contrast to everyone else in the room who has very white skin. Ravi is stiff, his limbs are at odd angles, his head is fixed, and he is silent except for occasional moans. Mom and Dad tell me they adopted Ravi after many in vitro attempts and know there is epilepsy in his African-American family of origin. They adore him and Mom talks about how articulate and talented he is. In terms of religious affiliation, Mom is of Jewish heritage and non-practicing. Dad was raised Catholic, but non-practicing, and has for some time sought spiritual expression in Buddhism.

As a chaplain, I am attuned to the different languages and styles people use to describe their values, the ways in which they cope, or do not. I am curious about how this couple navigates their different spiritual languages. These parents are at their wits' end and I feel like they are leaking out of the boundaries of their bodies. I am a witness to the leaks; and I am a bucket to catch and hold them. Perhaps the collection will be helpful for later reflection for Mom and Dad, but for now I am a bucket brigade with big ears. Over the course of an hour, Mom unfurls a rage aria; they hate the hospital and everyone in it and are furious at how long it is taking for a diagnosis. Next, she laments, revealing she is terrified that their boy will never be their boy again. She cannot bear considering this loss and she declares herself "desperate" for anything that will help, "even Jewish prayer". We both smile at "even Jewish prayer" as she tells me she never learned much about her Jewish heritage and is not sure what it might offer. I hear her curiosity expressed in the face of her desperation as a desire to connect to something, to claim something that is both a birth right and a tribal right, perhaps as intense as her desire to be a mother. I feel her words of anger and sorrow pierce my own body and consider the options. How to craft a communication from the depths of her soul to . . . God? She wants to regain her equanimity, but feels she cannot if she is going to continue to advocate effectively for Ravi. A prayer for healing, but for whom? I center the prayer on text written by a 19th century Moroccan rabbi because his origins are as far-flung as the circumstances. Dad is restrained, but cries when we pray in Hebrew and English around Ravi.

Board certified hospital chaplains are responsible for assessing and supporting the emotional, religious, and/or spiritual needs of patients, families, and staff. In addition to supporting these needs, we are trained to listen and to help people access, re-access, or even develop new coping resources regardless of religious or spiritual affiliations. Chaplains help people remember who they are when they are not in the hospital. The conversations can be confessional, investigative, witnessing, and always confidential unless there is potential harm to self or others. Formal research in evidence-based chaplaincy is still in its infancy, however, existing research points to the power of narrative [20] and the value of pastoral care interventions focused on supporting the spiritual needs of primary caregivers of children with life-limiting illnesses [21].

Some weeks later, Ravi has suffered a brain hemorrhage and cardiac arrest, and is in the ICU. He is sedated on a ventilator, his cognitive condition unknown. Over the weeks, Mom and Dad's spiritual engagement has consisted of meditation with a Buddhist chaplain and a perfunctory wave to the ICU chaplain. When I see them, their eyes are blank and their vitality is sapped. While Ravi has been steadily losing his muscle tone, his parents have begun to lose their person tone. They have so profoundly passed beyond the boundaries of their bodies that they have quietly imploded, and the outlines of who they are in the world as employees, co-workers, friends, and parents are slowly being erased. They tell me they are using meditation to have a moment to "shut down" their thinking and seek a moment of refuge "to not feel". They are no longer seeking refuge in spiritual resources because they see no purpose. Ravi has become a stranger to them, and they to themselves. They appear as shadows.

Pastoral care in the hospital setting is about identity recalibration. The chaplain looks for the shards of a shattered identity and the ways in which to help reunite them. The intention is to pause the chaos and co-create with the patient, or family, or staff a pathway through the obstacles to find and reclaim a sense of self.

In Ravi's case, however, there is no clear pathway to reunion, nor definitive resolution. The tragedy of this story is multi-layered. I cannot fix the situation. Instead, I listen to the loss and reflect back the confusion. I hold the myriad of desperate emotions flying around the room and help them to integrate this part of their life story while rebuilding their person tone through reflection of the unwanted emotions they are fiercely trying to shed. I intervene in the moment as each conversation unfolds and I can only hope that my practice in some way helps them to begin to find meaning in the shadows.

4. Art Therapy and the Practice of Mirroring Medical Trauma

"Ewww, Alan's toilet has that thing hanging there with his urine in it, that's gross". Alan's older brother was referring to the urinal. Alan is a tiny 10-year-old boy who speaks in a small inaudible voice, occupying little space in his room, contrary to his older brother and sister. His mother, nervous in nature, and his father, calm yet distant, routinely accompany him to the clinic where he receives treatments for his astrocytoma.

I was consulted to assess for and provide art therapy services throughout Alan's long and arduous treatment course. Initially he presented with flat affect, withholding of feelings and what appeared to be an absorption of his mother's anxiety that was present during every medical encounter.

The creative process of art making mirrors life itself. Both process and product serve as a bridge from an individual's inner world to the outside. Art therapists actively look and listen for imagery, symbols and metaphors, and use them to help explore pre-conscious content with patients. The process of exploring art media, creating and talking about the art offers patients increased opportunities to find more compatible relationships to potentially overwhelming thoughts and feelings [22,23].

Hospitalized children may not have the words to express what they are thinking or feeling, or these words may not do their experience justice. Art, then, serves as a translator to communicate internalized emotions to the important people in the room. Images offer children opportunities to externalize their content safely while the art therapist helps them find personal meaning in their work [24]. Finding meaning, in turn helps to alleviate feelings of anxiety, depression and pain that often accompany children with chronic illnesses [25–27].

Alan reported that his G-tube feedings resulted in "excruciating" pain, the primary symptom which led to his current hospitalization. In our first art therapy session, Alan approached the art making inauspiciously, carefully and with unwavering focus. He chose art materials with intention, requesting to work with non-traditional media, and repurposing mundane objects that he altered into a three-dimensional environment.

Typically, children select paints, pastels or clay to form their visual expressions. Alan used a paint brush container as the central sculptural component in his artwork where he used string to attach plastic aquatic figurines from the top allowing them to dangle inside. In art therapy, these two attributes of using non-traditional materials and repurposing objects (e.g., the process of transforming ordinary objects to significantly alter their appearance or use) indicate flexibility, creative problem solving and adaptability.

"That's not an art material Alan, choose something that is in her [my] basket". His mother's reprimands appeared to imply that Alan's behavior was impolite or defying the rules- in contrast to what I assessed to be a series of creative and resilient solutions. I wondered if this was a mother's instinct to protect her child and find control in this desperate situation.

Adhering a plastic transparent circular container (paint brush cleaner) to the center of a green painted circular cardboard base, Alan began to redefine and transform the objects.

Midway through the session, the oncology attending physician humbly entered the room. Alan's mother stood up to meet him at the foot of the bed, his words stacking like bricks in her arms as he delivered the unresolved news about Alan's G-tube infection. Upon his exit, Alan's mother and father murmured their discouragement and concern for Alan's unexplainable pain.

Shortly after this, the surgical team arrived. "Looks like fun", a resident commented to Alan about his art. Alan gave no response. Surrounded by the team, his infected G-tube site was examined. I transitioned to the back of the room to be with his siblings who were observing from a distance. "Ewwwww", exclaimed his sister, "I just saw Alan's feeding tube site, gross".

Alan remained quiet, frozen and naked.

As the team discussed their impressions with the parents, Alan continued with his art, selecting a variety of jungle animal figurines and gluing more than twenty tigers, elephants, giraffes and hippos around the perimeter of the circular base, encircling the large ominous container in the center.

"That's too many animals, save some for the other children", prompted Alan's mother once again. Alan's expressive non-verbal voice is scolded, minimized and criticized as if to say, 'Don't take up that much space, stop taking from others and use unforbidden objects. Stay quiet and unseen.'

Unexpectedly, Alan's roar pierced the room bringing everyone to a halt. "STOP!" He yelled in response to his brother's persistent attempt to look at his feeding tube site. "Why can't I see it?" he whined. He silenced the pervasive buzz in the room, "Because I don't trust you!"

"Whom do you trust?" I asked.

His mother and father stood frozen, holding their son's eyes with their own. Tears poured down Alan's cheeks, "I'm scared". His parents, like bookends, stood on alternate sides of him. "There's a hole in my side". Alan's fear, resounding and exposed, was now unavoidable.

Alan's art- a depiction of animals surrounding the 'watering hole'- communicated 'observation', 'vigilance' and 'feeding', all of which were prominent themes from his medical experience. In this moment he was surrounded by teams peering at his feeding tube, his family verbally and visually poking at an area which was the very hole that fed and sustained him. Throughout his exam he exhibited a hypervigilance to incoming danger (i.e., the medical team and his feeds). The container that water is poured into is the focal point in his art piece and a reflection of his own body. Occupying all dimensions of space, the animals' small stillness reflects the vulnerable unknown. The myriad of feelings elicited from the imagery mirror different aspects of Alan and his experience during this pre-surgical exam and a visit from his physician. Alan's voicelessness in his treatment was finally unleashed in this compelling moment, providing him an uncensored expression of his fears. Had the surgical team been in the room when Alan was able to clearly verbalize his fears, it's possible that the team may have listened and responded differently throughout the exam. And alternatively, the response, "Looks like fun" to Alan's 'watering hole' sculpture would not minimize his expression but rather validate it with "Looks like you have a lot to say".

As an art psychotherapist, I enter into symbolic and metaphoric language to meet the child in his/her inner world. It is humbling to be invited into this space and experience his/her story through imagery and expressive language. The presence of disease in the body can be without symptoms. So too, meaningful messages can exist in a child, and like that of disease, the meaning can be unknown until it is ready to be revealed. In the case of Alan, the unknown became a shared space for Alan, his illness, his art, and me.

5. Music Therapy and Interdisciplinary Co-treatments to Creatively Address Complex Medical Needs

"We can beat the bad man, make him go away, if we sing loud enough...All the way up to GOD!" Josiah was a typically developing vivacious seven-year-old boy with a history of prolonged hospitalization and chronic illness awaiting heart transplant. During the first month of his admission, Josiah appeared to exhibit increased signs of anxiety and regression so the interdisciplinary team asked me to assess him for music therapy services. Music therapy as defined by the American Music Therapy Association is "the clinical and evidence-based use of music interventions to accomplish individualized goals within a therapeutic relationship" [28].

In our first session, I quickly established rapport with Josiah through active music making and musical improvisation (e.g., playing extemporized musical rhythms, tempos, dynamics, and melodies composed in the moment without previous preparation on varied rhythmic and harmonic instruments, including drums, guitar, xylophones, and shakers). His initial improvisations presented as playful, melodic, and heavily percussive displaying steady, organized rhythms and lively tempos. His final musical improvisation, however, changed significantly. It became increasingly chaotic, displayed sharp contrasting rhythms in a disorganized pattern and was punctuated by strong accentuated beats. Mid-way into this improvisation Josiah stopped abruptly and pointed directly to a Halloween face mask adjacent to him on the bed. He placed his finger over his mouth and with wide-eyed affect whispered, "we need to be very quiet... so we don't wake the bad man". He then proceeded to sing softly in an effort to avoid being captured by this "bad man" monster who wanted to "silence" his music.

As a music psychotherapist, I use my modality to help patients explore, express, and discover their internal worlds by inviting ongoing musical and verbal dialogues between their conscious and unconscious selves [29]. During our first session, I assessed that Josiah's impromptu musical dialogue between his conscious self and a fictional "bad man" monster may have been prompted by a need to safely and creatively explore, express, and process difficult thoughts and feelings surrounding his chronic illness, prolonged hospitalization, isolation, and family separation. What was most interesting to me during our first encounter was that in calling out to a higher power at the conclusion of the session, Josiah appeared to achieve some kind of resolution. By singing "loudly, all the way up to God" he had triumphantly silenced the "bad man", holding him captive. Essentially, Josiah had discovered comfort, personal strength, power, and self-agency by engaging in musical prayer.

Pre-transplant, my clinical work with Josiah was predominantly psychodynamic in that I continued to invite him to engage in musical dialogues between his conscious and unconscious selves. In these ongoing dialogues, he explored a variety of recurring themes in the music, including 'silence/sound', 'dominance/submission', 'danger/safety', 'fear/courage', 'separation/reunion', 'helplessness/empowerment', and 'salvation'.

Mid-way through his admission, Josiah was successfully transplanted, however, postoperative complications led to a cardiac arrest that resulted in anoxic brain injury and substantial decompensation. Following this event, the family was in crisis and the team reported uncertainty as to Josiah's neurological outcome.

For me, the shift was just as dramatic. In many ways, Josiah's musical journey paralleled his cardiac journey; his music had stopped abruptly, unexpectedly, and without warning, leaving in its wake a painfully uncomfortable silence. Clinical music therapists are trained to create space in the music for our patients because rests are just as important as the notes. But how could I begin to honor Josiah's notes when his voice as I knew it had been silenced?

As a result of this experience, my clinical practice evolved to become more flexible, innovative, and creative. I began by increasing communication with team members to help identify common goals and innovative solutions aimed at addressing a variety of barriers to care. Josiah displayed extreme spasticity in his lower extremities, which created limited mobility, and he had difficulty maintaining autonomic stability. This was most evident during physical and occupational therapy sessions when he often became tachycardic and tachypneic. In these sessions, he also displayed visible and audible signs of distress and emotional dysregulation, including moaning, crying, contracted limbs, and a constricted, tearful affect.

In response to these barriers, I worked closely with the team to design individualized music therapy co-treatments. To encourage homeostasis during rehabilitation therapy sessions, I played improvised harmonies on the guitar, which emphasized regular, steady rhythms and slow tempos while singing improvised melodies with prolonged phrases or musical meter. This intervention known as *rhythmic entrainment* (a term used to describe the temporal locking process phenomenon in which two or more independent rhythmic processes synchronize with each other) [30] helped to stabilize Josiah's heart rate and respiration throughout sessions. Entrainment also proved a useful assessment tool for the team. The occupational therapist reported that she was able to more accurately assess his neurological capacity as a result of the musical accompaniment I provided that both activated and relaxed Josiah throughout our session. Because Josiah entrained easily to live music, the speech and language pathologist informed me that live music helped keep Josiah calm, which enabled her to successfully complete a visual, audial, and cognitive assessment to determine his altered baseline.

In physical therapy sessions, I used a sound and vibration intervention known as *vibroacoustic therapy* [31,32] to minimize pain and increase his limited range of motion. By placing a bass tuned buffalo drum near Josiah's lower extremities I was able to reduce his hypertonicity and spasticity [33]. Suddenly, the physical therapist was able to increase the passive range of motion and encourage active range of motion when Josiah was able to successfully reach for, grasp, hold, and shake a small bell in time to the music. As a result of increased integrative practice that targeted and treated both psychosocial and physiological symptoms of distress, Josiah's autonomic stability and emotional regulation slowly improved over time.

A final collaboration with pastoral care led to a co-treatment that provided Josiah's family the opportunity to give voice to overwhelming feelings of fear and anxiety. I played simple chord intervals (e.g., two sounds differing in pitch) on the guitar and sang an improvised melody to create a musical environment that was secure, contained, and predictable while the chaplain led the family in prayer. This technique known as *vocal holding* consists of the intentional use of playing two alternating chords on a harmonic instrument in combination with improvised singing in order to create a consistent and stable environment [34]. Initially, Josiah's mother expressed doubt and confusion surrounding the event, "Why would God let this happen?" Throughout the music her demeanor shifted. Toward the end of the session she presented as calm and hopeful, reporting, "I can't be upset at God . . . God has a plan. Even though it's bad, and it's dark ...We going to get through this. God's going to pull us through." In a way we had come full circle; once again, Josiah and his family were seeking comfort, empowerment, and strength in musical prayer.

At this point in the session, Josiah, who had been sleeping in a bed adjacent to our prayer circle, opened his eyes and his mother moved bedside to take his hand. Softly, she began to sing his favorite song, "Oh, the itsy, bitsy spider, went up the water spout..." I quietly fingered chords on my guitar to accompany her as she continued to sing, "Down came the rain, and washed the spider out..." Slowly, family members gathered around the bed holding hands, encircling Josiah as he held her gaze. "Out came the sun, and dried up all the rain..." Josiah opened his mouth slowly, hesitantly groping as his mother sang the last line, "and the itsy, bitsy spider went up the spout ah . . . " Josiah completed the song, penetrating the silence with his voice at last, "...gin".

My favorite thing about music therapy is that it is inherently collaborative. Unlike conversation, music happens concurrently offering participants an "I" and "Thou" [35] experience through "We" engagement [36]. 'We' engagement, however, can sometimes limit opportunities to unite 'us' in clinical practice. By expanding our practice to include multiple voices, we participate in a richer, more dynamic symphony. Ultimately, an integrated practice promotes true harmony in healthcare.

6. Yoga Therapy and Meditation: An Integrative Partnership with Patients and Families

The chemotherapy charge nurse texted, "Please come to the Infusion Center to meet a new patient who wants to talk to you about yoga therapy and meditation during her cancer treatment".

The patient, Stacey, had recently celebrated her 18th birthday. Soon after, she had felt a lump near her right armpit. The staggering diagnosis of stage IV breast cancer with metastases to the liver and spine literally took her breath away. Today was the first of an anticipated 180-day chemotherapy treatment plan to be delivered once every three weeks.

As I approached the infusion area, I paused to center myself so I could be fully present with Stacey—allowing her to be heard, to be seen; holding her in compassionate, loving space. Elizabeth Kubler-Ross said, "Telling your story often and in detail is primal to the grieving process. You must get it out. Grief must be witnessed to be healed [37] (p. 63)".

I washed my hands, focusing on my own breath: "Take three deep belly breaths, relax into the exhalation, allow your awareness to rest on the present moment". I continued to practice this deep breathing, and soon Stacey mirrored the gentle rise and fall of my abdomen. Her breathing slowed as I guided her through a 15-min meditation. She said she felt calmer and I saw on the monitor her systolic blood pressure had dropped 15 points. I showed her various breathing techniques to practice at home and during treatments to help manage anxiety and discomfort, and we began to create a plan for a daily meditation practice that was based on her personal preferences.

As a Yoga Therapist in Integrative Oncology, I work closely with Psycho-Oncology and Palliative Care. The cornerstone of our team's integrative approach is to partner with patients and families, providing attentive, empathic clinical care to address the needs of mind, body, and spirit. I was the first of our team to meet Stacey and immediately suggested she consult our Psychologist and Palliative Nurse Practitioner for help managing anxiety and prospective chemotherapy induced peripheral neuropathy. During her half-year of treatment, our team met regularly to discuss her case, and I supported my colleagues' behavioral and pharmaceutical interventions by customizing weekly sessions of conscious breathing, meditation, and mindful movement to address her evolving physical and emotional needs.

Mind-body interventions are important self-regulation practices that support psychosocial therapies by fostering general mental well-being, calmness, clarity, and concentration [38–40]. They promote sleep, and can ease anxiety and depression [41,42]. Mindfulness meditation, in particular, helps manage anxiety and improve quality of life [43]. It also helps patients reframe their relationship with pain by teaching them to rest in the present moment and observe sensations and thoughts without judgment. Jon Kabat-Zinn, the founder of Mindfulness Based Stress Reduction (MBSR), wrote, "It's possible to befriend your pain or your fear...rather than feeling that you can't get anywhere until this thing that bothers you is cut out or walled off or shut down" [44].

There is substantial evidence to support the efficacy of mind-body therapies in the outpatient clinical setting. At its June 2018 annual conference, the American Society of Clinical Oncology (ASCO) endorsed yoga and meditation as adjuvant therapy during conventional breast cancer treatment and survivorship to mitigate the sequelae of acute and late treatment side effects, including anxiety, mood disorder, depression, and to improve quality of life [45].

At the end of her treatment Stacey was declared with *no evidence of disease* and told us that our integrative care had "saved her life" by teaching her how to manage her fear and anxiety, and to help her keep physically active during her difficult treatment. In her mother's words, "Stacey's medical oncologists may have eradicated the disease and put her in remission, but her integrative support team gave her back a life worth living".

It is imperative that we, as integrative therapists, spearhead the effort to create a paradigm shift in the way our healthcare system treats our patients and their loved ones. Mind-body therapies are evidence-based, drug free, cost effective, and available to everyone regardless of cultural background and socioeconomic status. Let us listen closely to our patients and their families, see the elephant in its entirety, and commit to treating the individual, not the disease.

7. Results: Barriers to Integrative Therapy Practice

The above vignettes clearly illustrate how integrative therapies address the mental, emotional, functional, spiritual, social, and community domains of the patient, thereby improving the overall patient experience while supporting standard medical treatment outcomes. Despite the overwhelming evidence that points to the effectiveness of integrative healthcare, these writers encountered areas for further consideration.

7.1. Funding

Currently, in conventional medical settings, integrative therapy positions are funded in a variety of ways. While many creative arts therapy positions are typically donor funded, at this institution, art and music therapy and pastoral care positions are billed to the cost of room and board. Yoga therapy is funded by a private donor, and acupuncture services in the pediatric emergency department are currently not separately reimbursed. It remains clear that additional cost analysis research is needed to find sustainable solutions to increased integrative programming.

7.2. Misses in Appropriation, Placement, Classification, and Understanding

7.2.1. Misappropriation

In conventional medical settings, mind-body practices are often misplaced, misunderstood, and misclassified. This leads to a misappropriation of services, impaired practice and, ultimately, identity confusion regarding the role integrative therapists play within the treatment team. For this reason, clarifying the scope of practice and managing staff and family expectations is paramount.

7.2.2. Misplacement/Misclassification

Misplacement of integrative therapists creates confusion within the interdisciplinary team. Therapists are difficult to locate, often possessing job titles or embedded in departments unrelated to their discipline. For example, a pain specialist may have a hard time locating a mind-body therapist when he/she is identified on his/her identification badge as a recreational therapist and managed by a child life department.

7.2.3. Misunderstanding

Integrative therapists are trained to facilitate and process the expression of anxiety and fear that accompany medical encounters that are interwoven with pain symptomatology [46–49]. Not all healthcare providers understand the concrete benefits of mind-body interventions and may minimize the complementary benefits integrative therapies can provide. A better understanding of mind-body practices is necessary in order to achieve appropriate integration and promote a more holistic approach to care.

8. Discussion: Recommendations for Future Practice

Despite the aforementioned barriers, these writers were able to identify a number of innovative solutions to minimize siloed practice and help break down existing barriers. Through workshops, targeted in-services, interdisciplinary rounding, co-treatments, lectures, grand rounds, and hospital-wide educational forums, including conferences and workshops, medical professionals are provided with opportunities to learn and experience firsthand the benefits of integrative therapies, including art, music, yoga, pastoral care, and acupuncture.

Innovative Solutions to Promote Increased Integrative Practice

The advancement of integrative health care in a major academic hospital takes time and strategy to promote complementary practice. Below are suggested actions steps to help increase visibility, awareness, and accessibility to integrative services. The recommendations listed are from these writers' personal accounts and experiences of successful implementation of hospital-wide programs and initiatives.

- Create a customized website with a dedicated email address to promote understanding and classification of integrative therapies.
- Design and distribute educational brochures and marketing materials to staff detailing services and appropriate referral criteria.
- Facilitate weekly in-services for interdisciplinary staff, fellows, residents, medical students, and physicians that lead to better integration of mind-body services in treatment plans. This

practice also generates potential funding for additional positions, including expanding services to outpatient or satellite clinics.

- Obtain funding through grant support from established national organizations, such as the American Academy of Pediatrics, Virginia Apgar Academy, American Art Therapy Association, private donors, and foundations to support educational workshops and research.
- Conduct workshops, lectures, and grand rounds for nurses, students, residents, and faculty members, thereby gaining more acceptance and understanding from providers across the hospital on integrative therapists' role in medicine.
- Publish and present locally, nationally, and internationally on integrative therapy research and practices.
- Create an integrative rotation elective as part of residency training to educate and promote utilization of complementary practices located throughout the hospital.
- Involve integrative therapy students in the creation and co-facilitation of expressive therapy pilot programs for outpatient clinics, which increases complementary services to more patients and families in need.

9. Conclusions

A cultural shift in this conventional medical setting is growing as a result of increased visibility, education, understanding, and collaboration, but the need for increased integration of mind-body practices still remains. Barriers to true integrative health care include limited funding, misappropriation of services, misclassification, misunderstanding, and continued siloed practice. To affect global change, it is incumbent for all mind-body clinicians in conventional medical settings to join this cultural revolution. This publication is just the first step. A restructuring of conventional medical frameworks is necessary in order to see and treat the whole patient. From revolutionary paradigm shifts and innovative practices to eradicating siloed services, integrative, complementary "wholistic" health is the future.

Organizations that begin to successfully integrate humanistic medicine with evidence-based mind-body practices empower patients to become active partners in their treatment. Such integrative practice reduces harm, sustains ethical and legal professional standards, gives purposeful direction to therapeutic interventions, and enhances the efficacy of conventional treatment plans. It is the future of good medicine. This is the elephant that we can all see and heal.

Author Contributions: Conceptualization, M.H. and S.M.B.; Methodology, M.H. and S.M.B.; Writing—Original Draft Preparation, M.H., S.M.B., L.L., L.S.G. and S.-L.T.; Writing—Review & Editing, M.H., S.M.B., and L.L.; Visualization, M.H. and S.M.B.; Supervision, S.-L.T.; Project Administration, M.H. and S.M.B.

References

1. Saxe, J.G. *The Poems of John Godfrey Saxe*; University of Michigan: Ann Arbor, MI, USA, 2009.
2. Wen, J.; Shulman, K. Can team-based care improve patient satisfaction? A systematic review of randomized controlled trials. *PLoS ONE* **2014**, *9*, 7. [CrossRef] [PubMed]
3. Mitchell, P.; Matthew, W.; Golden, R.; McNellis, B.; Okun, S.; Webb, C.E.; Rohrbach, V.; Von Kohorn, I. Core Principles and Values of Effective Team-Based Health Care. Available online: https://nam.edu/wp-content/uploads/2015/06/VSRT-Team-Based-Care-Principles-Values.pdf (accessed on 9 November 2018).
4. Nolte, J. Enhancing Interdisciplinary Collaboration in Primary Healthcare in Canada. Available online: http://tools.hhrrhs.ca/index.php?option=com_mtree&task=att_download&link_id=5305&cf_id=68&lang=e (accessed on 9 November 2018).
5. National Center for Complementary and Integrative Health. Available online: https://nccih.nih.gov/health/integrative-health#integrative (accessed on 12 May 2018).

6. National Center for Complementary and Integrative Health. Available online: https://nccih.nih.gov/health/mindbody (accessed on 12 May 2018).
7. Tsai, S.-L.; Reynoso, E.; Shin, D.W.; Tsung, J. Acupuncture as a nonpharmacologic treatment for pain in a pediatric emergency department. *Pediatr. Emerg. Care* **2018**. under review. [CrossRef] [PubMed]
8. Deng, L. *Chinese Acupuncture and Moxibustion*, 3rd ed.; Foreign Languages Press: Beijing, China, 2010.
9. NIH Consensus Conference. Acupuncture. *JAMA* **1998**, *280*, 1518–1524. [CrossRef]
10. Han, J.S. Acupuncture and endorphins. *Neurosci. Lett.* **2004**, *361*, 258–261. [CrossRef] [PubMed]
11. Maeda, Y.; Kim, H.; Kettner, N.; Kim, J.; Cina, S.; Malatesta, C.; Gerber, J.; McManus, C.; Ong-Sutherland, R.; Libby, A.; et al. Rewiring the primary somatosensory cortex in carpal tunnel syndrome with acupuncture. *Brain* **2017**, *140*, 914–927. [CrossRef] [PubMed]
12. Langevin, H.M.; Bouffard, N.A.; Badger, G.J.; Churchill, D.L.; Howe, A.K. Subcutaneous tissue fibroblast cytoskeletal remodeling induced by acupuncture: Evidence for a mechanotransduction-based mechanism. *J. Cell. Physiol.* **2006**, *207*, 767–774. [CrossRef] [PubMed]
13. Li, Q.Q.; Shi, G.X.; Xu, Q.; Wang, J.; Liu, C.Z.; Wang, L.P. Acupuncture effect and central autonomic regulation. *Evid. Based Complement. Altern. Med.* **2013**, *2013*, 267959. [CrossRef] [PubMed]
14. Reindl, T.; Geilen, W.; Hartmann, R.; Wiebelitz, K.R.; Kan, G.; Wilhelm, I.; Lugauer, S.; Behrens, C.; Weiberlenn, T.; Gottschling, S.; et al. Acupuncture against chemotherapy-induced nausea and vomiting in pediatric oncology. Interim results of a multicenter crossover study. *Support Care Cancer* **2006**, *14*, 172–176. [CrossRef] [PubMed]
15. Dundee, J.W.; Ghaly, R.G.; Fitzpatrick, K.T.; Abram, W.P.; Lynch, G.A. Acupuncture prophylaxis of cancer chemotherapy-induced sickness. *J. R. Soc. Med.* **1989**, *82*, 268–271. [CrossRef] [PubMed]
16. Ezzo, J.M.; Richardson, M.A.; Vickers, A.; Allen, C.; Dibble, S.L.; Issell, B.F.; Lao, L.; Pearl, M.; Ramirez, G.; Shen, J.; et al. Acupuncture-point stimulation for chemotherapy-induced nausea or vomiting. *Cochrane Database Syst. Rev.* **2006**, CD002285. [CrossRef]
17. Tsai, S.L.; McDaniel, D.; Taromina, K.; Lee, M.T. Acupuncture for Sickle Cell Pain Management in a Pediatric Emergency Department, Hematology Clinic, and Inpatient Unit. *Med. Acupunct.* **2015**, *27*, 510–514. [CrossRef]
18. CDC Guideline for Prescribing Opioids for Chronic Pain—United States, 2016 [press release]. MMWR Recomm Rep; 2016. Available online: https://www.cdc.gov/mmwr/volumes/65/rr/rr6501e1.htm (accessed on 9 November 2018).
19. FDA. *Education Blueprint for Health Care Providers Involved in the Management or Support of Patients with Pain (May 2017)*; FDA: Silver Spring, MD, USA, 2017.
20. Charon, R. What to Do with Stories: The Sciences of Narrative Medicine. *Can. Fam. Phys.* **2007**, *53*, 1265–1267.
21. Kelly, J.A.; May, C.S.; Maurer, S. Assessment of the Spiritual Needs of Primary Caregivers of Children with Life-Limiting Illnesses Is Valuable Yet Inconsistently Performed in the Hospital. *J. Palliat. Med.* **2016**, *19*, 763–766. [CrossRef] [PubMed]
22. McNutt, J. Art therapy as a form of visual narrative in oncology care. In *Art Therapy and Healthcare*; Malchiodi, C.A., Ed.; Guilford Press: New York, NY, USA, 2012; pp. 127–135.
23. Favara-Scacco, C. Art therapy as perseus' shield for children with cancer. In *Art Therapy and Cancer Care*; Waller, D., Sibbett, C., Eds.; Open University Press: Berkshire, UK, 2005; pp. 119–127.
24. Council, T. Medical art therapy with children. In *Handbook of Art Therapy*, 2nd ed.; Malchiodi, C.A., Ed.; Guilford Publications: New York, NY, USA, 2012; pp. 222–240.
25. Aguilar, B.A. The efficacy of art therapy in pediatric oncology patients: An integrative literature review. *J. Pediatr. Nurs.* **2017**, *36*, 173–178. [CrossRef] [PubMed]
26. Varni, J.W.; Limbers, C.; Burwinkle, T.M. Literature review: Health-related quality of life measurement in pediatric oncology: Hearing the voices of the children. *J. Pediatr. Psychol.* **2007**, *32*, 1151–1163. [CrossRef] [PubMed]
27. Nainis, N.; Paice, J.A.; Ratner, J.; Wirth, J.H.; Lai, J.; Shott, S. Relieving symptoms in cancer: Innovative use of art therapy. *J. Pain Symptom Manag.* **2006**, *31*, 162–169. [CrossRef] [PubMed]
28. American Music Therapy Association. Available online: https://www.musictherapy.org (accessed on 9 November 2018).
29. Austin, D. The Role of Improvised Music in Psychodynamic Music Therapy with Adults. *Music Ther.* **1996**, *14*, 29–43. [CrossRef]

30. Thaut, M.H.; McIntosh, G.C.; Hoemberg, V. Neurobiological foundations of neurologic music therapy: Rhythmic entrainment and the motor system. *Front. Psychol.* **2014**, *5*, 1185. [CrossRef] [PubMed]
31. Kvam, M.H. The effect of vibroacoustic therapy. *Physiotherapy* **1997**, *83*, 290–295. [CrossRef]
32. Patrick, G. The Effects of Vibroacoustic Music on Symptom Reduction. *IEEE Eng. Med. Biol. Mag.* **1999**, *18*, 97–100. [CrossRef]
33. Boyd-Brewer, C.; McCaffrey, R. Vibroacoustic sound therapy improves pain management and more. *Holist. Nurs. Pract.* **2004**, *18*, 111–118. [CrossRef]
34. The Use of Vocal Holding Techniques with Adults Traumatized as Children. Available online: http://dianeaustin.com/pdfs/Traumaar.pdf (accessed on 9 November 2018).
35. Buber, M. *I and Thou*; Martino Publishing: Mansfield Centre, CT, USA, 2010.
36. Hall, M.M. Yes and: Discovering the Authentic Voice Through Integrated Improvisational Musical Play. Master's Thesis, New York University, New York, NY, USA, 2014.
37. Kubler-Ross, E.; Kessler, D. *On Grief and Grieving: Finding the Meaning of Grief Through the Five Stages of Loss*; Simon & Schuster UK Ltd.: London, UK, 2005.
38. Weitzner, M.A.; Meyers, C.A.; Stuebing, K.K.; Saleeba, A.K. Relationship between quality of life and mood in long-term survivors of breast cancer treated with mastectomy. *Support Care Cancer* **1997**, *5*, 241–248. [CrossRef] [PubMed]
39. Culos-Reed, S.N.; Mackenzie, M.J.; Sohl, S.J.; Jesse, M.T.; Zahavich, A.N.; Danhauer, S.C. Yoga & cancer interventions: A review of the clinical significance of patient reported outcomes for cancer survivors [serial online]. *Evid. Based Complement. Altern. Med.* **2012**, *2012*, 642576. [PubMed]
40. Lin, K.Y.; Hu, Y.T.; Chang, K.J.; Lin, H.F.; Tsauo, J.Y. Effects of yoga on psychological health, quality of life, and physical health of patients with cancer: A meta-analysis. *Evid. Based Complement. Altern. Med.* **2011**, *2011*, 659–876. [CrossRef] [PubMed]
41. Mustian, K.M.; Sprod, L.K.; Janelsins, M.; Peppone, L.J.; Palesh, O.G.; Chandwani, K.; Morrow, G.R. Multicenter, Randomized Controlled Trial of Yoga for Sleep Quality Among Cancer Survivors. *J. Clin. Oncol.* **2013**, *31*, 3233–3241. [CrossRef] [PubMed]
42. Taso, C.J.; Lin, H.S.; Lin, W.L.; Chen, S.; Huang, W.T.; Chen, S.W. The effect of yoga exercise on improving depression, anxiety, and fatigue in women with breast cancer: A randomized controlled trial. *J. Nurs. Res.* **2014**, *22*, 155–164. [CrossRef] [PubMed]
43. Kieviet-Stijnen, A.; Visser, A.; Garssen, B.; Hudig, W. Mindfulness-based stress reduction training for oncology patients: Patients' appraisal and changes in well-being. *Patient Educ. Couns.* **2008**, *72*, 436–442. [CrossRef] [PubMed]
44. The Healing Power of Mindfulness. Available online: https://www.mindful.org/the-healing-power-of-mindfulness/ (accessed on 29 May 2018).
45. Lyman, G.H.; Greenlee, H.; Bohlke, K.; Bao, T.; DeMichele, A.M.; Deng, G.E.; Fouladbakhsh, J.M.; Gil, B.; Hershman, D.L.; Mansfield, S.; et al. Integrative Therapies During and After Breast Cancer Treatment: ASCO Endorsement of the SIO Clinical Practice Guideline. *J. Clin. Oncol.* **2018**, *36*, 2647–2655.
46. Curry, A.N.; Kasser, T. Can coloring mandalas reduce anxiety? *Art Ther.* **2005**, *22*, 81–85. [CrossRef]
47. Lumley, M.A.; Cohen, J.L.; Borszcz, G.S.; Cano, A.; Radcliffe, A.M.; Porter, L.S.; Keefe, F.J. Pain and emotion: A biopsychosocial review of recent research. *J. Clin. Psychol.* **2011**, *67*, 942–968. [CrossRef] [PubMed]
48. University of California—Los Angeles. Putting Feelings into Words Produces Therapeutic Effects in the Brain. *Science Daily*, 22 June 2007. Available online: www.sciencedaily.com/releases/2007/06/070622090727.htm (accessed on 28 May 2018).
49. Landier, W.; Tse, A. Use of complementary and alternative medical interventions for the management of procedure related pain, anxiety, and distress in pediatric oncology: An integrative review. *J. Pediatr. Nurs.* **2010**, *25*, 566–579. [CrossRef] [PubMed]

10

Clinical Hypnosis, an Effective Mind–Body Modality for Adolescents with Behavioral and Physical Complaints

Anju Sawni [1,*] and Cora Collette Breuner [2]

1 Department of Pediatrics, Hurley Children's Hospital/Hurley Medical Center, Michigan State University College of Human Medicine, Flint, MI 48503, USA
2 Department of Pediatrics, Adolescent Medicine Division and Department of Orthopedics and Sports Medicine, Seattle Children's Hospital, University of Washington, Seattle, WA 98105, USA; Cora.Breuner@seattlechildrens.org
* Correspondence: Asawni1@hurleymc.com

Abstract: Mind–body medicine is a system of health practices that includes meditation/relaxation training, guided imagery, hypnosis, biofeedback, yoga, art/music therapy, prayer, t'ai chi, and psychological therapies such as cognitive behavioral therapy. Clinical hypnosis is an important mind–body tool that serves as an adjunct to conventional medical care for the adolescent patient. Clinical hypnosis specifically uses self-directed therapeutic suggestions to cultivate the imagination and facilitate the mind–body connection, leading to positive emotional and physical well-being. There are many similarities between clinical hypnosis and other mind–body/self-regulatory modalities such as visual imagery, mindfulness meditation, yoga, and biofeedback that incorporate experiential learning and mechanisms for change. They may be viewed as subtypes of the hypnotic experience and share the common experience of trance as the entrée into self-empowered change in physiologic and psychological states. Clinical hypnosis can be used by health care providers to teach adolescents coping skills to deal with a wide variety of conditions such as chronic headaches, recurrent abdominal pain, anxiety, depression, grief and bereavement, phobias, anger, family stressors, sleep disorders, or enuresis. Clinical vignettes are given to help illustrate the effectiveness of hypnosis in adolescents.

Keywords: mind–body therapies; adolescents; pain; headache; stress; anxiety; depression; hypnosis; guided imagery; mindfulness; emotional regulation

---

1. Introduction

Mind–body medicine is a philosophy and a system of health practices that enlist the mind in improving emotional well-being and physical health. These practices include meditation/relaxation training, guided imagery, hypnosis, biofeedback, yoga, art/music therapy, prayer, t'ai chi, and psychological therapies such as cognitive behavioral therapy.

Mind–body therapies focus on balancing the autonomic nervous system (ANS) by activating the parasympathetic branch of the ANS to reduce the sympathetic physiological response to stress and by regulating the hypothalamic pituitary adrenal axis, both of which are indicators of stress. This reduction of stress on the mind and body may help control or reverse certain underlying disease processes. Evidence suggests that the mind and body have constant bidirectional communication through neuro-endocrine, neuro-chemical, immunological, and energetic pathways.

Higher cognitive centers and limbic emotional centers are capable of regulating virtually all aspects of the immune system and therefore have a profound effect on health and illness-termed psychoneuroimmunology [1–3].

These therapies may improve the quality of life and reduce the physical symptoms for adolescents with various chronic diseases.

Data from the 2012 National Health Interview Survey show that mind–body therapies were used in adolescents aged 13 to 17 years, and more often among females versus males (5.7% vs. 1.7%). Children and youth were more likely to use mind–body therapies for pain-related conditions or emotional, behavioral, or mental conditions and if they received specialty or mental health care. The most common reasons for the use of mind–body therapies were to improve overall health/general wellness, to reduce stress levels or relax, and to feel better emotionally [4,5].

Mind–body therapies such as clinical hypnosis are considered safe and can be effective for adolescents with medical conditions such as tension or migraine headaches, enuresis, recurrent abdominal pain, constipation, sleep difficulties, acute or chronic pain, anxiety, and other emotional and stress-related symptoms [6,7].

2. Stress and the Developing Adolescent Brain

Adolescence is a period of rapid physical growth, intellectual and cognitive development, as well as a time for creating autonomy, and promoting both self-esteem and strong peer relationships. During adolescence, teens experience the ebb and flow of emotions between self-confidence, insecurity, invincibility, anxiety, worry, doubt, and self-worth as a result of rapid changes occurring in the brain and neuro-biological and neuro-endocrine systems.

The rapidly developing adolescent brain is sensitive to stress and adverse events due to changes in hormones and the plasticity in the structure and function of the brain [8].

Brain development during adolescence involves changes in the frontal and parietal cortices, the site of higher-order cognitive and socioemotional processes (i.e., executive function). The cortex is fine-tuned through synaptic pruning in areas that play a role in judgment, impulse control, planning, and emotion regulation [9–11].

Glucocorticoid receptors are found in the amygdala, hippocampus, and prefrontal cortex (PFC); exposure to stressful experiences (leading to increase in glucocorticoids) has been shown to alter the size and neuronal architecture of these areas as well as lead to functional differences in learning, memory, and other aspects of executive functioning. Specifically, chronic stress is associated with hypertrophy and over-activity in the amygdala and orbitofrontal cortex, and can lead to loss of neurons and neural connections in the hippocampus and medial PFC. The PFC turns off the cortisol response and regulates the autonomic balance (i.e., sympathetic versus parasympathetic effects), it also plays an important role in the development of executive functions, such as decision-making, working memory, behavioral self-regulation, and mood and impulse control [12]. The consequences of structural changes in the brain include more anxiety related to both hyper activation of the amygdala and less control as a result of PFC atrophy, as well as impaired memory and mood control due to hippocampal reduction [13].

The adolescent brain is particularly vulnerable to stressors in the youth's social and emotional environment. Executive functions, such as the ability to direct attention and solve problems efficiently, the awareness of threat, and effective fear processing are diminished when there are significant emotional stimuli during adolescence [14–17]. Rapid neurobiological changes during times of emotional stress may predispose adolescents to difficulties with emotion regulation [8]. Difficulties in emotion regulation are a feature of many emotional and behavioral problems seen in adolescents, including anxiety, depression, conduct problems, cutting, disordered eating, and substance abuse [18–20].

The prevalence of mental health disorders is 22% in adolescents 13 to 18 years old. Anxiety disorders are the most common condition (31.9%), followed by behavior disorders (19.1%), mood disorders (14.3%), and substance use disorders (11.4%). Approximately 40% of those with one class of disorder also meet criteria for another class of lifetime disorder [21,22].

With increasing exposure to technology and screen time (on smart phones, computers, television, and social media sites), more mental health concerns, and persistent economic, racial, and ethnic disparities in health status, we now have new morbidities in adolescents called the 'millennial morbidities'. These morbidities may lead to stress-related problems such as chronic headaches, abdominal pain, anxiety, depression, and other emotional problems [23].

Adolescents who experience emotional stress often complain of chronic physical symptoms that respond poorly to standard medications. Cognitive and emotion regulation, including the ability to modulate responses to stress, is increasingly found to contribute to overall adjustment, including social emotional development (e.g., peer relations). Mind–body/self-regulation therapies such as clinical hypnosis operate at the physiological, attentional, emotional, cognitive, and behavioral levels and teach adolescents' coping skills to control their inner wellbeing with respects to thoughts, emotions, attention, and performance [24,25]. Research shows that mind–body/self-regulation therapies can help develop appropriate connections between the relevant prefrontal structures in adolescents, thereby stabilizing arousal and reducing harmful risk-taking behaviors [26]. They may reduce the impact of stress-related conditions, lessen depression and anxiety, alleviate pain, improve quality of life, and increase emotion regulation and subjective well-being [27–34].

3. Clinical Hypnosis: An Effective Mind–body Modality for Adolescents

There are many similarities between clinical hypnosis and other mind–body/self-regulatory modalities such as visual imagery, mindfulness mediation, yoga, and biofeedback that incorporate experiential learning and mechanisms for change. They all have some overlap and may be viewed as subtypes of the hypnotic experience and share the common experience of trance (what happens when we engage in changing our mind) as the entrée into self-empowered change in physiological and psychological states. However, clinical hypnosis specifically uses self-directed therapeutic suggestions to cultivate the imagination and facilitate the mind–body connection, leading to positive physical, emotional, and behavioral change. Using brain imaging, cognitive neuroscientists have identified the power that therapeutic suggestions have on attention functions and associated brain networks and their impact on physical and mental experience [29,35].

Clinical hypnosis is a teachable coping skill that most adolescents (except those with moderate to severe mental retardation) are able to learn with minor effort, and it is safe, effective, and has no adverse side effects in trained hands.

Although there is no universally agreed-upon definition of hypnosis, it can be best described as the cultivation of the imagination in an altered state of consciousness (awareness and alertness) within a focused state (with or without physical relaxation), in which an individual is selectively focused, absorbed, and concentrating upon a particular idea or image aimed at improving mental or physical health. In adolescents, visual imagery/progressive muscle relaxation is often used to get into this altered state of awareness. It is an internal, imaginative process (similar in feeling to daydreaming and/or using the imagination to see, hear, touch, smell, and taste things) that is used to focus attention and become absorbed so that a hypnotic state/trance is entered into. In this state, perceptions and sensations can be enhanced, modified, or changed to inhibit and control reflexive actions, delay gratification, use problem-solving strategies, increase self-esteem, and decrease anxiety, stress, or discomfort. Hypnosis is a natural state and most adolescents move in and out of spontaneous hypnotic-like states as they focus their concentration, for example, while playing video games, "text-messaging", watching favorite movies, listening to music/stories, or otherwise engaging in fantasy/daydreaming [7].

Hypnosis in adolescents is more permissive and less directive than in adults, as it utilizes the natural hypnotic abilities that teens bring to the clinical encounter. Adolescents can enter into the hypnotic state easily and rapidly and, while in this state of deep concentration, are highly responsive to therapeutic suggestions/goals ("hypnotherapy"). Examples of therapeutic suggestions include decreasing or eliminating undesirable symptoms, reframing and rethinking distorted thoughts about situations and stressors, building positive expectations, re-enforcing control over reaction to problems/situations, and strengthening the concept/belief in the ability of the mind and body to work together to create desirable changes in behavior/outcome. Hypnotherapy allows the adolescent to gain a sense of control, increase self-esteem and competence, and reduce stress.

Clinical hypnosis is indicated when (1) an adolescent is responsive to hypnotic suggestions; (2) a problem is treatable with hypnosis; (3) good rapport exists between the adolescent and provider; (4) the adolescent is motivated to remedy the problem; and (5) no iatrogenic harm is anticipated by use. Caution is indicated in adolescents with a history of physical, sexual, or emotional abuse and those with post-traumatic stress disorder (PTSD), in which case coordination of care with a qualified mental health expert is strongly advisable.

Clinical hypnosis is an effective and powerful tool and with appropriate clinical pediatric hypnosis training (skills-based pediatric hypnosis workshops, www.nphti.org). Pediatric/adolescent health care providers' can help adolescents cope and deal with a wide variety of conditions such as chronic headaches/recurrent abdominal pain, anxiety, depression, grief and bereavement, phobias, anger, family stressors, sleep disorders, or enuresis [36–47].

Hypnosis can also be effective for managing procedure pain [48] and chronic pain related to disease—i.e., malignancy, sickle cell, chronic headaches, and abdominal pain (recurrent abdominal pain, inflammatory bowel disease) [49–54].

Clinical hypnosis/self-regulation therapies also can be helpful when integrated into a multimodal treatment plan for adolescents with Attention deficit hyperactivity disorder (ADHD). Hypnosis can be beneficial in teaching them to quiet their mind, slowing and focusing, so that they can sort out frustration or anger produced when the mind works faster than the ability to communicate, and direct them in a positive manner [55–58].

For more detailed descriptions and references of the wide range of clinical conditions for which hypnosis is applicable and effective in adolescents, readers can consult the two standard textbooks on clinical hypnosis by Kohen and Olness, Sugarman and Wester [59,60], as well as an excellent review article by Kohen and Kaiser [61].

4. Application of Clinical Hypnosis—Clinical Vignettes

Through clinical vignettes, this article illustrates common applications of clinical hypnosis in adolescent health care. These vignettes demonstrate the ease, value, and benefit of having pediatric/adolescent health care providers empower and teach clinical hypnosis strategies to adolescents.

The success of clinical hypnosis depends on establishing a strong rapport with the adolescent and individualizing the therapy to the specific goals and characteristics of the adolescent. During the initial visit, the clinician learns the adolescent's personal and family history, and assesses motivation, expectations, strengths, and other internal resources—such as capacity to self-regulate their emotions—the clinician should emphasize that the adolescent is in control. They should offer choices and options and teach the adolescent that they can use the skill (clinical hypnosis) when he/she chooses. The clinician should offer to be the teacher or coach, emphasize the adolescent's ability for control and mastery, and utilize the teen's language and imagery. They should reinforce whatever happens, get feedback from the teen, and address anxiety as well as pain. It is important to have a follow-up plan, such as emphasizing the importance of clinical-hypnosis practice and keeping a calendar of the practice and symptoms (this can easily be done on the teen's smart-phone; the majority of teens have a one). The provider should schedule a follow up appointment in a few weeks to reassess/reinforce progress. The use of other cognitive and behavioral strategies should be incorporated as well to address the symptom.

4.1. Clinical Vignette 1: Chronic Daily Headaches

A 16-year-old female was referred by her neurologist for chronic headaches. Her neurological work up for headaches was negative, with no anatomical or pathological etiology. She had a history of daily headaches, that did not wake her up from sleep but did cause her to miss school and not socialize with her friends. She took over-the-counter ibuprofen/acetaminophen with little relief. She would sleep to help her headaches.

Past medical history and social history were non-contributory. No history of depression, anxiety, or school problems. Family/home life was stable with no acute/chronic toxic stressors.

Mental status evaluation revealed normal cognition and no apparent psychiatric disorder such as a conversion disorder, psychosis, or thought disorder.

The initial session with her and her parents focused on obtaining a thorough history, performing a physical exam, and reviewing labs/imagery. Pain assessment scale using range of 0–10 was used (10 = worst imaginable headache, 0 = no headache, her average score was 8). When asked at which number she would be able to go to school/function so that the headache did not bother her, she replied ≤ 3.

The clinician then educated the patient and parents on the mind–body connection, with a more formalized introduction/discussion and demystification of hypnosis, emphasizing that learning strategies such as clinical hypnosis can be very effective in managing headache pain.

It was explained that clinical hypnosis could help her take control of her pain/headaches and she could do something so that her headaches would not bother her anymore. The patient and parents were receptive to learning clinical hypnosis. The patient was motivated to get rid of her headaches and resume her normal life.

A second visit was scheduled to teach the patient clinical hypnosis techniques. When designing a hypnotic or hypnosis/trance experience, the clinician utilizes the adolescent's imagination and perception of the symptom and how it affects them as well as probes into the adolescent's interests, strengths, and goals. The adolescent is taught to use techniques such as progressive muscle relaxation, focused breathing, and visual imagery to help them get into a relaxed and focused state (with or without physical relaxation). In this relaxed state, the brain is more focused and receptive to learning techniques to feel better and ultimately make the headache pain dissipate. Prior to incorporating visual imagery and giving a therapeutic suggestion to alleviate the symptom or problem, the clinician asks the adolescent what they would like to imagine that is fun and makes them happy (i.e., a favorite place or favorite things) and if they would like to imagine doing that to help them get into a deeper relaxed state (this reinforces that the teen is in control and empowers them). In this deeper relaxed state, the mind is open and receptive to ideas to help them with their symptoms. In this case the clinician asked the patient to draw a picture of what her headache felt like to her. She drew a picture of a hammer pounding her head. Then both the clinician and the patient devised a method to stop the hammer from pounding her head. The patient used her imagination to visualize having a stop sign come up before the hammer hit her head which would stop the hammer and thus would stop the headache. She then practiced visualizing the stop sign coming up and saying stop to the hammer before it hit her head (the therapeutic suggestion). The clinician then developed a concrete plan with the teen to help practice her clinical hypnosis techniques. Some clinicians ask their patients to keep a calendar of their practice (easy to do on their smartphone). The focus is on practicing clinical hypnosis, not on the symptoms. At the follow up visit a month later, she was practicing her clinical hypnosis, she had kept a calendar of when she practiced hypnosis and pain scale of the headaches. Her headaches were infrequent and not interfering with her daily activities or school.

4.2. Clinical Vignette 2: Needle Phobia

This was a 14-year-old male was referred by his primary care doctor to learn clinical hypnosis for needle phobia. He became very anxious and hysterical prior to obtaining any immunizations or blood draws and was therefore behind on immunizations and screening lab tests.

Past medical history was significant for attention deficit hyperactivity disorder, treated with methylphenidate. There was no history of other psychiatric diagnosis.

He was motivated to learn clinical hypnosis. He recognized that he needed immunizations to stay healthy but was afraid of shots. He was motivated and willing to overcome his "fear of shots". The clinician discussed mind–body/clinical hypnosis techniques with him and used a distraction technique (listening to his music on his iPod) and the hypnotic concept of disassociation i.e., dissociate body and mind, to encourage him to give his arm to the nurse to let her give him the shot so that he could stay healthy, and while she did what she needed to do, he could focus on something else like listening to his music. Also, exposure therapy with desensitization is the treatment of choice for phobias. He was exposed to the equipment (e.g., cleaning swab, syringe, needle) and procedure for injections, so those items no longer created panic symptoms. A "pretend needle" was used to do practice session. After rehearsing this for one session he then "practiced getting the shot" (exposure therapy), while listening to his music (distraction), "gave his arm to the nurse" (disassociation). He did well in the practice session. The patient came back two days later and went through the clinical hypnosis technique of distraction and disassociation and successfully received his immunizations.

4.3. Clinical Vignette #3: Primary Nocturnal Enuresis

A 14-year-old male was referred by his pediatrician for management of primary nocturnal enuresis. History revealed that he had nocturnal enuresis six/seven nights/week and never had a period of complete dryness. He was in the ninth grade and played hockey with practices late at night and quite a few games away from home. He was very embarrassed about his bedwetting and thus very motivated to stop.

Family history was positive for nocturnal enuresis in father until age 16.

He reported drinking a lot of fluids after each hockey practice and game. He had a difficult time unwinding and falling asleep and was a deep sleeper.

He denied drugs, alcohol, or tobacco use and did well in school. There were no other stressors at home or school.

He was motivated to learn clinical hypnosis and stop bedwetting. The clinician discussed the mind–body connection—i.e., the brain and bladder were communicating with each other. He was told that his brain and bladder talked to each other very well, and cooperated and worked well because during the day he never wet his pants even if he had to go really badly, he could hold his pee. He was shown a drawing of genitourinary anatomy and physiology, and was engaged in building curiosity about how the body works, thus helping him be in a spontaneous hypnotic state. The drawing showed how urine was sent from the kidneys to the bladder. The bladder was shown as a container with a muscle at the tip that has a gate that is closed and keeps the urine in the bladder until he goes to the bathroom and the mother computer (i.e., the brain) gives a signal to open the gate when it is full so he can pee. The drawing showed the brain and bladder connection, with bi-directional arrows communicating between the full bladder and the brain, keeping the gate closed until he gets the message from the brain to open it.

The clinician explained, that because he was a deep sleeper, his brain and bladder did not talk well/forgot at night so he had to remind them to talk to each other like they did during the day before he went to sleep.

Then the clinician had him imagine having this conversation in his head to practice how he would have the brain and bladder talk to each other. For example, the clinician coached the patient to say "bladder, tonight let the brain know when you are full. Brain, you have a choice. When the bladder says its full, tell me to wake up, walk to the bathroom, open the gate, pee in the toilet, close the gate, and go back to my comfortable dry bed, or, instead tell the bladder gate to stay closed and locked all night until morning, when I get up from my nice, warm, dry bed and go to the bathroom".

With either choice, the bed is dry in the morning. The patient then wanted to sleep through the night and decided to send a message to brain to keep the gate closed to his bladder till he woke up in the morning. Other behavior modification techniques such as no fluids 1 hour before bed, and bladder

Kegel strengthening exercises during the day were taught. The patient kept a calendar of his clinical hypnosis practice and of dry nights.

He focused on dry nights, positive behaviors, feeling proud and good when his bed was dry, which gave him positive messages of success. He went through two sessions and at a two-month follow up his enuresis had resolved completely.

4.4. Clinical Vignette 4: Anxiety with Sleep Disturbance

A 13-year-old female was referred by her pediatrician for concerns regarding palpitations/panic attacks and sleep problems that started a few months earlier. The patient reported symptoms of shortness of breath, sharp chest pain, and hyperventilation. Extensive medical evaluation by a pediatrician and a cardiologist were negative for physical/anatomical abnormalities.

Patient continued experiencing palpitations and felt as if she "could not catch her breath, and her throat was closing".

She also reported having trouble sleeping, and frequently watched scary movies on her iPad at night to help her sleep. She occasionally took melatonin to help her sleep.

Her mom reported that she was a "worrier" thought often about her safety, as well as her parents' safety, and was concerned that something was wrong with her.

There were no recent illness/stressors in the family and no acute life changes. Family history was positive for anxiety in the father. She lived at home with parents, was an only child and got along well with both parents. She was in the eighth grade, doing virtual home schooling for past two years and was doing well. She did not like crowds and school, so parents decided to do home/virtual school. She had one close friend and cousins with whom she socialized. She liked to play the piano and do arts and crafts. She was referred to a psychologist and also saw a psychiatrist once. She was diagnosed with "social anxiety" by psychiatrist after one visit and told to take sertraline but she never started as her mother did not want to give her medications.

The clinician educated the patient and mom on the benefits of learning mind–body techniques such as focused breathing/visual imagery/clinical hypnosis, to help her cope with her panic attacks/anxiety/worried thoughts.

The patient was open and motivated to learning clinical hypnosis/relaxation techniques. She was taught focused breathing, progressive muscle relaxation, and visual imagery techniques to help her relax and get into a state of focused concentration. The clinician discussed imagining something that made her happy or feel good; her favorite imagery was being up at a lake on the boat. While in this relaxed state the clinician gave her therapeutic suggestions to notice that her breathing was calm, strong, and comfortable; her heart was beating normally and was strong and well; and she was healthy. Her parents were fine and she did not have to worry about her health or her parents' health.

The clinician also discussed other behavioral modification techniques when she felt anxious such as coloring and journaling to help her worry less and distract her when her worry thoughts were taking over her mind. She was shown smart phone e apps (e.g., calm, breathe & relax, mind shift, stop, breathe & think) that helped her practice her breathing.

The patient was told to schedule regular practice time and instructed to keep a calendar of her clinical hypnosis exercise breathing practice and to note the days she felt good/less worried. It was recommended that she continue therapy with a psychologist. She was also advised on proper sleep hygiene techniques (i.e., no screen time one hour before bed, no TV). At a one-month follow-up she was doing better. She was practicing her clinical hypnosis/breathing/visual imagery exercises before bed, two to three times a week. Her mom noticed her overall mood was better and she had fewer panic attacks although she still got anxious, especially when she had to go to new places or places with crowds. She practiced her focused breathing when she would get anxious and she reported sleeping better. At the two month follow up, she had no more panic attacks or excessive worrying.

4.5. Clinical Vignette 5: Substance Abuse

A 17-year-old male was referred by his primary care doctor for management of substance abuse, anxiety, and panic attacks. The patient experienced his first acute panic attack one week prior to his visit which resulted in an emergency room (ED) visit. He was started on short acting alprazolam for acute panic attacks in ED. Was prescribed escitalopram but did not take it because he "(did not) want to take medication". The patient had a history of smoking marijuana (MJ) daily for past four months and weekly for the past year and more recently admitted to smoking a more potent form of MJ oil called "wax/butane hash oil". He denied any other illicit drug use or any prescription drug abuse except for an occasional beer.

He had a past history of mild depressive symptoms/anxiety which was progressively getting worse the past year. For the past several months, he was more socially isolated and stayed in his room and smoked marijuana. He denied self-harm or suicidal thoughts.

He had a lot of worry/concerns/anxiety about his physical health especially the negative effects of marijuana on his health.

He had a lot of psychosomatic complaints, chest pain, numbness and tingling in hands/arms, nonspecific abdominal pain, back pain, and musculoskeletal pain. Since the acute panic episode, he was motivated to stop marijuana and any illicit drug use. He recognized that when he smoked the more potent marijuana "wax", he would be more anxious, feel panicky, heart beating fast, chest hurting, nausea, abdominal pain, and numbness.

Past medical history was significant for attention deficit disorder for which he was prescribed methylphenidate for a few months but stopped two years prior. He currently reported having difficulty focusing at school and declining grades. Family history was positive for anxiety in sister.

He was a senior in high school. His hobbies included making music on his computer and playing in a band. He admitted to peer pressure to smoke marijuana. He denied being sexually active. He worked part time at a fast food restaurant.

A complete physical and neurological exam was normal. Vital signs were all normal.

He needed a lot of reassurance that physically he was fine.

He was open to learning clinical hypnosis/focused breathing/to help with panic attacks/anxiety. He was taught progressive muscle relaxation/focused breathing/visual imagery to help him get into a relaxed alter state of focused consciousness. He visualized himself playing his electronic music/making music. While in this relaxed state, he was given therapeutic suggestions of noting that his body was healthy, that his heart, lungs, hands, and chest were all fine.

He was told he did not need drugs to make good music. He was reminded that when he smoked marijuana he did not feel good. Smoking MJ made him anxious and it was not good for his health, it made his heart beat fast, chest hurt, and nauseous. The clinician discussed the importance of regular practice of clinical hypnosis/breathing exercises. At three week follow up, he was practicing his clinical hypnosis daily and had no further panic attacks or ED visits.

He was followed monthly and for several months he continued to be pre-occupied about his physical health and have vague physical complaints. At each visit he was reassured that physically he was healthy.

He did admit to occasionally smoking marijuana on weekends with his friends but only a few hits as he noted that when he smoked too much he would feel his heart beat fast and get anxious. He was also started on Concerta for his ADHD.

4.6. Clinical Vignette 6: Crohn's Disease with Abdominal Pain

A 17-year-old female with Crohn's disease was referred by her gastroenterologist with severe abdominal pain after multiple hospitalizations for relapse. It was hoped that clinical hypnosis would help her as she was going away to college in the fall and prior to going away was scheduled for small bowel resection/with colostomy.

Mom and patient were interested in "holistic therapies" to help her with the surgery as well as with management of her abdominal discomfort/Crohn's disease while away at college. Mom took herbs/nutritional supplements. Clinician discussed nutrition/healthy eating with patient and mother and added probiotics and omega-3 essential fatty acid supplements to her daily medication regimen.

Patient was very motivated to feel better and manage her Crohn's disease. The clinician taught her clinical hypnosis prior to surgery using progressive muscle relaxation/visual imagery (going to her favorite place in her imagination), then gave her therapeutic suggestions to notice how well the surgery went and how well she was healing, how healthy her gut was, and she could eat healthy foods.

She chose the suggestion "that she wanted to send a message (via text messaging) from her brain to her gut that it was healing well. The clinician reinforced that if her stomach bothered her she could breathe and go to her favorite place and imagine herself feeling good. The surgery was successful and she recovered without complications and was having less abdominal pain. She left for college feeling more confident that she could manage her distress/pain and Crohn's disease.

The above case studies are an example of the benefits of using clinical hypnosis to help adolescents manage common medical conditions. However, it is important to keep in mind that not every adolescent will respond so quickly and positively and that proper certification is essential when applying pediatric hypnosis. Certified pediatric hypnosis training is provided by National Pediatric Hypnosis Training Institute-Inaugural Annual Skill Development Workshops in Pediatric Clinical Hypnosis (Introductory, Intermediate, and Advanced; www.nphti.org).

Not only is a trained clinical provider important for success but so is building a positive rapport with the teen and family with ongoing re-assessment, flexibility, and brainstorming for problem resolution, good outcomes, and healing. As with any skill, regular practice of clinical hypnosis by the teen enhances competence, confidence, and positive outcomes, whereas absence of regular practice is more likely to result in slower and/or less positive results. Homework assignments for the adolescent and their parents involves practice of clinical hypnosis—i.e., keeping a calendar of practice and specifying when they will practice—counseling parents about their level of involvement, and encouraging/motivating adolescents to take charge and control of their symptoms and life in order to have a positive outcome.

5. Conclusions

Clinical hypnosis is a natural state that can be cultivated, with permission from the adolescent and builds on the adolescent's existing strengths and interests. It is an altered state of consciousness (awareness and alertness) within a focused state (with or without physical relaxation), in which an individual is selectively focused, absorbed, and concentrating upon a particular idea or image aimed at improving mental or physical health. Clinical hypnosis is a teachable skill that most adolescent patients are able to learn with minor effort, and is safe, effective, and free of adverse side effects in trained hands. Hypnosis promotes the cultivation of imagination and patients' positive expectations and motivation for success.

Hypnosis in adolescents is more permissive and less directive than in adults, as it utilizes the natural hypnotic abilities that teens bring to the clinical encounter. As a result, adolescents can enter into the hypnotic state quicker and easier than adults and are highly responsive to therapeutic suggestions/goals (hypnotherapy).

Examples of therapeutic suggestions include decreasing or eliminating undesirable symptoms, reframing and rethinking distorted thoughts about situations and stressors, building positive expectations, and re-enforcing control over reaction to problems/situations, and strengthening the concept/belief in the ability of the mind and body to work together to create desirable changes in behavior/outcome. Clinical hypnosis allows the adolescent to gain a sense of control, increase self-esteem and competence, and reduce stress, therefore helping them to manage their physical and emotional well-being. For some problems, hypnosis may be the treatment of choice (e.g., enuresis, headaches, abdominal pain, procedural pain/anxiety, and adjustment reaction to stress).

For more complex problems/conditions, hypnosis may be more adjunctive but a highly effective and important modality in the overall management.

6. Suggested Training

(1) American Society for Clinical Hypnosis. http://www.asch.net.
(2) National Pediatric Hypnosis Training Institute. http://www.nphti.org.

Author Contributions: Anju Sawni was the lead author of this review article. She provided contributions to this article through organizing, writing, literature review, case presentations and editing of the major sections. Cora Collette Breuner provided contributions to the article through, literature review, editing, writing and advising of the article.

References

1. Pert, C. *Molecules of Emotion*; Simon and Schuster: New York, NY, USA, 1997.
2. Chiarmonte, D.R. Mind–body therapies for primary care physicians. *Prim. Care* **1997**, *24*, 787–807. [CrossRef]
3. *Psychoneuroimmunolgy*, 4th ed.; Ader, R. (Ed.) Academic Press: Cambridge, MA, USA, 2007.
4. Clarke, T.C.; Black, L.I.; Stussman, B.J.; Barnes, P.M.; Nahin, R.L. *Trends in the Use of Complementary Health Approaches among Adults: United States, 2002–2012*; National health Statistics Reports, no 79; National Center for Health Statistics: Hyattsville, MD, USA, 2015.
5. Child and Adolescent Health Measurement Initiative. *What's New in the 2012 NHIS Child Complementary and Alternative Medicine Supplemen?* Data Resource Center for Child & Adolescent Health: Washinton, DC, USA, 2013; Available online: www.childhealthdata.org (accessed on 25 January 2017).
6. Sussman, D.; Culbert, T. Pediatric Self-regulation. In *Developmental-Behavioral Pediatrics*, 3rd ed.; Levine, M.D., Carey, W.B., Crocker, A.C., Eds.; W.B. Saunders: Philadelphia, PA, USA, 1999; pp. 843–850.
7. Kohen, D.P. A pediatric perspective on mind–body medicine. In *Integrative Pediatrics*; Culbert, T., Olness, K., Eds.; Oxford University Press: New York, NY, USA, 2009; pp. 267–301.
8. Romeo, R.D. Adolescence: A central event in shaping stress reactivity. *Dev. Psychobiol.* **2010**, *52*, 244–253. [CrossRef] [PubMed]
9. Giedd, J.N.; Blumenthal, J.; Jeffrie, N.O.; Castellanos, F.X.; Liu, H.; Zijdenbos, A.; Rapoport, J.L. Brain development during childhood and adolescence: A longitudinal MRI study. *Nat. Neurosci.* **1999**, *2*, 861–863. [CrossRef] [PubMed]
10. Stroud, L.; Foster, E.; Handwerger, K.; Papandonatos, G.D.; Granger, D.; Kivilighan, K.T.; Niaura, R. Stress response and the adolescent transition: Performance versus peer rejection stress. *Dev. Psychobiol.* **2009**, *21*, 47–68. [CrossRef] [PubMed]
11. Sumter, S.R.; Bokhorsta, C.L.; Miersa, A.C.; Van Pelt, J.; Westenberg, P.M. Age and puberty differences in stress responses during a public speaking task: Do adolescents grow more sensitive to social evaluation? *Psychoneuroendocrinology* **2010**, *35*, 1510–1516. [CrossRef] [PubMed]
12. Shonkoff, J.P.; Garner, A.S. Committee on psychosocial aspect of child and family health, Committee on early childhood adoption and dependent care and Section on Developmental and Behavioral Pediatrics. The Lifelong Effects of Early Childhood Adversity and Toxic Stress. *Pediatrics* **2011**, *29*, e232–e246.
13. McEwen, B.S.; Gianaros, P.J. Stress- and allostasis-induced brain plasticity. *Ann. Rev. Med.* **2011**, *62*, 431–445. [CrossRef] [PubMed]
14. Silk, J.S.; Siegel, G.J.; Whalen, D.J.; Ostapenko, L.J.; Ladoucer, C.D.; Dahl, R.E. Pubertal changes in emotional information processing: Pupillary, behavioral, and subjective evidence during emotional work identification. *Dev. Psychopathol.* **2009**, *21*, 7–26. [CrossRef] [PubMed]
15. Blakemore, S.J. Development of the social brain during adolescence. *Q. J. Exp. Psychol.* **2008**, *61*, 40–49. [CrossRef] [PubMed]
16. Arnsten, A.F.T.; Shansky, R.M. Adolescent vulnerable period for stress-induced prefrontal cortical function? Introduction to Part IV. *Ann. N. Y. Acad. Sci.* **2004**, *1021*, 143–147. [CrossRef] [PubMed]
17. Andersen, S.L.; Teicher, M.H. Stress, sensitive periods and maturational events in adolescent depression. *Trends Neurosci.* **2008**, *31*, 183–191. [CrossRef] [PubMed]

18. Beato-Fernández, L.; Rodríguez-Cano, T.; Pelayo-Delgado, E.; Calaf, M. Are there gender-specific pathways from early adolescence psychological distress symptoms toward the development of substance use and abnormal eating behavior? *Child Psychiatry Hum. Dev.* **2007**, *37*, 193–203. [CrossRef] [PubMed]
19. Cisler, J.M.; Olatunji, B.O.; Felder, M.T.; Forsyth, J.P. Emotion regulation and the anxiety disorders: An Integrative Review. *J. Psychopathol. Behav. Assess.* **2010**, *32*, 68–82. [CrossRef] [PubMed]
20. Andersen, S.L.; Teicher, M.H. Desperately driven and no brakes: Developmental stress exposure and subsequent risk for substance abuse. *Neurosci. Biobehav. Rev.* **2009**, *33*, 516–524. [CrossRef] [PubMed]
21. U.S. Department of Health and Human Services; Centers for Disease Control and Prevention. *Mental Health Surveillance among Children—United States, 2005–2011*; MMWR: Atlanta, GA, USA, 2013; Volume 62, pp. 1–35. Available online: http://www.cdc.gov/mmwr/preview/mmwrhtml/su6202a1.htm (accessed on 25 January 2017).
22. Merikangas, R.; He, J.P.; Burstein, M.; Swanson, S.A.; Avenevoli, S.; Cui, L.; Benjet, C.; Georgiades, K.; Swendsen, J. Lifetime prevalence of mental disorders in U.S. adolescents: Results from the National Comorbidity Survey Replication–Adolescent Supplement (NCS-A). *J. Am. Acad. Child Adolesc. Psychiatry* **2010**, *49*, 980–989. [CrossRef] [PubMed]
23. Palfrey, J.S.; Tonniges, T.F.; Green, M.; Richmond, J. Introduction: Addressing the millennial morbidity—The context of community pediatrics. *Pediatrics* **2005**, *115*, 1121–1123. [CrossRef] [PubMed]
24. Bell, M.A.; Deater-Deckard, K. Biological systems and the development of self-regulation: Integrating behavior, genetics, and psychophysiology. *J. Dev. Behav. Pediatr.* **2007**, *28*, 409–420. [CrossRef] [PubMed]
25. Greenberg, M.T. Promoting resilience in children and youth: Preventive interventions and their interface with neuroscience. *Ann. N. Y. Acad. Sci.* **2006**, *1094*, 139–150. [CrossRef] [PubMed]
26. Atkins, S.M.; Bunting, M.F.; Bolger, D.J.; Dougherty, M.R. Training the adolescent brain: Neural plasticity and the acquisition of cognitive abilities. In *The Adolescent Brain: Learning, Reasoning, and Decision Making*; Reyna, V.F., Chapman, S.B., Dougherty, M.R., Confrey, J., Eds.; American Psychological Association: Washington, DC, USA, 2012; pp. 211–242.
27. Pascoea, M.C.; Bauerb, I.E. A systematic review of randomized control trials on the effects of yoga on stress measures and mood. *J. Psychiatr. Res.* **2015**, *68*, 270–282. [CrossRef] [PubMed]
28. Hölzel, B.K.; Lazar, S.W.; Gard, T.; Schuman-Olivier, Z.; Vago, D.R.; Ott, U. How Does Mindfulness Meditation Work? Proposing Mechanisms of Action from a Conceptual and Neural Perspective. *Perspect. Psychol. Sci.* **2011**, *6*, 537–559. [CrossRef] [PubMed]
29. Baijal, S.; Jha, A.P.; Kiyonaga, A.; Singh, R.; Srinivasan, N. The influence of concentrative meditation training on the development of attention networks during early adolescence. *Front. Psychol.* **2011**, *12*, 153. [CrossRef] [PubMed]
30. Cahn, B.R.; Polich, J. Meditation states and traits: EEG, ERP, and neuroimaging studies. *Psychol. Bull.* **2006**, *132*, 180–211. [CrossRef] [PubMed]
31. Britton, W.B.; Bootzin, R.R.; Cousins, J.C.; Hasle, B.P.; Peck, T.; Shapiro, S.L. The contribution of mindfulness practice to a multicomponent behavioral sleep intervention following substance abuse treatment in adolescents: A treatment-development study. *Subst. Abus.* **2010**, *31*, 86–97. [CrossRef] [PubMed]
32. Tang, Y.Y.; Holzel, B.K.; Posner, M.I. The neuroscience of mindfulness meditation. *Nat. Rev. Neurosci.* **2015**, *16*, 213–225. [CrossRef] [PubMed]
33. Sibinga, E.M.; Kerrigan, D.; Stewart, M.; Johnson, K.; Magyari, T.; Ellen, J.M. Mindfulness-based stress reduction for urban youth. *J. Altern. Complement. Med.* **2011**, *17*, 213–218. [CrossRef] [PubMed]
34. Sibinga, E.M.; Webb, L.; Ghazarian, S.R.; Ellen, J.M. School-based mindfulness instruction: An RCT. *Pediatrics* **2016**, *137*, 1–8. [CrossRef] [PubMed]
35. Raz, A. Does neuroimaging of suggestion elucidate hypnotic trance? *Int. J. Clin. Exp. Hypn.* **2011**, *59*, 363–377. [CrossRef] [PubMed]
36. Kaiser, P. Chlldhood Anxiety, Worry, and Fear: Individualizing Hypnosis Goals and Suggestions for Self-Regulation. *Am. J. Clin. Hypn.* **2011**, *54*, 16–31. [CrossRef] [PubMed]
37. Cyr, L.R.; Culbert, T.; Kaiser, P. Helping children with stress and anxiety: An integrative medicine approach. *Biofeedback* **2003**, *31*, 12–17.
38. Yapko, M. *Mindfulness and Hypnosis: The Power of Suggestion to Transform Experience*; W.W. Norton & Co.: New York, NY, USA, 2011.
39. Kaiser, P. Childhood anxiety and psychophysiological reactivity: Hypnosis to build discrimination and self-regulation skills. *Am. J. Clin. Hypn.* **2014**, *56*, 343–367. [CrossRef] [PubMed]

40. Kuttner, L.; Friedrichsdorf, S.J. Hypnosis and palliative care. In *Therapeutic Hypnosis with Children and Adolescents*, 2nd ed.; Sugarman, L.I., Wester, W.C., Eds.; Crown House Publishing: Carmarthen, UK, 2014; pp. 491–509.
41. Golden, W. Cognitive Hypnotherapy for Anxiety Disorders. *Am. J. Clin. Hypn.* **2012**, *54*, 263–274. [CrossRef] [PubMed]
42. Kerns, C.M.; Read, K.L.; Klugman, J.; Kendall, P.C. Cognitive-behavioral therapy for youth with social anxiety: Differential short and long-term treatment outcomes. *J. Anxiety Disord.* **2013**, *27*, 210–215. [CrossRef] [PubMed]
43. Yapko, M.D. *Applying Hypnosis in Treating Depression: Innovations in Clinical Practice*; Routledge Press: New York, NY, USA, 2006.
44. Kohen, D.P.; Murray, K. Depression in Children and Youth: Applications of Hypnosis to Help Young People Help Themselves. In *Applying Hypnosis in Treating Depression: Innovations in Clinical Practice*; Yapko, M.D., Ed.; Routledge Press: New York, NY, USA, 2006; pp. 189–216.
45. Kohen, D.P. Depression. In *Therapeutic Hypnosis with Children and Adolescents*; Sugarman, L.I., Wester, W.C., II, Eds.; Crown House Publishing: Carmarthen, UK, 2014; Chapter 9; pp. 187–208.
46. Kuttner, L. Treating pain, anxiety and sleep disorders with children and adolescents. In *Advances in the Use of Hypnosis in Medicine, Dentistry, Pain Prevention and Management*; Brown, D.C., Ed.; Crown House Publishers: Bethel, CT, USA, 2009; Chapter 11; pp. 177–194.
47. Schlarb, A.A.; Liddle, C.C.; Hautzinger, M. JuST—A multimodal treatment program for treatment of insomnia in adolescents: A pilot study. *Nat. Sci. Sleep* **2011**, *3*, 13–20. [PubMed]
48. Curtis, S.; Wingert, A.; Ali, S. The Cochrane Library and Procedural Pain in Children: An Overview of Reviews. *Evid. Based Child Heal. A Cochrane Rev. J.* **2012**, *7*, 1363–1399. [CrossRef]
49. Eccleston, C.; Palermo, T.M.; Williams, A.C.; Lewandowski, A.; Morley, S. Psychological therapies for the management of chronic and recurrent pain in children and adolescents. *Cochrane Database Syst. Rev.* **2009**. [CrossRef]
50. Hammond, D.C. Review of the efficacy of clinical hypnosis with headaches and migraines. *Int. J. Clin. Exp. Hypn.* **2007**, *55*, 207–219. [CrossRef] [PubMed]
51. Kohen, D.P.; Zajac, R. Self-hypnosis training for headaches in children and adolescents. *J. Pediatr.* **2007**, *150*, 635–639. [CrossRef] [PubMed]
52. Shaoul, R.; Sukhotnik, I.; Mogilner, J. Hypnosis as an adjuvant treatment for children with inflammatory bowel disease. *J. Dev. Behav. Pediatr.* **2009**, *30*, 268. [CrossRef] [PubMed]
53. Anbar, R.D. Self-hypnosis for the treatment of functional abdominal pain in childhood. *Clin. Pediatr.* **2001**, *40*, 447–451. [CrossRef] [PubMed]
54. Vlieger, A.M.; Rutten, J.M.; Govers, A.M.; Frankenhuis, C.; Benninga, M.A. Long-term follow-up of gut-directed hypnotherapy vs. standard care in children with functional abdominal pain or irritable bowel syndrome. *Am. J. Gastroenterol.* **2012**, *107*, 627–631. [CrossRef] [PubMed]
55. Bogels, S.; Hopgstad, B.; van Dun, L.; de Schutter, S. Mindfulness training for adolescents with externalizing disorders and their parents. *Behav. Cogn. Psychother.* **2008**, *36*, 193–209. [CrossRef]
56. Van der Oord, S.; Bögels, S.M.; Peijnenburg, D. The Effectiveness of Mindfulness Training for Children with ADHD and Mindful Parenting for their Parents. *J. Child Fam. Stud.* **2012**, *21*, 139–147. [CrossRef] [PubMed]
57. Zylowska, L.; Ackermann, D.L.; Yang, M.H.; Futrell, J.L.; Horton, N.L.; Hale, S.T.; Pataki, C.; Smalley, S.L. Mindfulness meditation training in adults and adolescents with ADHD. A feasibility study. *J. Attent. Disord.* **2007**, *11*, 737–746. [CrossRef] [PubMed]
58. Culbert, T.; Banez, G.; Reiff, M. Children who have Attentional disorders: Interventions. *Pediatr. Rev.* **1994**, *15*, 5–15. [CrossRef] [PubMed]
59. Kohen, D.P.; Olness, K.N. *Hypnosis and Hypnotherapy with Children*, 4th ed.; Routledge Publications, Taylor'& Francis: New York, NY, USA, 2011.

60. Sugarman, L.I.; Wester, W.C. *Therapeutic Hypnosis with Children and Adolescents*, 2nd ed.; Crown House Publishing: Carmarthen, UK, 2014.
61. Kohen, D.P.; Kaiser, P. Clinical hypnosis with children and adolescents—What? Why? How? Origins, applications, and efficacy. *Children* **2014**, *1*, 74–98. [CrossRef] [PubMed]

11

Pharmacological Strategies for Decreasing Opioid Therapy and Management of Side Effects from Chronic Use

Genevieve D'Souza [1], Anava A. Wren [2], Christina Almgren [1], Alexandra C. Ross [1], Amanda Marshall [1] and Brenda Golianu [1,*]

1 Department of Anesthesia, Perioperative and Pain Medicine, Stanford University, Palo Alto, CA 94304, USA; gdsouza@stanford.edu (G.D.); calmgren@stanfordchildrens.org (C.A.); alexandra.cram.ross@gmail.com (A.C.R.); 11am203@queensu.ca (A.M.)

2 Department of Pediatrics, Division of Pediatric Gastroenterology, Hepatology and Nutrition, Stanford University, Palo Alto, CA 94304, USA; awren2@stanford.edu

* Correspondence: bgolianu@stanford.edu

Abstract: As awareness increases about the side effects of opioids and risks of misuse, opioid use and appropriate weaning of opioid therapies have become topics of significant clinical relevance among pediatric populations. Critically ill hospitalized neonates, children, and adolescents routinely receive opioids for analgesia and sedation as part of their hospitalization, for both acute and chronic illnesses. Opioids are frequently administered to manage pain symptoms, reduce anxiety and agitation, and diminish physiological stress responses. Opioids are also regularly prescribed to youth with chronic pain. These medications may be prescribed during the initial phase of a diagnostic workup, during an emergency room visit; as an inpatient, or on an outpatient basis. Following treatment for underlying pain conditions, it can be challenging to appropriately wean and discontinue opioid therapies. Weaning opioid therapy requires special expertise and care to avoid symptoms of increased pain, withdrawal, and agitation. To address this challenge, there have been enhanced efforts to implement opioid-reduction during pharmacological therapies for pediatric pain management. Effective pain management therapies and their outcomes in pediatrics are outside the scope of this paper. The aims of this paper were to: (1) Review the current practice of opioid-reduction during pharmacological therapies; and (2) highlight concrete opioid weaning strategies and management of opioid withdrawal.

Keywords: opioid therapy; weaning of opioids; withdrawal; assessment of withdrawal

---

1. Introduction

There is growing public concern regarding the use and risks related to prescription opioid therapy [1]. Historically, opioid therapy has been a central component to clinical pain management in most pediatric hospitals. Opioids are frequently prescribed for the management of pain related to acute conditions, as well as for sedation and management of agitation among patients receiving intensive care. Research in both adults and children has demonstrated that opioids are effective and potent in the acute management of pain [2,3]. Opioids increase descending modulation, and reduce descending facilitation in pain pathways of the central nervous system [4]. Opioids also target affective centers of the brain that impact emotional states, which can alter pain perception [5].

With long term use, however, physiological dependence and tolerance increase due to internalization of receptors and other adaptive processes [6]. Efficacy of clinical pain control decreases requiring increasing doses of analgesic agents, corresponding to increases in side effect profiles [6]. The range of side effects include respiratory depression, constipation, cognitive dysfunction, and psychiatric comorbidities such as anxiety and depression [7–10]. Additionally, chronic opioid use can lead to physical tolerance and dependence, and carries the risk of addiction [11]. Opioid use can also have the unexpected result of increased sensitization to pain (i.e., opioid induced hyperalgesia), though this is a rare phenomenon [12].

Understanding the appropriate use and side effect profiles of opioids, and effective tapering strategies, is vital to delivering safe pain management to pediatric patients. A search in Pubmed was performed on the following topics in both pediatric and adult literature: Opioid dependence, tolerance, withdrawal, and weaning from 2000 to 2018. Articles focused on pediatric data were chosen. Adult data was reviewed and utilized when pediatric data was lacking. Where data was pediatric-focused, specific references were made in the text. All other references refer to adult data.

The aims of this paper were to: (1) Review the current practice of opioid-reduction during pharmacological therapies; and (2) highlight concrete opioid weaning strategies, and management of opioid withdrawal. We reviewed and defined opioid dependence, withdrawal, tolerance and addiction, assessment of opioid withdrawal utilizing age appropriate withdrawal scales, and utilization of wean strategies and pharmacological aids to assist in safe reduction in therapy. This article did not address the use of opioids for pain management specifically or aim to assess pain management outcomes of opioid therapy.

2. Opioid-Reduction Weaning Protocols in Pediatric Patients

Effective medical management of patients receiving opioids can be addressed by appropriate assessment of pain, an accurate understanding of opioids and related side effects and withdrawal, and implementation of opioid reduction strategies including opioid weaning protocols and opioid-sparing adjuvants. Opioid withdrawal may occur in 0–100% of children who are exposed to opioids. Prevalence ranged from 45 to 86% in one recent review [13], while in another study 68% of patients experienced withdrawal [14].

Pediatric weaning protocols are highly variable. In a recent survey of pediatric healthcare providers, only 27% of respondents utilized a written protocol for opioid tapering, 22% consulted a pain management team regarding weaning of opioids, and the majority seldom or never consulted a pharmacist [15]. In another survey of pediatric congenital heart disease centers, only 25% of sites used a standardized clinical pathway when weaning opioid medications [16]. In the RESTORE study—a randomized controlled multicenter study of protocolized sedation of 1225 pediatric patients—Curley et al. demonstrated that the use of protocolized weaning of opioid medication was associated with shorter durations of opioid treatment (9 vs. 10 days, $p = 0.01$), and more study days spent in the calm and awake states (86% vs. 75%, $p = 0.004$) [14].

Common management strategies described in small pediatric studies include the use of methadone, addition of alpha 2 agonists, and protocolized reduction in dosing [17]. The most common weaning strategies involved decreases of 10–20% per day [13]. Identification of high-risk patients can help prevent iatrogenic withdrawal [18]. These include young age, pre-existing cognitive impairment, higher mean preweaning opioid dose, duration of opioid treatment, use of three or more sedative medications, and higher nurse to patient ratio.

The developmental aspects of opioid therapy deserve some consideration. The endogenous opioid system is highly expressed by developing neural cells, and can influence both neuronal as well as glial maturation [19]. While opioids do not directly trigger maturational events, they modulate ongoing cellular processes. These potentially detrimental effects must be balanced against the effects of untreated pain and physiologic stress, which have been associated with adverse outcomes and may also affect subsequent development [20], as well as ongoing clinical care of critically ill children [21]. Research on long-term neurocognitive effects of opioids on children is limited, and confounded by multiple co-existing morbidities [22].

The use of synthetic or short acting opioids may cause greater tolerance in preterm and term neonates. For example, patients receiving fentanyl while on extracorporeal membrane oxygenation (ECMO) require longer durations of opioid weaning compared to neonates who have received morphine during their treatment [23]. Additionally, neonates have immature kidney and liver functions leading to the accumulation of morphine metabolites, notably morphine-3-glucuronide, which can lead to antagonism of analgesia, as well as morphine-6-glucuronide, which is a more potent analgesic in comparison to morphine and may lead to excessive sedation [24].

Therefore, the treating physician must be aware of developmental concerns from pharmacokinetic to pharmacodynamic perspectives, as well as the developmental needs of the child from a neurological and psychological perspective at each phase of the treatment, and weaning processes. The use of appropriate and well timed adjuvant therapies, both pharmacological and nonpharmacological, may help minimize the need for sedatives and analgesics at various stages of the treatment process [25].

3. Opioids and Common Side Effects

The mechanisms of opioid analgesia include inhibiting the transmission of noxious input from the periphery to the central nervous system, and facilitating the descent of the inhibitory system that can decrease noxious input and affective modulation [26,27]. While opioids are very effective at the acute management of pain, some pediatric patients develop physiologic dependence or withdrawal following as little as seven days of opioid therapy [28]. Tolerance and addiction are other potential physiological effects of opioids. See Table 1 for a summary of potential physiological effects described below.

Table 1. Summary of physiological effects [29–31].

Term	Definition	Causative Mechanism
Dependence	A physiologic and biochemical adaptation of neurons such that removing a drug precipitates withdrawal or abstinence syndrome	Activation of second-messenger protein kinases; changes in neurotransmitter levels; changes in neuronal networks
Withdrawal	A clinical syndrome that manifests after stopping or reversing a drug after prolonged exposure to that drug	Superactivation of AC; opioid receptor coupling to G_s protein; activation of excitatory amino acid receptors
Tolerance	Decreasing clinical effects of a drug after prolonged exposure to it	Upregulation of the cAMP pathway; desensitization of opioid receptors
Addiction	A chronic, relapsing syndrome of psychological dependence and craving a drug for its psychedelic, sedative, or euphoric effects; characterized by compulsion, loss of control, and continued use of a substance despite harmful effects	Activation of dopaminergic reward systems in nucleus accumbens; mechanisms associated with tolerance and dependence

3.1. Dependence and Withdrawal

Dependence is an involuntary physiological response that occurs when there is an adaptation to the opioid, which is manifested by withdrawal symptoms when the opioid is abruptly discontinued [30,32]. Common neurologic signs of dependence in children include anxiety, agitation, grimacing, insomnia, increased muscle tone, abnormal tremors, and choreoathetoid movements. Gastrointestinal symptoms include vomiting, diarrhea, and poor appetite, while autonomic signs include tachypnea, tachycardia, fever, sweating, and hypertension [21].

In children, there are still many unanswered questions regarding the long term effects of opioid tolerance and withdrawal [33]. Sirnes et al., in a preliminary study, found that school-age children who had been exposed to prenatal opioids, showed Functional Magnetic Resonance Imaging (fMRI) changes and possible impaired executive function task performance [34]. Although some preliminary animal data suggests that there may be a faster onset of dependence in younger rats, it is unclear whether this applies to pediatric patients, and more studies are needed in this area [21].

The onset of withdrawal is dependent on the characteristics of the opioid the child was exposed to. For shorter acting opioids, such as oxycodone or hydrocodone, the symptoms may start as soon as 12 h after the last dose and peak over the next one or two days. In contrast, when stopping a longer acting opioid such as methadone, the signs of withdrawal may not be seen for more than 24 h and can last up to 10 days [35].

Studies have shown that children at increased risk of iatrogenic withdrawal syndrome include those who are less than six months old, have had a higher cumulative opioid dose or longer duration of exposure, have been exposed to three or more sedative classes (e.g., opioids, benzodiazepines, dexmedetomidine, and ketamine), or have a pre-existing cognitive impairment [18]. Of note, in neonatal abstinence syndrome, newborn infants may be dependent on opioids or benzodiazepines due to in-utero exposure. Following birth, they must be closely observed for signs of withdrawal, and treated as appropriate [18].

In older children, symptoms of delirium—a neurocognitive disorder due to a somatic illness or its treatment—can mimic those of withdrawal such as tachycardia, tachypnea, agitation, irritability, muscle tension, and sleep disturbances [36]. Children who are critically ill or in the Intensive Care Unit (ICU) are at risk of delirium secondary to the multiple sedative agents used, the severity of illness, changes in metabolic dysfunction or infection. Environmental factors such as changes in sleep can be additive [37,38]. One study found that children who received benzodiazepines were at a five-times greater risk of developing delirium than those that did not receive benzodiazepines [39]. Several delirium scoring tools have been developed, such as the Pediatric Confusion Assessment Method for ICU in children over five years of age (modified version of the adult assessment tool) [37]. Several symptoms of delirium such as tachycardia, tachypnea, and agitation are scored on both the withdrawal and delirium scales making definitive diagnostic determination difficult. Appropriate treatment of delirium may include, but is notlimited to, the treatment of any underlying withdrawal.

3.2. Tolerance

Tolerance is a state of physiological adaptation that occurs after prolonged exposure to an opioid. With tolerance, the patient requires progressively larger doses of the opioid to achieve the same effect. Complex intracellular neural mechanisms, including opioid receptor desensitization and down-regulation, are believed to be key mechanisms underlying opioid tolerance [40]. Tolerance can occur as soon as three days after opioid exposure [41]. In critically ill children, the effects can be profound. One multicenter study found that 16% of mechanically ventilated children required doubling of their opioid doses after seven days, and 20% doubled their requirement after 14 days [42]. In spite of potentially rapid development of tolerance in the pediatric population, especially in the case of life-limiting illnesses such as oncologic conditions or other severe illnesses, the rapid escalation and resultant tolerance to keep severely ill pediatric patients comfortable is often justified. [43,44].

3.3. Opioid Induced Hyperalgesia

Research has shown that the administration of higher doses of opioids over longer periods of time does not always lead to improved pain control, rather it can result in hyperalgesia. A recent study found that the regular use of opioids for more than 90 days led to increased pain sensitivity [45]. The exact mechanisms by which patients developcentral sensitization found in opioid induced hyperalgesia is still unknown, but possible contributing factors include characteristics of the opioids being used, changes in corticotrophin releasing factors, suppressed reuptake or increased release of excitatory neurotransmitters, changes in glial cells, and genetic variability [46,47]. Opioid induced hyperalgesia (OIH) is less commonly addressed in pediatric literature. One case report from 2012 noted the development of OIH in a nine year-old receiving opioids for flare of polyarticular juvenile idiopathic arthritis. The child was treated by stopping the opioid. Subsequently, pain and hyperalgesia decreased [48]. Treatment for OIH often involves the reduction or elimination of the opioid to monitor for resolution of symptoms. Ongoing adult research is evaluating ketamine and methadone, which have NMDA receptor antagonist activity, to determine if these medications decrease the likelihood of developing OIH or help resolve symptoms [12].

3.4. Addiction

Chronic opioid use also has the potential to lead to addiction. Addiction, as defined by the American Pain Society and the American Society of Addiction Medicine, is a chronic neurobiological disease with genetic, psychosocial, and environmental factors contributing to its development and presentation [31]. Addiction is characterized by the inability to consistently abstain from an addictive stimulus, impairment in behavioral control, craving, diminished recognition of significant problems with one's behaviors and interpersonal relationships, and a dysfunctional emotional response.

Research has demonstrated that approximately one in four adults receiving chronic opioid therapy in a primary care setting suffers from opioid addiction [49–51]. To our knowledge, there are no published data detailing rates of opioid addiction among youth. Interestingly, in a Canadian study examining methadone maintenance therapy, initial age of opioid use was associated with increased physical and psychological comorbidities. Individuals with an age-of-onset of opioid use younger than 18 years were found to be at higher odds of having a physical or psychiatric comorbid disorder, compared to individuals with an age-of-onset of 31 years or older [52]. Future research should explore rates and risk factors of opioid addiction among pediatric populations, as well as risk factors for addiction. Appropriate treatment of comorbid disorders in patients who are being considered for opioid therapy is recommended to minimize the risk of opioid addiction.

4. Assessment of Opioid Withdrawal

Assessment of opioid withdrawal is central to developing and applying effective opioid-reduction during pharmacological treatments. A number of scales have been developed to help providers distinguish between signs of neonatal withdrawal and iatrogenic withdrawal, and to help determine when treatment might be required. The Finnegan neonatal abstinence scale, and its recent modification, allows clinicians to accurately assess clinical symptoms of neonatal withdrawal [53]. Scores >8 indicate the necessity for further evaluation for treatment.

The Withdrawal Assessment Tool-1 (WAT-1) scores youth on symptoms of withdrawal including tremors, increased muscle tone, repetitive movements, loose stools, and vomiting. This tool was originally validated for children six months to eight years of age [32]; however, more recent studies have found WAT-1 to be reliable for youth up to 17 years of age [54].

The Sophia Observation withdrawal Symptoms scale scores infants and children three months or older on withdrawal symptoms within a four-hour period. Scores >4 should be evaluated further for withdrawal. This scale was found to have a sensitivity of 83%, and specificity of 95% in critically ill children in the Pediatric Intensive Care Unit (PICU) [55]. Only the Sophia Observation withdrawal scale and WAT-1 have been specifically developed to evaluate iatrogenic withdrawal in a range of ages and settings [54].

5. Opioid Weaning Treatments

Although there is no certainty about whether an individual patient will experience symptoms of withdrawal, some general guidelines are helpful for the clinician to consider in developing an individualized opioid-reduction program.

For opioid therapy lasting less than seven days, no gradual reduction in dose is necessary as patients are at a lower risk of withdrawal. The opioid infusion may be discontinued without a taper, and patients should be monitored for signs and symptoms of withdrawal. Additional factors placing a patient at increased risk for withdrawal following opioid therapy lasting less than seven days include higher cumulative dose of opioids and prior exposure to opioids.

When opioid therapy has been delivered for more than seven days, or symptoms of withdrawal are present, gradual opioid weaning is usually necessary. Opioid weaning protocols aim to gradually decrease plasma concentrations of the drug to prevent symptoms of opioid withdrawal syndrome. As no definite outcome-based evidence exists to support an ideal weaning protocol, therapy should be based on the individual treatment response, and should consider the length of opioid exposure and the total daily opioid dose (TDD) [56]. One suggested weaning schedule is to decrease the TDD by 10–20% everyday, while monitoring for signs and symptoms of withdrawal. Oral morphine, methadone, clonidine, and transdermal fentanyl have all been used in opioid weaning programs.

Methadone is often the most suitable medication for weaning due to the long half-life and convenience of oral dosing [57,58]. To account for cross tolerance, the converted methadone dosage may need to be reduced by 30–50%. The total daily dose of methadone is then divided into four equal doses to be given every 6 h (q6hr). Initial q6hr dosing is for 24 h only—this is functionally a "loading dose" to rapidly increase serum levels of methadone. Due to the long half-life of methadone, the dosing interval will change to every 12 h after the initial 24 h period, with close observation for possible sedation. Once a steady state is reached, methadone can then be tapered by 10–20% every other day, observing for symptoms of withdrawal. Of note, methadone is not suitable for children with prolonged QT corrected (QTc). A baseline EKG is recommended prior to initiating therapy with methadone. In these critically ill children, the TDD of their current opioid may be decreased by 10–20% daily until the wean is accomplished, or the patient may be transitioned to another oral or intravenous opioid (e.g., morphine, hydromorphone). See Table 2 for sample opioid weaning schedules.

Table 2. Sample Opioid Weaning Schedules.

Weaning schedules	
IV morphine dose	Methadone total daily dose
<0.05 mg/kg/h	0.3 mg/kg/day
0.05–0.1 mg/kg/h	0.4 mg/kg/day
0.11–0.2 mg/kg/h	0.6 mg/kg/day
0.21–0.4 mg/kg/h	0.8 mg/kg/day
>0.4 mg/kg/h	1 mg/kg/day
IV fentanyl dose	Methadone total daily dose
1 µg /kg/h	0.05 mg/kg/day
2 µg/kg/h	0.1 mg/kg/day
3 µg/kg/h	0.15 mg/kg/day
4 µg/kg/h	0.2 mg/kg/day

Transitioning to enteral methadone should be considered as early as clinically feasible. The bioavailability of enteral methadone is 75–80% that of intravenous methadone, thus it is not usually necessary to adjust dosing for this difference. If converting from high doses of opioid infusions, it is recommended that intravenous infusions be tapered to lower doses (e.g., ≤0.2 mg/kg/h morphine equivalent) before transitioning to methadone.

When weaning patients from opioids, withdrawal and related symptoms often occur and can be distressing for children. Clonidine can be useful in treating these symptoms of opioid withdrawal.

Duffet et al. performed a prospective randomized control trial (RCT) on 50 pediatric patients undergoing reduction of opioid therapy and studied the use of parenteral clonidine 5 µg/kg, administered every 6 h [59]. No significant effect on withdrawal symptoms was observed. Thirteen patients experienced hypotension or bradycardia requiring intervention; however, the relationship to the study group was unclear.

The use of clonidine as a prophylactic for withdrawal syndromes was studied in 10 consecutive patients undergoing single-state laryngotracheal reconstruction [60]. No significant side effects were noted. A study of plasma concentrations of whole vs. cut patches showed that the delivered dose from whole patches was found to be 7 ± 1.7 μg/kg/day (plasma concentration 0.55 ± 0.3 ng/mL), while cut patches delivered a lower dose but with increased variability, 6.4 ± 3 μg/kg/day (plasma concentration 1 ± 1.1 ng/mL) [61]. A recent review suggested that, while oral and transdermal clonidine have a potential role in the management of sedation and withdrawal in critically ill infants and children, and were relatively well tolerated, the use of cut transdermal patches should be avoided [62]. Further prospective studies were recommended. No data exists on the weaning of clonidine dose following its use as an adjuvant for opioid withdrawal [53]. The recommendations noted below are a result of developed clinical practice at our institution.

Sample Clonidine Dosing and Weaning Schedule

1. Start with clonidine 4–8 μg/kg/day oral (per os (PO)) divided every 4 h. If not taking oral intake (nil per os (NPO)), give clonidine 1 μg/kg IV q4h.
2. Concurrently initiate opioid weaning by reducing daily opioid dose by 5–10% of baseline dose.
3. After 48 h on oral or parenteral clonidine without adverse blood pressure effects, convert to clonidine patch 5–10 μg/kg/day, rounding up or down to nearest 50 μg increment.
4. The minimum patient weight for patch use is typically about 5 kg. Although doses as high as 2 μg/kg may be tolerated, the physical patch size makes it difficult to use in smaller children. Therefore, for children ≤5 kg, use oral or intravenous (i.v.) clonidine.
5. Once ready to wean, reduce the clonidine patch size by 50 μg/day two times a week until the dose is reduced to the 100 μg/day patch size for children >10 kg, or 50 μg/day patch size for children <10 kg. Then leave this last patch on for 14 days and discontinue afterwards.
6. Clonidine weaning may occur concomitantly with opioid weaning, provided the opioid parenteral morphine equivalent dose is less than 0.3 mg/kg/day.

For excessive withdrawal (WAT-1 > 3), the total as needed (pro re nata (PRN)) morphine requirement may be added to the daily methadone dose, and the taper resumed once symptoms are controlled consistently. For excessive sedation, a dose of methadone should be held, and the total daily methadone dose decreased by 10–20%. Ondansetron 0.1 mg/kg up to 4 mg every 6 h may be used to treat nausea related to withdrawal [63]. Patients should be assessed for QT prolongation, particularly if other QT-prolonging medications are being used [64]. Co-administration of benzodiazepines with opioids is frequently practiced in the context of intensive care sedation or in acute postoperative pain management settings. When discontinuation is planned, the benzodiazepines may need concurrent weaning, often alternating with the opioid wean, as described in a recent review by Fenn et al. [13]. Care should be taken due to the risk of over sedation when opioids and benzodiazepines are co-administered. Conversely, when benzodiazepines are reduced rapidly, withdrawal, agitation, and other potentially life-threatening side effects such as seizures may occur. The use of a flexible patient-centered approach is important where weaning of multiple medications is needed [65].

6. Adjuvant Therapies for Opioid Reduction Therapy

When implementing opioid-reduction pharmacological treatments, adjuvant therapies are regularly considered for possible integration into treatment regimens. Adjuvant analgesics target specific aspects of nociceptive and neuropathic pain physiology, reducing pain and opioid consumption [25]. Nociceptive analgesics include acetaminophen, non-steroidal anti-inflammatory drugs (NSAIDS), and glucocorticoids. Neuropathic analgesics commonly include gabapentinoids, lidocaine, ketamine, alpha-2-agonists, and rare use of tricyclic antidepressants and serotonin and norepinephrine reuptake inhibitors. Low dose ketamine may be helpful as an adjuvant to assist in weaning off opioid therapy [66].

Cannabidiol (CBD) is another adjuvant therapy that is increasingly considered for chronic pain management treatments. CBD is one of the active cannabinoids identified in cannabis. CBD does not appear to have the hallucinogenic/intoxication side effects of another major component of cannabis, tetrahydrocannabinol (THC) [67]. Randomized controlled studies are needed to further examine the efficacy of medical cannabis and its potential use in opioid weaning therapy.

Integrating adjuvant therapies with nonpharmacological therapies such as cognitive behavioral therapy, mindfulness, hypnosis, and acupuncture is commonly employed during opioid-reduction pharmacological treatments to optimize patient comfort, functional well-being, and quality of life. Consultation with a pain management specialists can facilitate this integrative opioid reduction approach.

7. Conclusions

Opioid use has risen significantly in the past two decades. Although opioids are an effective means of managing acute pain, risks associated with opioids are plentiful and may outweigh such benefits, especially when treating chronic pain. Having an accurate understanding of opioid-related side effects, age appropriate tools for assessment of withdrawal, and opioid reduction strategies, may help to minimize symptoms of withdrawal and safely reduce or discontinue opioid therapy.

As outlined above, opioids can be safely tapered in both acute and chronic settings by gradually reducing the total opioid dose or, if appropriate, transitioning to a long acting opioid such as methadone, followed by a gradual weaning protocol and close observation for symptoms of withdrawal. Opioid-sparing adjuvants, including acetaminophen, non-steroidal agents, gabapentinoids, benzodiazepines, ketamine and alpha-1-agonists, can also provide safe and effective analgesia and sedation, and may reduce the necessity and/or dose of opioid therapy. Alpha-1-agonists in particular may help in management of withdrawal symptoms. Opioid reduction utilizingpharmacological protocols provides a safe and efficacious way to decrease opioid therapy when this is appropriate, and minimizes related adverse side effects.

Author Contributions: Conceptualization, All; Methodology, All; Investigation, All; Tables, G.D.; Writing-Original Draft Preparation, All; Writing-Review & Editing, All; Supervision, B.G.

References

1. Blendon, R.J.; Benson, J.M. The public and the opioid-abuse epidemic. *N. Engl. J. Med.* **2018**, *378*, 407–411. [CrossRef] [PubMed]
2. Fields, H.L. The doctor's dilemma: Opiate analgesics and chronic pain. *Neuron* **2011**, *69*, 591–594. [CrossRef] [PubMed]
3. Krane, E.J.; Weisman, S.J.; Walco, G.A. The national opioid epidemic and the risk of outpatient opioids in children. *Pediatrics* **2018**, *142*. [CrossRef] [PubMed]
4. Ossipov, M.H.; Morimura, K.; Porreca, F. Descending pain modulation and chronification of pain. *Curr. Opin. Support. Palliat. Care* **2014**, *8*, 143–151. [PubMed]
5. Nummenmaa, L.; Tuominen, L. Opioid system and human emotions. *Br. J. Pharmacol.* **2017**, *175*, 2737–2749. [CrossRef]
6. Koch, T.; Hollt, V. Role of receptor internalization in opioid tolerance and dependence. *Pharmacol. Ther.* **2008**, *117*, 199–206. [CrossRef]
7. Berde, C.; Nurko, S. Opioid side effects—Mechanism-based therapy. *N. Engl. J. Med.* **2008**, *358*, 2400–2402. [CrossRef]
8. Moore, R.A.; McQuay, H.J. Prevalence of opioid adverse events in chronic non-malignant pain: Systematic review of randomised trials of oral opioids. *Arthritis Res. Ther.* **2005**, *7*, R1046–R1051. [CrossRef]
9. Gomes, T.; Mamdani, M.M.; Dhalla, I.A.; Paterson, J.M.; Juurlink, D.N. Opioid dose and drug-related mortality in patients with nonmalignant pain. *Arch. Intern. Med.* **2011**, *171*, 686–691. [CrossRef] [PubMed]
10. Grunkemeier, D.M.; Cassara, J.E.; Dalton, C.B.; Drossman, D.A. The narcotic bowel syndrome: Clinical features, pathophysiology, and management. *Clin. Gastroenterol. Hepatol.* **2007**, *5*, 1126–1139. [CrossRef]

11. Fudin, J.; Raouf, M.; Wegrzyn, E.L. *Opioid Dosing Policy: Pharmacological Considerations Regarding Equianalgesic Dosing*; American Academy of Integrative Pain Management: Lenexa, KS, USA, 2017.
12. Lee, M.; Silverman, S.M.; Hansen, H.; Patel, V.B.; Manchikanti, L. A comprehensive review of opioid-induced hyperalgesia. *Pain Phys.* **2011**, *14*, 145–161.
13. Fenn, N.E., 3rd; Plake, K.S. Opioid and benzodiazepine weaning in pediatric patients: Review of current literature. *Pharmacotherapy* **2017**, *37*, 1458–1468. [CrossRef]
14. Curley, M.A.; Wypij, D.; Watson, R.S.; Grant, M.J.; Asaro, L.A.; Cheifetz, I.M.; Dodson, B.L.; Franck, L.S.; Gedeit, R.G.; Angus, D.C.; et al. Protocolized sedation vs. usual care in pediatric patients mechanically ventilated for acute respiratory failure: A randomized clinical trial. *JAMA* **2015**, *313*, 379–389. [CrossRef]
15. Deborah, F.; Ameringer, S.W. Survey of opioid tapering practices of pediatric healthcare providers: A national perspective. *J. Opioid Manag.* **2017**, *13*, 59–64.
16. O'Connell, C.; Ziniel, S.; Hartwell, L.; Connor, J. Management of Opioid and Sedative Weaning in Pediatric Congenital Heart Disease Patients: Assessing the State of Practice. *Dimens. Crit. Care Nurs.* **2017**, *36*, 116–124.
17. Chiu, A.W.; Contreras, S.; Mehta, S.; Korman, J.; Perreault, M.M.; Williamson, D.R.; Burry, L.D. Iatrogenic Opioid Withdrawal in Critically Ill Patients: A Review of Assessment Tools and Management. *Ann. Pharmacother.* **2017**, *51*, 1099–1111. [CrossRef]
18. Best, K.M.; Wypij, D.; Asaro, L.A.; Curley, M.A. Randomized evaluation of sedation titration for respiratory failure study investigators. Patient, process, and system predictors of iatrogenic withdrawal syndrome in critically ill children. *Crit. Care Med.* **2017**, *45*, e7–e15. [CrossRef]
19. Hauser, K.F.; Knapp, P.E. Opiate drugs with abuse liability hijack the endogenous opioid system to disrupt neuronal and glial maturation in the central nervous system. *Front. Pediatr.* **2017**, *5*, 294. [CrossRef]
20. Holsti, L.; Weinberg, J.; Whitfield, M.F.; Grunau, R.E. Relationships between adrenocorticotropic hormone and cortisol are altered during clustered nursing care in preterm infants born at extremely low gestational age. *Early Hum. Dev.* **2007**, *83*, 341–348. [CrossRef]
21. Anand, K.J.; Willson, D.F.; Berger, J.; Harrison, R.; Meert, K.L.; Zimmerman, J.; Carcillo, J.; Newth, C.J.; Prodhan, P.; Dean, J.M.; et al. Tolerance and withdrawal from prolonged opioid use in critically ill children. *Pediatrics* **2010**, *125*, e1208–e1225. [CrossRef]
22. Jain, G.; Mahendra, V.; Singhal, S.; Dzara, K.; Pilla, T.R.; Manworren, R.; Kaye, A.D. Long-term neuropsychological effects of opioid use in children: A descriptive literature review. *Pain Phys.* **2014**, *17*, 109–118. [CrossRef]
23. Franck, L.S.; Vilardi, J.; Durand, D.; Powers, R. Opioid withdrawal in neonates after continuous infusions of morphine or fentanyl during extracorporeal membrane oxygenation. *Am. J. Crit. Care* **1998**, *7*, 364–369.
24. Suresh, S.; Anand, K.J. Opioid tolerance in neonates: A state-of-the-art review. *Paediatr. Anaesth.* **2001**, *11*, 511–521. [CrossRef]
25. Brooks, M.R.; Golianu, B. Perioperative management in children with chronic pain. *Paediatr. Anaesth.* **2016**, *26*, 794–806. [CrossRef]
26. Bannister, K.; Kucharczyk, M.; Dickenson, A.H. Hopes for the future of pain control. *Pain Ther.* **2017**, *6*, 117–128. [CrossRef]
27. D'Mello, R.; Dickenson, A.H. Spinal cord mechanisms of pain. *Br. J. Anaesth.* **2008**, *101*, 8–16. [CrossRef]
28. Best, K.M.; Boullata, J.I.; Curley, M.A. Risk factors associated with iatrogenic opioid and benzodiazepine withdrawal in critically ill pediatric patients: A systematic review and conceptual model. *Pediatr. Crit. Care Med.* **2015**, *16*, 175–183. [CrossRef]
29. Heit, H.A. Addiction, physical dependence, and tolerance: Precise definitions to help clinicians evaluate and treat chronic pain patients. *J. Pain Palliat. Care Pharmacother.* **2003**, *17*, 15–29. [CrossRef]
30. Galinkin, J.; Koh, J.L.; Committee on Drugs; Section On Anesthesiology and Pain Medicine; American Academy of Pediatrics. Recognition and management of iatrogenically induced opioid dependence and withdrawal in children. *Pediatrics* **2014**, *133*, 152–155. [CrossRef]
31. American Society of Addiction Medicine. Public Policy Statement: Definition of Addiction. Available online: https://www.asam.org/advocacy/find-a-policy-statement/view-policy-statement/public-policy-statements/2011/12/15/the-definition-of-addiction (accessed on 14 June 2018).
32. Franck, L.S.; Scoppettuolo, L.A.; Wypij, D.; Curley, M.A. Validity and generalizability of the Withdrawal Assessment Tool-1 (WAT-1) for monitoring iatrogenic withdrawal syndrome in pediatric patients. *Pain* **2012**, *153*, 142–148. [CrossRef]

33. Maguire, D.J.; Taylor, S.; Armstrong, K.; Shaffer-Hudkins, E.; Germain, A.M.; Brooks, S.S.; Cline, G.J.; Clark, L. Long-term outcomes of infants with neonatal abstinence syndrome. *Neonatal Netw.* **2016**, *35*, 277–286. [CrossRef]
34. Sirnes, E.; Griffiths, S.T.; Aukland, S.M.; Eide, G.E.; Elgen, I.B.; Gundersen, H. Functional MRI in prenatally opioid-exposed children during a working memory-selective attention task. *Neurotoxicol. Teratol.* **2018**, *66*, 46–54. [CrossRef]
35. American Society of Addiction Medicine. National Practice Guideline for the Use of Medications in the Treatment of Addiction Involving Opioid Use. Available online: https://www.asam.org/docs/default-source/practice-support/guidelines-and-consensus-docs/asam-national-practice-guideline-supplement.pdf?sfvrsn=24 (accessed on 5 September 2018).
36. Harris, J.; Ramelet, A.S.; van Dijk, M.; Pokorna, P.; Wielenga, J.; Tume, L.; Tibboel, D.; Ista, E. Clinical recommendations for pain, sedation, withdrawal and delirium assessment in critically ill infants and children: An ESPNIC position statement for healthcare professionals. *Intensive Care Med.* **2016**, *42*, 972–986. [CrossRef]
37. Madden, K.; Burns, M.M.; Tasker, R.C. Differentiating delirium from sedative/hypnotic-related iatrogenic withdrawal syndrome: Lack of specificity in pediatric critical care assessment tools. *Pediatr. Crit. Care Med.* **2017**, *18*, 580–588. [CrossRef]
38. Thorn, R.P. Pediatric delirium. *Am. J. Psychiatry Resid. J.* **2017**, *12*, 6–8.
39. Traube, C.; Silver, G.; Gerber, L.M.; Kaur, S.; Mauer, E.A.; Kerson, A.; Joyce, C.; Greenwald, B.M. Delirium and mortality in critically ill children: Epidemiology and outcomes of pediatric delirium. *Crit. Care Med.* **2017**, *45*, 891–898. [CrossRef]
40. Williams, J.T.; Ingram, S.L.; Henderson, G.; Chavkin, C.; von Zastrow, M.; Schulz, S.; Koch, T.; Evans, C.J.; Christie, M.J. Regulation of mu-opioid receptors: Desensitization, phosphorylation, internalization, and tolerance. *Pharmacol. Rev.* **2013**, *65*, 223–254. [CrossRef]
41. Jenkins, I.A. Tolerance and addiction; the patient, the parent or the clinician? *Paediatr. Anaesth.* **2011**, *21*, 794–799. [CrossRef]
42. Anand, K.J.; Clark, A.E.; Willson, D.F.; Berger, J.; Meert, K.L.; Zimmerman, J.J.; Harrison, R.; Carcillo, J.A.; Newth, C.J.; Bisping, S.; et al. Opioid analgesia in mechanically ventilated children: Results from the multicenter Measuring Opioid Tolerance Induced by Fentanyl study. *Pediatr. Crit. Care Med.* **2013**, *14*, 27–36. [CrossRef]
43. Slater, M.E.; De Lima, J.; Campbell, K.; Lane, L.; Collins, J. Opioids for the management of severe chronic nonmalignant pain in children: A retrospective 1-year practice survey in a children's hospital. *Pain Med.* **2010**, *11*, 207–214. [CrossRef]
44. McCulloch, R.; Collins, J.J. Pain in children who have life-limiting conditions. *Child. Adolesc. Psychiatr. Clin. N. Am.* **2006**, *15*, 657–682. [CrossRef]
45. Samuelsen, P.J.; Nielsen, C.S.; Wilsgaard, T.; Stubhaug, A.; Svendsen, K.; Eggen, A.E. Pain sensitivity and analgesic use among 10,486 adults: The Tromso study. *BMC Pharmacol. Toxicol.* **2017**, *18*, 45. [CrossRef]
46. Weber, L.; Yeomans, D.C.; Tzabazis, A. Opioid-induced hyperalgesia in clinical anesthesia practice: What has remained from theoretical concepts and experimental studies? *Curr. Opin. Anaesthesiol.* **2017**, *30*, 458–465. [CrossRef]
47. Bannister, K.; Dickenson, A.H. Opioid hyperalgesia. *Curr. Opin. Support. Palliat. Care* **2010**, *4*, 1–5. [CrossRef]
48. Vijayan, V.; Moran, R.; Elder, M.E.; Sukumaran, S. Acute-onset opioid-induced hyperalgesia in a child with juvenile idiopathic arthritis. *J. Clin. Rheumatol.* **2012**, *18*, 349–351. [CrossRef]
49. Banta-Green, C.J.; Merrill, J.O.; Doyle, S.R.; Boudreau, D.M.; Calsyn, D.A. Opioid use behaviors, mental health and pain—Development of a typology of chronic pain patients. *Drug Alcohol. Depend.* **2009**, *104*, 34–42. [CrossRef]
50. Boscarino, J.A.; Rukstalis, M.; Hoffman, S.N.; Han, J.J.; Erlich, P.M.; Gerhard, G.S.; Stewart, W.F. Risk factors for drug dependence among out-patients on opioid therapy in a large US health-care system. *Addiction* **2010**, *105*, 1776–1782. [CrossRef]
51. Fleming, M.F.; Balousek, S.L.; Klessig, C.L.; Mundt, M.P.; Brown, D.D. Substance use disorders in a primary care sample receiving daily opioid therapy. *J. Pain* **2007**, *8*, 573–582. [CrossRef]

52. Naji, L.; Dennis, B.B.; Bawor, M.; Varenbut, M.; Daiter, J.; Plater, C.; Pare, G.; Marsh, D.C.; Worster, A.; Desai, D.; et al. The association between age of onset of opioid use and comorbidity among opioid dependent patients receiving methadone maintenance therapy. *Addict. Sci. Clin. Pract.* **2017**, *12*, 9. [CrossRef]
53. Zimmermann-Baer, U.; Notzli, U.; Rentsch, K.; Bucher, H.U. Finnegan neonatal abstinence scoring system: Normal values for first 3 days and weeks 5-6 in non-addicted infants. *Addiction* **2010**, *105*, 524–528. [CrossRef]
54. Hardesty, A.; Letzkus, L.; Miller, J.; Turner, L.; Conaway, M. Determining the reliability of the Withdrawal Assessment Tool-1 incomparison to the Neonatal Drug Withdrawal Scoring System. *Clin. Nurs. Stud.* **2015**, *3*, 66–71.
55. Ista, E.; de Hoog, M.; Tibboel, D.; Duivenvoorden, H.J.; van Dijk, M. Psychometric evaluation of the Sophia Observation withdrawal symptoms scale in critically ill children. *Pediatr. Crit. Care Med.* **2013**, *14*, 761–769. [CrossRef]
56. Dervan, L.A.; Yaghmai, B.; Watson, R.S.; Wolf, F.M. The use of methadone to facilitate opioid weaning in pediatric critical care patients: A systematic review of the literature and meta-analysis. *Paediatr. Anaesth.* **2017**, *27*, 228–239. [CrossRef]
57. Siddappa, R.; Fletcher, J.E.; Heard, A.M.; Kielma, D.; Cimino, M.; Heard, C.M. Methadone dosage for prevention of opioid withdrawal in children. *Paediatr. Anaesth.* **2003**, *13*, 805–810. [CrossRef]
58. Giby, K.; Vaillancourt, R.; Varughese, N.; Vadeboncoeur, C.; Pouliot, A. Use of methadone for opioid weaning in children: Prescribing practices and trends. *Can. J. Hosp. Pharm.* **2014**, *67*, 149–156. [CrossRef]
59. Duffett, M.; Choong, K.; Foster, J.; Cheng, J.; Meade, M.O.; Menon, K.; Cook, D.J. Clonidine in the sedation of mechanically ventilated children: A pilot randomized trial. *J. Crit. Care* **2014**, *29*, 758–763. [CrossRef]
60. Deutsch, E.S.; Nadkarni, V.M. Clonidine prophylaxis for narcotic and sedative withdrawal syndrome following laryngotracheal reconstruction. *Arch. Otolaryngol. Head Neck Surg.* **1996**, *122*, 1234–1238. [CrossRef]
61. Zuppa, A.F.; Tejani, S.M.; Cullen, E.J., Jr.; Nadkarni, V.M. Plasma Concentrations Following Application of Whole versus Cut Transdermal Clonidine Patches To Critically Ill Children. *J. Pediatr. Pharmacol. Ther.* **2004**, *9*, 43–48. [CrossRef]
62. Capino, A.C.; Miller, J.L.; Johnson, P.N. Clonidine for Sedation and Analgesia and Withdrawal in Critically Ill Infants and Children. *Pharmacotherapy* **2016**, *36*, 1290–1299. [CrossRef]
63. Gan, T.J.; Diemunsch, P.; Habib, A.S.; Kovac, A.; Kranke, P.; Meyer, T.A.; Watcha, M.; Chung, F.; Angus, S.; Apfel, C.C.; et al. Consensus guidelines for the management of postoperative nausea and vomiting. *Anesth. Analg.* **2014**, *118*, 85–113. [CrossRef]
64. Tobias, J.D. Tolerance, withdrawal, and physical dependency after long-term sedation and analgesia of children in the pediatric intensive care unit. *Crit. Care Med.* **2000**, *28*, 2122–2132. [CrossRef]
65. Siden, H.B.; Collin, K. Three patients and their drugs: A parallel case paper on paediatric opiate use and withdrawal. *Paediatr. Child. Health* **2005**, *10*, 163–168. [CrossRef]
66. Quinlan, J. The use of a subanesthetic infusion of intravenous ketamine to allow withdrawal of medically prescribed opioids in people with chronic pain, opioid tolerance and hyperalgesia: Outcome at 6 months. *Pain Med.* **2012**, *13*, 1524–1525. [CrossRef]
67. Jensen, B.; Chen, J.; Furnish, T.; Wallace, M. Medical marijuana and chronic pain: A review of basic science and clinical evidence. *Curr. Pain Headache Rep.* **2015**, *19*, 50. [CrossRef]

12

Do Mothers Benefit from a Child-Focused Cognitive Behavioral Treatment (CBT) for Childhood Functional Abdominal Pain?

Claudia Calvano [1], Martina Groß [2] and Petra Warschburger [1,*]

[1] Counseling Psychology, University of Potsdam, Potsdam 14469, Germany; calvano@uni-potsdam.de
[2] Deutsche Morbus Crohn/Colitis ulcerosa Vereinigung (DCCV e.V.), Berlin 10179, Germany; mgross@dccv.de
* Correspondence: warschb@uni-potsdam.de

Abstract: While the efficacy of cognitive-behavioral treatment (CBT) approaches for childhood functional abdominal pain (FAP) is well-established for child outcomes, only a few studies have reported on parent-specific outcomes. This randomized controlled pilot trial analyzed effects of a group CBT on maternal variables (i.e., pain-related behavior, worries and self-efficacy, as well as general psychosocial strain). *Methods*: The sample constituted of 15 mothers in the intervention group (IG) and 14 mothers in the waitlist control group (WLC). Outcome measures were assessed pre-treatment, post-treatment and at three months follow-up. *Results*: Analyses revealed significant, large changes in maladaptive maternal reactions related to the child's abdominal pain in the IG compared to the WLC—i.e., reduced attention (d = 0.95), medical help-seeking (d = 0.92), worries (d = 1.03), as well as a significant increase in behaviors that encourage the child's self-management (d = 1.03). In addition, maternal self-efficacy in dealing with a child's pain significantly increased in the IG as well (d = 0.92). Treatment effects emerged post-treatment and could be maintained until three months follow-up. There were no effects on general self-efficacy and maternal quality of life. *Conclusion*: While these results are promising, and underline the efficacy of the CBT approach for both the child and mothers, further studies, including long-term follow-ups, are warranted.

Keywords: functional abdominal pain; parents; CBT; behavior; self-efficacy; RCT; waitlist control

---

1. Introduction

Functional abdominal pain (FAP) is very prevalent in childhood [1], highly impairing [2] and persistent when untreated [3]. Not only do the children suffer from increased psychological distress [4,5] and a poor health-related quality of life [6,7], childhood FAP also affects the family functioning and is commonly associated with parental stress [8]. Furthermore, literature suggests that parents often influence a child's coping and course of abdominal pain [8,9] therefore a parent's reaction when the child experiences pain can be pivotal. This is especially true for parental protective behaviors, such as excusing the child from school or household chores and increased attention when their child is in pain—which are often seen as maladaptive behaviors—and can be associated with a child's impairment [10–12] and increased healthcare use due to abdominal pain [13].

Current literature reports that a significant number of parents experience high psychological strain and a poor quality of life [14–16]. Taking this into account, analyses of treatment effects on parents' psychosocial well-being should be of interest to researchers as well. The efficacy of cognitive behavioral treatment (CBT) approaches for FAP, in reducing a child's pain and disability, is well-established [17–20]. Despite the critical role parents play in pediatric pain, comparatively few data exist focusing on parent-specific outcomes in relation to these approaches [21,22]. Results from controlled trials have suggested that significant effects on parental protective behavior and threat beliefs can be seen up to 12 months post-intervention [23–25]. A short-term improvement of maladaptive parental responses was also reported [25]. However, thus far, there is no data analyzing the effects on parents' self-efficacy, which can be an important mediating mechanism underlying behavioral changes [26,27]. In pediatric pain research, self-efficacy refers to the perceived competence in dealing with pain in everyday life [28]. Analyzing this construct may extend current knowledge on parent-specific treatment effects [22] and could identify possible mediators for long-term sustenance of change.

This report aims to fill these gaps by analyzing the effects of an outpatient, manualized CBT group for children suffering from FAP (described in [29]), on the mothers' behavior, worries, self-efficacy and quality of life. Data are derived from a randomized controlled trial (RCT) that included a waitlist control group (WLC) and three months follow-up. Positive, large-sized effects on self-reported pain, coping and health-related quality of life were observed in the children's outcomes [30,31]. In line with these favorable effects on the affected children, we hypothesize that the mothers in the intervention group (IG) compared to the WLC, will report a more pronounced reduction of child's pain and gastrointestinal (GI) symptoms.

Additionally, we hypothesize that mothers in the IG compared to the WLC will show a more pronounced reduction in: (1) attention, protective behavior, medical help-seeking; in (2) pain-related worries; and a more pronounced increase in (3) behavior encouraging child's self-management; and in (4) their self-efficacy in dealing with the child's pain. In an exploratory manner, we will analyze whether positive changes will also be observed in the mothers' general self-efficacy and quality of life.

2. Materials and Methods

2.1. Study Design and Procedure

The study is a prospective RCT with a parallel waitlist design for the evaluation of a group cognitive behavioral program for children aged 6–12 years suffering from FAP (Current Controlled Trials registration ISRCTN 69830258). Figure 1 displays the RCT flow chart, which follows CONSORT guidelines. The complete CONSORT checklist is provided (Table S1) as an online supplementary document. Eligible families were recruited from an epidemiological study on the psychological well-being of primary school children over a 15-month period (recruitment: April 2008–July 2009). Eligibility criteria for further medical and psychological examination referred to the children, and were defined as the occurrence of chronic abdominal pain at least once a week and lack of organic findings which could account for the symptoms. The 144 eligible cases were invited for further examination to confirm self-reported questionnaire data. This included referring the child for a medical examination for the diagnosis of pediatric FAP and a psychological examination by a standardized diagnostic parent interview [32] to eliminate the possibility that the child fulfills criteria for a psychiatric disorder, according to ICD-10. For pain symptomatology, Rome-III diagnosis of Functional Abdominal Pain Syndrome (FAPS) [33] had to be fulfilled. Diagnosis of FAPS, according to Rome III, requires abdominal pain at least once per week for at least two months, along with associated impairment in everyday life or occurrence of other bodily complaints. A detailed description of the study design can be found in previous publications by the authors [30,31].

In total, 29 families were included and randomized to either the IG (n = 15) or the WLC (n = 14), applying a 1:1 allocation ratio. A computer-assisted randomization sequence was generated, with no restriction, and conducted by a person not involved in the study, and one of the authors enrolled the participants and assigned them to interventions based on the randomization results. Due to the waitlist control design, blinding was not possible. Data were collected at diagnostic examination (T0), two weeks pre-treatment (T1), 2 weeks post-treatment (T2) and 3 months post-treatment (T3). Data collection, as well as the intervention, took place in the outpatient Patient Training Center (PTC) for chronically ill children and their parents, associated with the Counseling Psychology Department of the University of Potsdam, over a 20-month period (interventions: April 2008–December 2009). In the IG, four groups were conducted consecutively. One child in the IG dropped out after the second child session due to an injury (broken leg) and the family did not participate any longer in the training program (the parents did not take part in the parent session, which was scheduled after the third child session) [29]. The participants in the WLC were offered a participation in the training program, only after completion of T3 assessments, which was approximately five months after inclusion. The study was approved by the Ethics Committee of the University of Potsdam.

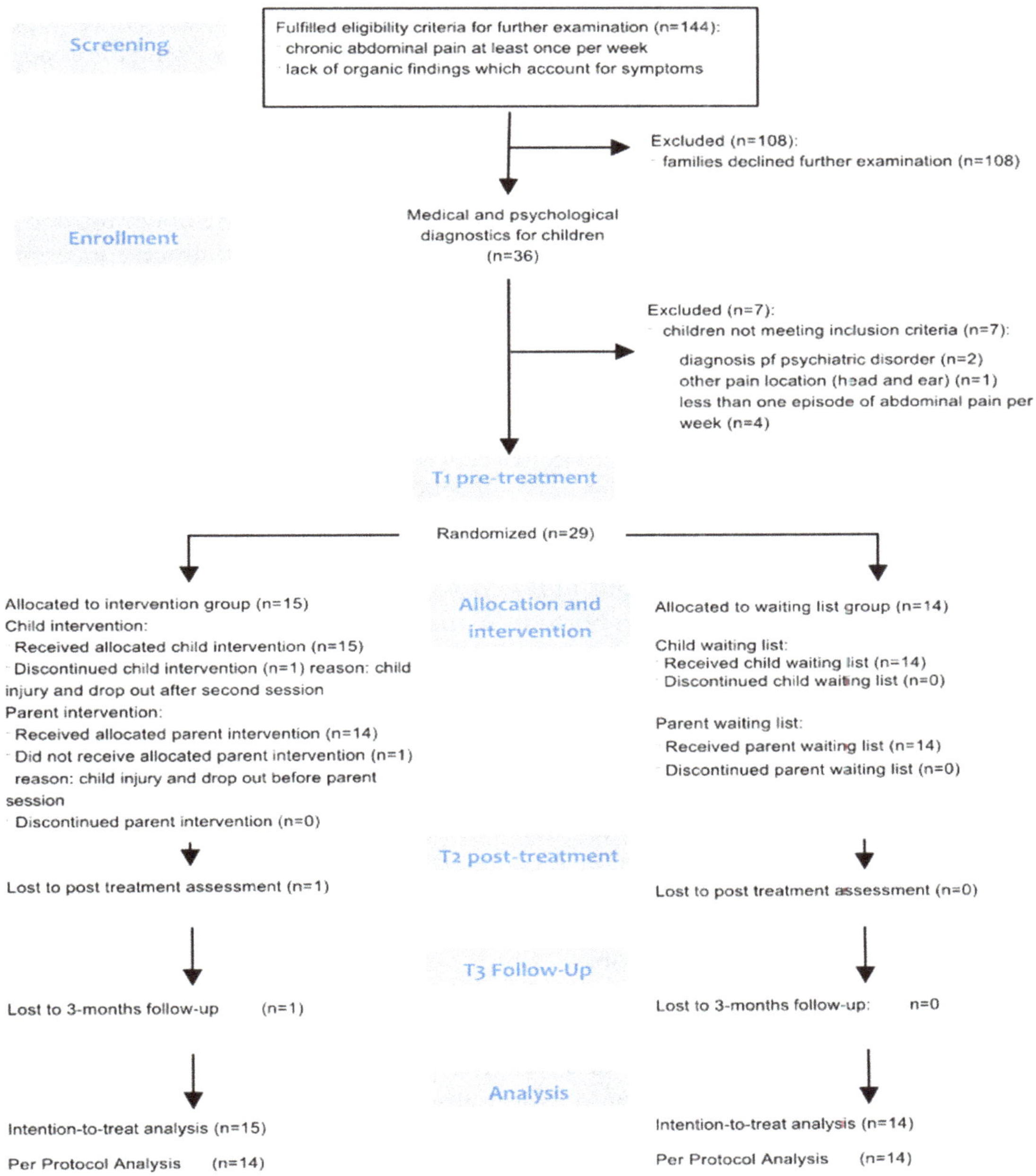

Figure 1. Trial flow chart. Adapted and extended for parent analysis from [31].

2.2. *Intervention*

Families assigned to the IG received the manualized, cognitive-behavioral, child-centered group intervention entitled "Stop the pain with Happy Pingu" [29], including six group sessions for the children (weekly; each 90 min) and one parent group session (90 min). The primary aim of the training was to enhance the children's self-management skills to cope with their pain. In order to attain this goal, children participated alone in the sessions without their parents, learned different skills to cope with their pain and were encouraged to do their regular homework (relaxation and practice of coping skills) on their own. In particular, children were instructed to apply cognitive-behavioral techniques, such as progressive muscle relaxation, distraction, cognitive restructuring and stopping negative thoughts [29,31].

The main goal of the parent session was to foster trust in the new competencies that the child had acquired. Parents received detailed information about the contents of the preceding sessions with the children and the biopsychosocial disease model underlying the intervention. Thereby, parents were asked to reflect on their own role in maintaining the disorder. The group training allowed the mutual exchange of personal experiences and the discussion of potential maladaptive reactions. In particular, parents were encouraged to rely on the competencies the child had learned and to support their child to implement these skills in their pain-coping activities. This was based on a mutual exchange led by the trainer, not on practices of behavioral responses. In addition, parents were informed how to recognize clinical alarm signals, according to the recommendations of the Subcommittee on Chronic Abdominal Pain in Children [34]. Since carbohydrate malabsorptions are common concerns in children suffering from FAP, nutritional guidelines were discussed, with the focus on a balanced diet [29]. This part of the parent session was conducted by a nutrition scientist, with the remaining contents, as well as the child sessions, conducted by one of the authors.

2.3. *Measures*

For this study, primary outcomes refer to pain-related measures (i.e., parental perception of pain and GI symptoms, parent's behavior, worries and self-efficacy). Secondary outcomes refer to general self-efficacy and the parent's quality of life. In addition, treatment satisfaction in the IG was also assessed. Except for the demographic and socioeconomic measures (T0), primary and secondary outcome data were assessed pre-treatment (T1), post-treatment (T2) and at 3 months follow-up (T3). Parents of the intervention group reported on treatment satisfaction for the intervention at post-treatment (T2).

2.3.1. Demographic and Socioeconomic Measures

Child age, gender and number of siblings were reported by the mothers. In addition, child psychological distress was assessed in the parent report of the validated German version of the Strengths and Difficulties Questionnaire (SDQ) [35]. To evaluate its clinical impact, the total problem score was compared with German normative values; scores were classified as normal, borderline and abnormal psychological distress. Socioeconomic status (SES) was assessed according to the procedure defined by Blossfeld [36], which was a validated and broadly used measure to include the parent's educational level and current work situation.

2.3.2. Treatment Satisfaction

To assess treatment satisfaction, we adapted the parent version of the Therapy Evaluation Questionnaire [37], a validated questionnaire originally developed for the psychotherapy setting. In our study, 15 of the 21 items were adapted to properly fit to our context (i.e., "therapy"/"therapist" was replaced by "training"/"trainer" and "problem" was replaced by "pain"). The 21 items were split into two scales: treatment success (7 items, e.g., "I got a better understanding of child's pain"; "I was able to positively change my behavior in the course of training") and treatment process (14 items, e.g., "The trainer understood our situation"; "I was able to openly talk to the trainer about the problems which made us come here"). Answer format was on a 5-point scale: (1) not at all/never; (2) hardly/seldom; (3) partly/sometimes; (4) predominantly/mostly; (5) exactly/always. According to the manual, we also calculated the total score as the mean of all items. The questionnaire was administered to the mothers of the IG at the T2 session post-treatment (n = 14). The raw scores and total score had good internal consistencies (treatment success: $\alpha = 0.83$; treatment process: $\alpha = 0.81$; total score: $\alpha = 0.89$). Scale scores and the total score were compared with normative data.

2.3.3. Parental Perceptions of Changes in Abdominal Pain

Mothers were asked about changes in their child's abdominal pain symptoms (i.e., intensity, duration and frequency) in short, standardized interviews conducted by a psychologist at T1, T2 and T3. Answers were recorded on graded scales for a standardized recording of answers. Data from pre-intervention assessment (T1) referred to the last seven days and included pain location, intensity, frequency and duration. T1 data were then analyzed for a sample description. At post-intervention (T2) and follow-up (T3), parents were asked to rate the change of pain since the end of the intervention ("How did the abdominal pain change since the end of the intervention?") with respect to the overall change of pain (very much improved; somewhat improved; not changed; somewhat worsened; very much worsened), perceived changes in pain intensity (intensity decreased; not changed; intensity increased), perceived changes in pain frequency (frequency decreased; not changed; frequency increased), and perceived changes in duration of pain (duration decreased; not changed; duration increased). These T2 and T3 data were analyzed descriptively and presented in the results section.

2.3.4. Parent-Reported Outcome Measures

The following parent-reported outcome measures were assessed at all three points of measurement (T1–T3).

(1) Gastrointestinal Symptoms: Mothers were asked to report on their child's GI symptoms in accordance with the current Rome-III classification ("My child was suffering during the last month from ... "; six items: abdominal pain, diarrhea, constipation, nausea, vomiting, bloating; [33]). Items of this symptom list were answered on a five-point frequency scale (never, almost never, sometimes, often, almost always). We calculated a mean score as an indicator of GI symptom severity, which yielded an acceptable internal consistency (Cronbach's alpha = 0.72).

(2) Parental pain-related behavior: A self-developed 24-item questionnaire was administered, covering different adaptive and maladaptive aspects of parental behavior and worries related to their child's abdominal pain. Following the introductory sentence, "When my child has abdominal pain, ... " mothers rated their reactions on a five-point Likert scale (never, seldom, sometimes, often, always). The inventory comprises the following six subscales: "protection" (five items, e.g., "let him/her stay home from school"; "allow things which are usually forbidden"; $\alpha = 0.77$), "attention" (6 items, e.g., "I comfort my child"; $\alpha = 0.77$), "medical help-seeking and home remedies" (4 items, e.g., "I consult a doctor"; "I give him a hot water bottle"; $\alpha = 0.72$), "support child's coping" (3 items, e.g., "I support my child to distract on his own"; "I support my child to relax on his own"; $\alpha = 0.86$) , and "worries" (6 items, e.g., "I am worried"; "I am concerned about my child's future"; $\alpha = 0.83$). Compilation of the items was based on literature of parent behavior [38,39] and pre-tested in another pilot-study [40]. Psychometric properties were sufficient with internal consistencies >0.70 for all scales and sufficient selectivity for all items (part-whole-correlations >0.30). As hypothesized, the scale "protection" showed significant positive correlations to attention ($r_{T1} = 0.406$, $p = 0.029$), medical help-seeking ($r_{T1} = 0.404$, $p = 0.030$) and worries ($r_{T1} = 0.436$, $p = 0.018$). The negative correlation to the scale "support child's coping" was not statistically significant ($r_{T1} = -0.189$, $p = 0.327$).

(3) Parental pain-related self-efficacy: We adapted a validated, illness-specific self-efficacy scale for parents with children suffering from atopic dermatitis or asthma [41,42] to measure pain-specific self-efficacy expectations. The pain-specific self-efficacy scale was preceded by a short introduction ("Dealing with abdominal pain challenges you. We would like to know how confident you are about dealing with those challenges."). The nine-item scale covers self-efficacy

expectations with respect to preventive actions (two items; e.g., "My child spontaneously wants to do something that could worsen the pain. I am able to refuse his/her wish."), being consequent (two items; e.g., "My child is in pain in the morning and doesn't want to go to school. I am able to encourage my child to go to school."), as well as intervening actions when the child is in acute pain (Five items; e.g., "My child is in hard pain. I am able to distract my child."). The items were answered on a six-point Likert scale ("very unsure"–"very sure"). Internal consistency of the total score for parental pain-specific self-efficacy was acceptable (Cronbach's alpha = 0.72).

(4) General self-efficacy: Self-efficacy was measured by the validated and broadly used General Self-Efficacy Scale (GSES; [43]). Schwarzer and Jerusalem [44] report internal consistencies from 0.82–0.93 and a 2-year retest-reliability of 0.47 (men) and 0.63 (women). The GSES total score is positively associated with self-esteem and optimism, and negatively correlated with anxiety and depression [43]. The GSES covers 10 items, enquiring about the subjective evaluation of one's ability to cope with new or difficult demands in life (e.g., "When there are obstacles, I find my way to assert myself"; "I can find a solution for every problem"). Answer format was four-point ("not true", "hardly true", "somewhat true", "exactly true"). Higher raw scores are associated with higher perceived self-efficacy. Internal consistency in our sample was excellent (Cronbach's alpha = 0.92).

(5) Parental quality of life: We used the "Ulm Quality of Life Inventory for Parents of Chronically Ill Children" (ULQUIE) [45] to assess mothers' self-reported quality of life. The questionnaire was developed for parents of chronically ill children and has been shown to discriminate between clinical and non-clinical groups, as well as different stages of illness [45]. The authors had reported acceptable to good internal consistency for the total score in the validation study on 244 parents of chronically ill children [45]. The 29 items have a five-point answer format (never, seldom, sometimes, often, always) and refer to the last seven days. The wording was adapted to our study and "chronic illness" was replaced by "abdominal pain". We used the total score as a global measure for mothers quality of life, which yielded excellent internal consistency in our sample (Cronbach's $\alpha = 0.91$).

2.4. Data Analysis

Statistical analyses were carried out using SPSS Statistics (Version 22). All scale scores were transformed to the range of 0–100 to enhance comparability of measures within the study. Effects for primary and secondary outcomes were analyzed by two-factorial analysis of variance for repeated measures, using group (IG × WLC) and the factor time (T1 × T2 × T3) as a repeated measurement factor. Hypotheses refer to a significant group × time interaction (i.e., an increase or decrease of measures in mothers of the IG compared to the WLC over the three measurement points). In case of significant overall effects, changes from T1–T2, T1–T3 and T2–T3 in the outcome measure will be analyzed by post hoc tests, applying Bonferroni correction of alpha-level. Main effects for group and time will be reported as well. In case the assumption of sphericity is violated (Mauchly-Test), the Greenhouse–Geisser correction of degrees of freedom and significance level will be applied [46]. In an exploratory fashion, changes in child pain will be correlated with changes in maternal outcomes. For this, results with at least a statistical trend ($p < 0.100$) will be reported. Change will be measured by the mean difference in the outcomes between T1–T2 and T1–T3.

As previously mentioned, one child dropped out from the IG due to a physical injury after the second of six sessions. No other adverse events occurred. For this one case, the mother did not participate in the parent session and the parent report of the post-intervention and their 3 month follow-up is consequently missing. We replaced the missing data of this case for T2 and T3 according to the last observation carried forward (LOCF) method for an intention to treat (ITT) analysis (Figure 1). Besides the ITT analysis, data were also analyzed by per protocol analysis (PPA). Besides this one dropout, we were able to report a full retention rate. There was no a priori power calculation for this study, as power calculation was performed for child's self-reported abdominal pain, which was our main outcome of the trial [31]. For the current analysis on maternal effects, we performed a post hoc power calculation and defined a power of 1-β >0.80 as sufficient. For each effect, Cohen's *d* was used as a measure for effect size. Cohen's *d* represents the treatment effect in units of standard deviations (*SDs*), with interpretation of Cohen's $d = 0.20$ as a low, $d = 0.50$ as a moderate and $d = 0.80$ as a high effect. Significance level was set at alpha = 0.05.

3. Results

3.1. Sample and Baseline Pain Characteristics

The 29 randomized children were between 6.6 and 11.9 years old ($M = 9.59$, $SD = 1.54$), and predominantly girls ($n = 25$; 86.2%). All 29 children were suffering from abdominal pain for three months or longer. For the parents in the IG, all mothers participated in the parent sessions and in two cases, the fathers participated as well. With respect to the data analysis, only the mothers of the IG and WLC participated in the assessment sessions T1–T3. There were no missing data, except for the one dropout, and therefore 14/15 randomized mothers in the IG participated in the parent session. A summary of demographic and baseline pain characteristics can be found in Table 1.

Table 1. Demographic data and baseline pain characteristics of the sample ($n = 29$).

Variables	IG ($n = 15$)	WLC ($n = 14$)	*p*-Value
Single parent			
yes	14	11	0.280
no	1	3	
Educational level mother			
≤10 years	5	7	0.362
>10 years	10	7	
Educational level father			
≤10 years	4	4	0.909
>10 years	11	10	
Job situation mother			
not employed	1	1	0.960
(self-) employed	14	13	
Job situation father			
not employed	0	0	NA
(self-) employed	15	14	
Number of siblings			
M (SD)	1.79 (1.67)	1.50 (0.76)	0.566
range	0–7	1–3	
Psychological distress of the child [1]			
Total problem score			
Normal	8	11	
Borderline	5	2	0.415
Abnormal	1	1	
Abdominal pain intensity (last 7 days)			
M (SD)	3.00 (1.00)	2.64 (1.28)	0.407
range	1–4	1–5	
Abdominal pain frequency *			
M	9.13	11.61	0.396
SD	(4.91)	(9.55)	
range	2–20	3–30	
Abdominal pain duration **			
M (SD)	57.13 (34.41)	61.79 (73.00)	0.826
range	15–120	10–300	

All variables were collected from the mother's report. All frequencies are depicted for the number of cases *n*; for metric variables, mean (*M*), standard deviation (*SD*) and range are depicted. *p*-value refers to the significance value according to χ^2/t-test when $p < 0.05$. NA, not applicable (as there were no cases of unemployed fathers, group comparisons were not conducted); IG, intervention group; WLC, wait list control group. [1] data on psychological distress ($n = 14$ in the IG due to missing item) are based on German normative values [35] and are published for the total sample in [30]; * number of days last month; ** minutes on average.

3.2. *Initial Analyses*

All outcome measures were tested for a priori baseline differences between groups. There was a significantly higher baseline value in the IG only for the total score of quality of life ($t(27) = 2.187$, $p = 0.038$), which is included as a covariate in the repeated measures analysis for this outcome. Between mothers in the IG versus WLC, there were no baseline differences at T1 in the sum score of GI symptoms ($t(27) = 1.111$, $p = 0.276$), pain-related self-efficacy ($t(27) = -1.725$, $p = 0.096$) and general self-efficacy ($t(27) = 0.297$, $p = 0.789$). Mothers did also not differ on the baseline measures of pain-related behavior and worries (attention $t(27) = -0.938$, $p = 0.357$; protection $t(27) = -1.678$, $p = 0.105$; support child's coping $t(27) = -1.427$, $p = 0.165$; medical help-seeking $t(27) = -0.346$, $p = 0.732$; worries $t(27) = 0.683$, $p = 0.500$).

Treatment Satisfaction

For the IG, the mothers' evaluation of the intervention yielded high scores on the different scales of treatment success ($M = 74.75$, $SD = 13.54$, range 53.57–92.86) and treatment process ($M = 96.05$, $SD = 4.49$, range 87.50–100). The total score for treatment satisfaction was therefore high ($M = 88.95$, $SD = 7.16$, range 76.19–97.62). Taking the German cutoff values (percentile ranks: 0–10 clearly under average; 11–25 under average; 26–75 average; 76–90 over average; 91–100 clearly over average; [37]), treatment success was rated under average in 21.4% of participants; as average in 7.1%; as over average in 14.3% and as clearly over average in 57.1%. For the scale treatment process, 100% of ratings were over average. Taking the total score, 100% of ratings were categorized as clearly over average.

3.3. *Primary Outcomes*

3.3.1. Maternal Perceptions of Changes in Pain

Analysis of the mother's evaluation of changes in pain revealed highly significant differences between the groups, both for post-intervention T2 and for the follow-up assessment T3. As items were not assessed at T1, the dropout data could not be replaced in this analysis, resulting in 14 participants analyzed in the IG. For the overall change of pain at T2, 13/14 mothers in the IG reported that pain had very much improved ($n = 1$ reported somewhat improved), whereas in the WLC, 10/14 reported no change ($n = 3$ reported somewhat improved and $n = 1$ worsened; $\chi^2(3) = 25.00$, $p < 0.001$). Results at T3 were comparable. For the overall change at T3, 13/14 mothers in the IG reported that pain had very much improved ($n = 1$ reported somewhat improved), whereas in the WLC, 12/14 reported no change ($n = 1$ reported very much improved and $n = 1$ very much worsened; $\chi^2(3) = 24.29$, $p < 0.001$). A similar pattern was found when analyzing the data for pain intensity, frequency and duration (data not shown).

Table 2 summarizes the results of repeated measures ANOVA for the outcomes GI symptoms, pain-related self-efficacy, general self-efficacy and maternal quality of life. Results for maternal pain-related behavior and worries are summarized in Table 3.

Table 2. Outcome measures (means, *SDs*) with results of repeated measures ANOVA (main effects for group, time, and group × time interaction).

	IG $n = 15$		WLC $n = 14$		Main Effect Time	Main Effect Group	Group × Time Interaction			
							p^a/d^a	Post Hoc Test [b]		
	M	SD	*M*	SD	*p/d*	*p/d*		*F*	*p*	*d*
Gastrointestinal Symptoms										
Baseline	32.22	11.72	26.49	15.90				1.722 (1–2)	0.201 (1–2)	0.51 (1–2)
Post	18.61	11.12	20.24	12.43	<0.001/1.36	0.492/0.27	0.003/0.97	5.390 (2–3)	0.028 (2–3)	0.89 (2–3)
Follow-up	11.67	9.61	23.81	16.24				13.128 (1–3)	0.001 (1–3)	1.39 (1–3)
Pain-related self-efficacy										
Baseline	65.33	12.79	72.22	7.98				5.483 (1–2)	0.027 (1–2)	0.90 (1–2)
Post	73.63	11.93	70.00	9.58	0.059/0.70	0.730/0.13	0.011/0.92	1.101 (2–3)	0.303 (2–3)	0.40 (2–3)
Follow-up	77.63	13.92	70.79	10.38				7.496 (1–3)	0.011 (1–3)	1.05 (1–3)
General self-efficacy										
Baseline	70.44	15.78	69.74	13.84				NA	-	-
Post	73.33	12.60	70.25	13.43	0.030/0.76	0.705/0.16	0.818/0.18	-	-	-
Follow-up	76.22	15.47	74.10	16.79				-	-	-
Quality of life										
Baseline	76.03	6.73	67.86	12.70				-	-	-
Post	71.55	11.40	65.70	10.96	0.278/0.43	0.886/0.06	0.487/0.28	-	-	-
Follow-up	77.87	11.25	72.29	14.78				-	-	-

p, significance level; *d*, effect size. All scores were transformed to a range of 0–100. [a] for group × time interaction; when violated sphericity, df and *p*-value correction (Greenhouse–Geisser); [b] test of within-subject contrasts for interaction, with 1 = T1; 2 = T2; 3 = T3. NA, post-hoc analyses not applicable due to non-significant group × time interaction.

Table 3. Mothers' pain-related behavior and worries (means, *SDs*) with results of repeated measures ANOVA (main effects for group, time, and group × time interaction).

	IG $n = 15$		WLC $n = 14$		Main Effect Time	Main Effect Group	Group × Time Interaction			
							p^{a}/d^{a}	Post Hoc Test [b]		
	M	SD	*M*	SD	*p/d*	*p/d*		*F*	*p*	*d*
Attention										
Baseline	51.39	19.71	57.14	12.17	0.001/1.04	<0.001/1.59	0.004/0.95	9.746 (1–2)	0.004 (1–2)	1.20 (1–2)
Post	34.72	12.27	58.93	16.00				0.044 (2–3)	0.835 (2–3)	0.09 (2–3)
Follow-up	31.39	13.81	54.46	12.71				7.320 (1–3)	0.012 (1–3)	1.04 (1–3)
Protection										
Baseline	17.67	17.61	28.93	18.52	0.109/0.59	0.0004/1.21	0.466/0.34	NA	–	–
Post	12.33	15.34	29.29	17.41				–	–	–
Follow-up	8.00	9.60	26.07	16.66				–	–	–
Support coping										
Baseline	51.67	19.21	60.12	11.40	<0.001/1.17	0.0342/0.37	0.002/1.03	8.147 (1–2)	0.008 (1–2)	1.10 (1–2)
Post	69.44	17.16	59.52	15.28				0.276 (2–3)	0.603 (2–3)	0.20 (2–3)
Follow-up	75.56	17.10	62.50	17.30				11.994 (1–3)	0.002 (1–3)	1.33 (1–3)
Help-seeking										
Baseline	28.75	15.99	30.80	15.97	<0.001/1.46	0.032/0.87	0.005/0.92	5.891 (1–2)	0.022 (1–2)	0.93 (1–2)
Post	12.08	10.94	25.00	13.31				1.100 (2–3)	0.304 (2–3)	0.40 (2–3)
Follow-up	11.67	11.54	28.57	16.39				8.108 (1–3)	0.008 (1–3)	1.10 (1–3)
Worries										
Baseline	41.11	19.79	36.01	20.39	<0.001/1.69	0.222/0.48	0.002/1.03	7.133 (1–2)	0.013 (1–2)	1.03 (1–2)
Post	21.11	17.21	32.44	16.19				0.444 (2–3)	0.511 (2–3)	0.26 (2–3)
Follow-up	14.72	13.90	28.87	13.02				10.120 (1–3)	0.004 (1–3)	1.23 (1–3)

p, significance level; *d*, effect size. All scores were transformed to a range of 0–100. "support coping" refers to the scale "support child's coping"; "help-seeking" refers to the scale "medical help-seeking and home remedies"; [a] for group × time interaction; when violated sphericity, df and *p*-value correction (Greenhouse–Geisser); [b] test of within-subject contrasts for interaction, with 1 = T1; 2 = T2; 3 = T3. NA, post-hoc analyses not applicable due to non-significant group × time interaction.

3.3.2. Gastrointestinal (GI) Symptoms

In line with our hypothesis, we found a significant decrease in the occurrence of child's GI symptoms overtime, as perceived by the mothers, in the IG compared to the WLC (interaction $F(2, 54) = 6.345$, $p = 0.003$, $d = 0.97$). Of note, there was also an overall main time-effect (Table 2) and both groups showed a decrease from study inclusion to the T2 assessment (time effect $F_{1\text{-}2}(1, 27) = 12.871$, $p_{1\text{-}2} = 0.001$, $d_{1\text{-}2} = 1.38$).

However, there was a significant decrease of GI symptoms in the IG during the follow-up time span between T2–T3 (interaction $F_{2\text{-}3}(1, 27) = 5.390$, $p_{2\text{-}3} = 0.028$, $d_{2\text{-}3} = 0.89$) and overall from T1 to T3 (interaction $F_{1\text{-}3}$ $(1, 27) = 13.128$, $p_{1\text{-}3} = 0.001$, $d_{1\text{-}3} = 1.39$), with large effect sizes.

3.3.3. Pain-Related Self-Efficacy

In line with our hypothesis, we found a significant and large-sized increase in maternal pain-related self-efficacy in dealing with child's abdominal pain in the IG over time (group × time interaction $F(1.58, 42.78) = 5.660$, $p = 0.011$, $d = 0.92$). Post hoc analyses for the interaction term revealed significant changes with large effect sizes from T1 to T2 and overall from T1 to T3 (Table 2). While from T2 to T3 the scores further increased in the IG, the interaction term was not significant ($F_{2\text{-}3}(1, 27) = 1.101$, $p_{2\text{-}3} = 0.303$, $d_{2\text{-}3} = 0.40$).

3.3.4. Maternal Pain-Related Behavior

We found significant, large treatment effects ($d = 0.92$–$d = 1.03$) consistent with all hypotheses for attention, medical help-seeking, support child's coping and worries. Post hoc analyses revealed that all changes were significant from T1 to T2 as well as overall from T1 to T3, with large effect sizes from $d = 0.93$–$d = 1.33$. Detailed results for the main effects (time, group) and treatment effect (group × time interaction, including post-hoc analyses for interaction) are summarized in Table 3. For the follow-up time span, the changes in the IG could be maintained and significant group differences with large effect sizes emerged, consistent with the direction of hypotheses ($d_{2\text{-}3} = 2.10$ for significant less attention in the IG, $d_{2\text{-}3} = 1.22$ for less medical help-seeking and home remedies, $d_{2\text{-}3} = 0.94$ for less worries and $d_{2\text{-}3} = 0.80$ for more support of child's coping).

The scale "protection" was the only one for which results were not consistent with hypotheses, as the interaction term was not significant ($F(2, 54) = 0.775$, $p = 0.466$, $d = 0.34$). On a descriptive level, scores were reduced in the IG by on average 9.67 points, however, there were also large-sized differences on group level overall and at all time points ($F_{1\text{-}2}(1, 27) = 6.437$, $p_{1\text{-}2} = 0.017$, $d_{1\text{-}2} = 0.98$; $F_{2\text{-}3}(1, 27) = 12.494$, $p_{2\text{-}3} = 0.001$, $d_{2\text{-}3} = 1.37$); $F_{1\text{-}3}$ $(1, 27) = 8.331$, $p_{1\text{-}3} = 0.008$, $d_{1\text{-}3} = 1.11$).

3.4. Secondary Outcomes

3.4.1. General Self-Efficacy

Analysis of variance revealed a significant increase of general self-efficacy in both groups over time (main effect time $F(2, 52) = 3.747$, $p = 0.030$, $d = 0.76$). Scores increased from T1 to T3 on average by 5.78 (IG) respectively 4.36 (WLC) points. Changes in time were significant from T2 to T3 ($F_{2\text{-}3}(1, 26) = 5.078$, $p_{2\text{-}3} = 0.033$, $d_{2\text{-}3} = 0.88$) and T1–T3 ($F_{1\text{-}3}(1, 26) = 5.438$, $p_{1\text{-}3} = 0.028$, $d_{1\text{-}3} = 0.92$). There was no significant main effect for group ($F(1, 26) = 0.146$, $p = 0.705$), nor group × time interaction ($F(2, 52) = 0.201$, $p = 0.818$; Table 2).

3.4.2. Maternal Quality of Life

Analysis of covariance controlling for the baseline T1 value did not show significant effects for time ($F(1, 26) = 1.228$, $p = 0.278$), group ($F(1, 26) = 0.021$, $p = 0.886$) or for group × time interaction ($F(1, 26) = 0.497$, $p = 0.478$). However, statistical power was insufficient, ranging from $1\text{-}\beta = 0.05$–0.37 for the ULQUIE analyses (Table 2).

All presented results were derived from an ITT analysis. Result patterns of the PPA were similar, with increased effect sizes.

In an exploratory manner, we analyzed whether changes in the child's pain corresponded with changes in maternal outcomes. Only results with $p < 0.100$ were reported. For the child's pain, we used both the GI symptom score as perceived by the mother, as well as the child's self-reported pain as a mean score covering pain intensity, frequency and duration per day. Data for the pain diary were derived from a previous publication [31] and are based on a 14 day pain diary. Bivariate correlations within the IG showed that for changes between T1 and T2, a pronounced decrease of self-reported abdominal pain was positively correlated with a pronounced decrease of maternal attention ($r = 0.519$, $p = 0.047$). A pronounced decrease of mother-reported GI symptoms corresponded with a higher increase in the support of child's coping ($r = -0.509$, $p = 0.052$) and higher decrease in help-seeking ($r = 0.464$, $p = 0.082$), although not statistically significant. For the overall change between T1 and T3, a pronounced decrease in GI symptoms was significantly correlated with a pronounced decrease in help-seeking ($r = 0.596$, $p = 0.088$).

4. Discussion

While the efficacy of CBT on a child's pain has been confirmed in several studies [17,18,20,47,48], only a few studies have reported on changes in parent outcomes [23–25]. This paper aimed to analyze whether any effects on the mothers of children suffering from FAP were noticeable, after participation in a group CBT focusing on their child's self-management. We observed significant, large-sized effects, even though only one parent session was included. We first analyzed changes in the mother's perception of her child's symptom load. Mothers in the IG reported a clear improvement of abdominal pain and GI symptoms, which is in line with results for proxy reported pain in other treatment trials for FAP [23,24,49,50] and also corresponds to previously reported positive effects reported by the children [31].

We also assessed a broad range of pain-related maternal behaviors. According to the cognitive-behavioral pain model, hypotheses differentially referred to an increase of adaptive behavior, defined as supporting the child's coping skills (i.e., distraction and relaxation), and a decrease of maladaptive behavior, defined as attention to pain, protective behavior and medical help-seeking. With the exception of protective reactions, all treatment effects on maternal behavior were significant, with large effect sizes and even maintained over the follow-up span. These results suggest that a broad range of maternal behavior can be influenced by even a short intervention. Palermo et al. [25] also reported similar significant, medium sized effects on parent's encouragement of their child's activities. In addition, in an uncontrolled study, Frerker et al. [51] observed long-term reductions in solicitous behavior and short-term increases in distraction after treatment. Contrary to hypotheses and other trials [23–25], no significant decrease of protective reactions in the IG compared to the WLC was observed. A floor effect might explain this result, since despite the fact that scores halved from pre-intervention to follow-up in the IG, the IG displayed very low scores already at pre-treatment, impeding further improvement.

Consistent with our hypothesis, the mothers in the IG also reported significantly less worries concerning their child's abdominal pain at follow-up, which might imply that psychoeducation was successful ("pain is real, but not dangerous"). These results are promising, as there is evidence that the parent's conceptual pain model is critical for their child's prognosis [52]. Other CBT trials also report effects on parental cognitive-affective variables, like the reduction of perceived threats [24] and reduction of self-blame [25]. Participation in the training program also led to significant improvements in the mother's pain-related self-efficacy, which is in line with research on other chronic diseases [41,42]. Thus far, no trial in childhood FAP research has included parent's pain-specific self-efficacy as an outcome measure. As perceived self-efficacy constitutes an important variable in the context of chronic illness, explaining and predicting the implementation of treatment [28,42] and behavior change [27], further investigations of the parent's pain-specific self-efficacy might give additional insight into other mechanisms of change.

Taking recent systematic reviews into account [21,22,53], evidence for treatment efficacy on parent and child outcomes, may also depend on the degree to which the parents are involved. Recent studies have reported that parental involvement varies between 25%–50% of total therapy time [53] and also varies with respect to the setting. In our intervention, parental involvement was comparably low, with a 6:1 ratio of child to parent therapy time (14% of total therapy time)—despite the young age of the children in our sample. Of note, trials can differ greatly with respect to the age range of participants. While we focused on younger children aged 6–12 years, others included a broader age range (e.g., aged 7–17 years [23] or only older children and adolescents aged 11–17 years [25]). However, the specific contents of these parent interventions are quite similar, covering, for instance, psychoeducation on FAP, the cognitive-behavioral model and discussions of parental behavior [23,49]. Since all other interventions have included more comprehensive parent sessions [22,53], the large-sized effects on parent outcomes are especially of interest. Perhaps parent involvement in FAP treatment does not need to be very extensive, as our results indicate that the approach of one accompanying parent session is still very effective.

In accordance with integrative views on childhood chronic pain [8,54], the effects of our intervention effect the child as well as the parent—which probably interact with one another in a self-reinforcing circle of positive effects. The improvement of maternal behavior might positively influence changes on the child level, while the reduction of child's pain and impairment may be a motor for change in the mother's behavior and worries. Levy et al. [55] found that changes in a parent's threat perception significantly mediates changes in the child's pain. Although these conclusions are limited due to the small sample size, exploratory correlation analyses provided promising first results on the mutual benefits of a child's pain and maternal behavior. Future trials should systematically analyze both the child and parent effects of CBT interventions and mediational pathways, in order to gain further insight into possible reciprocal effects of treatment.

One further conclusion of this trial is that while we observed large-sized treatment effects on almost all abdominal pain-related measures, the constructs conceptualized on an unspecific, general level were not affected by treatment.

With respect to general self-efficacy, we did not observe an intervention effect. To put this in context with the level of self-efficacy, we compared the score of our total sample (n = 29) at baseline (M = 30.90, SD = 4.38; range 19–40) with the score of the normative sample derived from the validation study [56]. Paired t-test revealed that our sample reported even significantly higher general self-efficacy than the normative population-based score for adult women (M = 28.8, SD = 4.9; p = 0.015). Based on these results, the non-significant effects on general self-efficacy could be attributed to a ceiling effect. We can only speculate that the comparatively high level of self-efficacy might have catalyzed the significant changes found in pain-specific measures of self-efficacy and behavior in the IG. However, the potentially positive effects of general self-efficacy pointed out by other studies [57] needs to be analyzed in larger samples. In general, the different treatment responses of pain-specific versus general self-efficacy, as found in this study, are in line with the current literature. Since for chronic conditions, disease-specific measures are more sensitive to change [58,59] and accordingly, treatment effects for parents in the context of other pediatric chronic conditions have also been reported [60].

We also did not observe significant changes in the mother's quality of life in our sample. This might be attributable to the fact that treatment content of the parent session was focused on pain-specific issues like the disease model and the child's coping with pain, and therefore changes in the parent's general well-being were not primarily focused on. One other reason might also be that for the mother's quality of life, we already observed high levels at baseline. Exploratory comparisons to other ULQUIE data show that our sample, with M = 72.09 and SD = 10.72 for the total score in both groups at baseline, not only showed significantly higher scores than reported for parents of children with other chronic pediatric conditions [61,62], but also that values did not significantly differ from a healthy control sample ($M = 74.0$, $SD = 28.6$, $p = 0.345$; [61]). These data might suggest that parents in our trial were not severely strained to begin with. This is in line with results from a study on parental quality of life in a sample of parents with children suffering from inflammatory bowel disease who also reported higher quality of life scores in most of the domains [63]. On the other side, this observation contradicts other evidence on increased maternal psychosocial strain in FAP samples (e.g., [14–16]). It can be assumed that the relatively high scores on maternal quality of life in our study are attributable to the fact that recruitment for this trial took place in the general population, not in a clinical setting. To the best of our knowledge, there are few data on the quality of life of parents with children with FAP; therefore further studies with more representative samples are warranted.

This trial also has to be reviewed in the context of methodological strengths and limitations. We included various dimensions of parental experience and behavior as outcome measures and we were consequently able to draw differentiated conclusions, not only regarding maladaptive maternal reactions, but also regarding adaptive reactions and pain-specific self-efficacy. While the measure for parent behavior was a self-developed questionnaire based on clinical experience and literature, psychometric properties were satisfactory. Assessment of changes in child pain was conducted by an interview, which was standardized, but did not include established measures for pain assessment like a Numeral Rating Scale. Of note, the data on changes in pain are the mother's subjective perception of her child's pain level and not meant to be a validated proxy marker for the child's pain experience. However, maternal perceptions of child's pain are considered as important pathways for change and pain-related outcomes like healthcare seeking [23,64]. Additionally, this RCT was conducted according to CONSORT guidelines. The retention rate over the follow-up time span was excellent (96.6%) and there were no missing data on the questionnaires. The intervention was standardized and is available as manualized treatment program [29]. However, one should mention the comparably low sample size, with <20 individuals in each treatment arm, which can be traced back to the calculation of the sample size for the primary study outcome [31]; however, statistical power was sufficient for the main analyses in this paper ($1-\beta > 0.80$). As a common problem in pediatric pain research, only mothers participated in the assessment sessions and therefore we unfortunately do not have data of the fathers. However, Frerker et al. [51] did not find different changes in parental behavior after treatment in mothers versus fathers. Nonetheless, RCTs including a sufficient number of fathers are warranted to enable conclusions with respect to gender-related treatment effects. In addition, interpretation and generalizability of results may be constrained due to the selectivity of the non-treatment-seeking sample with a high rate of decliners for further examination and single-site conduction of this trial. Replication of results, including a multi-site approach with a one-year follow-up and active control group, is currently ongoing [65].

The evaluations of our CBT program gave not only promising evidence for its efficacy, but it also identified possible decisive catalysts for improvement, which should be targeted in further clinical practice. Of note, we cannot imply the degree of parent involvement which is needed, or whether we need a child or a parent focus. Nonetheless, child's self-management, together with parent interventions such as psychoeducation on FAP, and taking parental concerns seriously, such as discussing everyday demands and working on adaptive alternatives, seem to constitute promising strategies for improvement of the psychosocial situation of both children and parents. Identification of the mechanisms at work in the circle of positive effects can deliver valuable implications for management of FAP in pediatric practice and also amend integrative parent-child approaches in childhood FAP [8].

5. Conclusions

Functional abdominal pain in children is a common and impairing condition, affecting not only the children themselves but also the parents. Taking into account the growing evidence on parent-specific changes in pediatric pain management, as well as the positive effects of our CBT program on the child level that have recently been published, this study aimed to analyze whether the mothers randomized to the CBT IG for their child's FAP, may benefit from participation in the program as well. Despite a strong focus on child's self-management, large-sized effects on mother's behavior, worries and self-efficacy in dealing with child's pain were observed in the IG, whereas for the mothers in the waitlist control group, no changes were observed. Of note, despite these pain-specific effects, the mother's perception of their self-efficacy in everyday life and their quality of life was not significantly affected.

These results add to the current knowledge on treatment changes experienced by mothers of children suffering from FAP. The fact that, in our sample, the mothers strongly benefited from the training program, together with previously reported child benefits, implies that the circle many families find themselves in can be broken with these interventions. Extending this line of research and taking a broader family perspective [8,9], a thorough investigation of treatment effects on the family level are also warranted. Therefore, additional studies are needed to gain a better understanding of mechanisms of FAP treatment.

Acknowledgments: C.C. is supported by a grant of the German Research Foundation (DFG; WA 1143/9-1). M.G. was supported by a grant of Potsdam Graduate School.

Author Contributions: M.G. and P.W. conceived the study and the study design; M.G. recruited patients and collected data; C.C. was responsible for data analysis and together with P.W. for interpretation of data; C.C. drafted the article; and C.C., M.G. and P.W. critically revised the article. All authors were given the opportunity to discuss the results and comment on the manuscript. C.C. and P.W. take responsibility for the work as whole. All authors approved the final manuscript.

References

1. Korterink, J.J.; Diederen, K.; Benninga, M.A.; Tabbers, M.M. Epidemiology of pediatric functional abdominal pain disorders: A meta-analysis. *PLoS ONE* **2015**, *10*, e0126982. [CrossRef] [PubMed]
2. Warschburger, P.; Hänig, J.; Friedt, M.; Posovszky, C.; Schier, M.; Calvano, C. Health-related quality of life in children with abdominal pain due to functional or organic gastrointestinal disorders. *J. Pediatr. Psychol.* **2014**, *39*, 45–54. [CrossRef] [PubMed]
3. Lisman-van Leeuwen, Y.; Spee, L.A.A.; Benninga, M.A.; Bierma-Zeinstra, S.M.A.; Berger, M.Y. Prognosis of abdominal pain in children in primary care—A prospective cohort study. *Ann. Fam. Med.* **2013**, *11*, 238–244. [CrossRef] [PubMed]
4. Gulewitsch, M.D.; Enck, P.; Schwille-Kiuntke, J.; Weimer, K.; Schlarb, A.A. Rome III criteria in parents' hands: Pain-related functional gastrointestinal disorders in community children and associations with somatic complaints and mental health. *Eur. J. Gastroenterol. Hepatol.* **2013**, *25*, 1223–1229. [CrossRef] [PubMed]
5. Campo, J.V.; Bridge, J.; Ehmann, M.; Altman, S.; Lucas, A.; Birmaher, B.; Di Lorenzo, C.; Iyengar, S.; Brent, D.A. Recurrent abdominal pain, anxiety, and depression in primary care. *Pediatrics* **2004**, *113*, 817–824. [CrossRef] [PubMed]
6. Petersen, S.; Hägglöf, B.L.; Bergström, E.I. Impaired health-related quality of life in children with recurrent pain. *Pediatrics* **2009**, *124*, e759–e767. [CrossRef] [PubMed]
7. Varni, J.W.; Bendo, C.B.; Nurko, S.; Shulman, R.J.; Self, M.M.; Franciosi, J.P.; Saps, M.; Pohl, J.F. Health-related quality of life in pediatric patients with functional and organic gastrointestinal diseases. *J. Pediatr.* **2015**, *166*, 85–90. [CrossRef] [PubMed]
8. Palermo, T.M.; Chambers, C.T. Parent and family factors in pediatric chronic pain and disability: An integrative approach. *Pain* **2005**, *119*, 1–4. [CrossRef] [PubMed]
9. Palermo, T.M.; Valrie, C.R.; Karlson, C.W. Family and parent influences on pediatric chronic pain: A developmental perspective. *Am. Psychol.* **2014**, *69*, 142–152. [CrossRef] [PubMed]
10. Walker, L.; Claar, R.; Garber, J. Social consequences of children's pain: When do they encourage symptom maintenance? *J. Pediatr. Psychol.* **2002**, *27*, 689–698. [CrossRef] [PubMed]

11. Levy, R.L.; Whitehead, W.E.; Walker, L.S.; von Korff, M.; Feld, A.D.; Garner, M.; Christie, D. Increased somatic complaints and health-care utilization in children: Effects of parent IBS status and parent response to gastrointestinal symptoms. *Am. J. Gastroenterol.* **2004**, *99*, 2442–2451. [CrossRef] [PubMed]
12. Peterson, C.C.; Palermo, T.M. Parental reinforcement of recurrent pain: The moderating impact of child depression and anxiety on functional disability. *J. Pediatr. Psychol.* **2004**, *29*, 331–341. [CrossRef] [PubMed]
13. Walker, L.S.; Levy, R.L.; Whitehead, W.E. Validation of a measure of protective parent responses to children's pain. *Clin. J. Pain* **2006**, *22*, 712–716. [CrossRef] [PubMed]
14. Campo, J.V.; Bridge, J.; Lucas, A.; Savorelli, S.; Walker, L.; Di Lorenzo, C.; Iyengar, S.; Brent, D.A. Physical and emotional health of mothers of youth with functional abdominal pain. *Arch. Pediatr. Adolesc. Med.* **2007**, *161*, 131–137. [CrossRef] [PubMed]
15. Eccleston, C.; Crombez, G.; Scotford, A.; Clinch, J.; Connell, H. Adolescent chronic pain: Patterns and predictors of emotional distress in adolescents with chronic pain and their parents. *Pain* **2004**, *108*, 221–229. [CrossRef] [PubMed]
16. Lipani, T.A.; Walker, L.S. Children's appraisal and coping with pain: relation to maternal ratings of worry and restrictions in family activities. *J. Pediatr. Psychol.* **2006**, *31*, 667–673. [CrossRef] [PubMed]
17. Palermo, T.M.; Eccleston, C.; Lewandowski, A.S.; Williams, A.C.; Morley, S. Randomized controlled trials of psychological therapies for management of chronic pain in children and adolescents: An updated meta-analytic review. *Pain* **2010**, *148*, 387–397. [CrossRef] [PubMed]
18. Sprenger, L.; Gerhards, F.; Goldbeck, L. Effects of psychological treatment on recurrent abdominal pain in children—A meta-analysis. *Clin. Psychol. Rev.* **2001**, *31*, 1192–1197. [CrossRef] [PubMed]
19. Eccleston, C.; Palermo, T.M.; Williams, A.C.; Lewandowski Holley, A.; Morley, S.; Fisher, E.; Law, E. Psychological therapies for the management of chronic and recurrent pain in children and adolescents. *Cochrane Database Syst. Rev.* **2012**, *12*, CD003968. [CrossRef] [PubMed]
20. Eccleston, C.; Palermo, T.M.; Williams, A.C.; Lewandowski Holley, A.; Morley, S.; Fisher, E.; Law, E. Psychological therapies for the management of chronic and recurrent pain in children and adolescents. *Cochrane Database Syst. Rev.* **2014**, *5*, CD003968. [CrossRef]
21. Eccleston, C.; Palermo, T.M.; Fisher, E.; Law, E. Psychological interventions for parents of children and adolescents with chronic illness. *Cochrane Database Syst. Rev.* **2012**, *8*, CD009660. [CrossRef]
22. Eccleston, C.; Fisher, E.; Law, E.; Bartlett, J.; Palermo, T.M. Psychological interventions for parents of children and adolescents with chronic illness. *Cochrane Database Syst. Rev.* **2015**, *4*. [CrossRef]
23. Levy, R.L.; Langer, S.L.; Walker, L.S.; Romano, J.M.; Christie, D.L.; Youssef, N.; DuPen, M.M.; Feld, A.D.; Ballard, S.A.; Welsh, E.M.; et al. Cognitive-behavioral therapy for children with functional abdominal pain and their parents decreases pain and other symptoms. *Am. J. Gastroenterol.* **2010**, *105*, 946–956. [CrossRef]
24. Levy, R.L.; Langer, S.L.; Walker, L.S.; Romano, J.M.; Christie, D.L.; Youssef, N.; DuPen, M.M.; Ballard, S.A.; Labus, J.; Welsh, E.; et al. Twelve-month follow-up of cognitive behavioral therapy for children with functional abdominal pain. *JAMA Pediatr.* **2013**, *167*, 178–184. [CrossRef] [PubMed]
25. Palermo, T.M.; Law, E.F.; Fales, J.; Bromberg, M.H.; Jessen-Fiddick, T.; Tai, G. Internet-delivered cognitive-behavioral treatment for adolescents with chronic pain and their parents: A randomized controlled multicenter trial. *Pain* **2016**, *157*, 174–185. [CrossRef] [PubMed]
26. Bandura, A. *Self-Efficacy: The Exercise of Self-Control*; W.H. Freeman: New York, NY, USA, 1997.
27. Jones, V.; Whitehead, L.; Crowe, M.T. Self-efficacy in managing chronic respiratory disease: Parents' experiences. *Contemp. Nurse* **2016**, *52*, 341–351. [CrossRef] [PubMed]
28. Bursch, B.; Tsao, J.C.I.; Meldrum, M.; Zeltzer, L.K. Preliminary validation of a self-efficacy scale for child functioning despite chronic pain (child and parent versions). *Pain* **2006**, *125*, 35–42. [CrossRef] [PubMed]
29. Groß, M.; Warschburger, P. *Chronische Bauchschmerzen im Kindesalter: Das "Stopp-den-Schmerz-mit-Happy-Pingu"-Programm*; Hogrefe: Göttingen, Germany, 2011.
30. Groß, M.; Warschburger, P. Chronic abdominal pain: Psychosocial strain and treatment-associated changes in coping. *Verhaltenstherapie* **2013**, *23*, 80–89. [CrossRef]
31. Groß, M.; Warschburger, P. Evaluation of a cognitive-behavioral pain management program for children with chronic abdominal pain: A randomized controlled study. *Int. J. Behav. Med.* **2013**, *20*, 434–443. [CrossRef] [PubMed]
32. Schneider, S. *Kinder-DIPS: Diagnostisches Interview bei psychischen Störungen im Kindes- und Jugendalter*, 2nd ed.; Springer: Heidelberg, Germany, 2009.

33. Rasquin, A.; Di Lorenzo, C.; Forbes, D.; Guiraldes, E.; Hyams, J.S.; Staiano, A.; Walker, L.S. Childhood functional gastrointestinal disorders: Child/adolescent. *Gastroenterology* **2006**, *130*, 1527–1537. [CrossRef] [PubMed]
34. SCAP. Chronic abdominal pain in children: Clinical Report. *Pediatrics* **2005**, *115*, 812–815.
35. Woerner, W.; Becker, A.; Rothenberger, A. Normative data and scale properties of the German parent SDQ. *Eur. Child. Adolesc. Psychiatry* **2004**, *13* (Suppl. 2), ii3–ii10. [CrossRef] [PubMed]
36. Blossfeld, H.-P. Berufseintritt und Berufsverlauf: Eine Kohortenanalyse über die Bedeutung des ersten Berufs in der Erwerbsbiographie. *Mitt. Arb.- Berufsforsch.* **1985**, *18*, 177–197.
37. Mattejat, F.; Remschmidt, H. *Fragebögen zur Beurteilung der Behandlung (FBB)*; Hogrefe: Göttingen, Germany, 1999.
38. Lohaus, A.; Klein-Heßling, J. Problemlösungen sind erlernbar. Zur Evaluation von Stressbewältigungs- und Entspannungstrainings für Kinder im Grundschulalter. *Rep. Psychol.* **2003**, *28*, 95–102.
39. Sharrer, V.W.; Ryan-Wenger, N.M. Measurements of stress and coping among school-aged children with and without recurrent abdominal pain. *J. Sch. Health* **1991**, *61*, 86–91. [CrossRef] [PubMed]
40. Groß, M. *Recurrent Abdominal Pain in Childhood. Development and Evaluation of Cognitive-Behavioral Pain Management Program—A Pilot Study*; Diploma Psychology, University of Potsdam: Potsdam, Germany, May 2007.
41. Buchholz, H.T.; Warschburger, P.; von Schwerin, A.-D.; Petermann, F. SEND: Eine Skala zur Erhebung der spezifischen Selbstwirksamkeit für Eltern neurodermitiskranker Vorschulkinder. *Z. Med. Psychol.* **2003**, *12*, 63–68.
42. Warschburger, P.; von Schwerin, A.-D.; Buchholz, T.; Petermann, F. Eine Skala zur Erfassung von elterlichen Selbstwirksamkeitserwartungen im Umgang mit dem Asthma ihres Kindes. *Z. Klin. Psychol. Psychother.* **2003**, *32*, 184–190. [CrossRef]
43. Schwarzer, R.; Jerusalem, M. *Skalen zur Erfassung von Lehrer- und Schülermerkmalen: Dokumentation der Psychometrischen Verfahren im Rahmen der Wissenschaftlichen Begleitung des Modellversuchs Selbstwirksame Schulen*; Freie Universität Berlin: Berlin, Germany, 1999.
44. Schwarzer, R.; Jerusalem, M. Generalized Self-Efficacy scale. In *Measures in Health Psychology: A User's Portfolio*; Weinman, J., Wright, S., Johnston, M., Eds.; NFER-NELSON: Windsor, UK, 1995; pp. 35–37.
45. Goldbeck, L.; Storck, M. ULQIE: A quality-of-life inventory for parents of chronically ill children. *Z. Klin. Psychol. Psychother.* **2002**, *31*, 31–39. [CrossRef]
46. Field, A.P. *Discovering Statistics Using SPSS (and Sex and Drugs and Rock 'n' Roll)*, 3rd ed.; SAGE Publications: Los Angeles, SC, USA, 2009.
47. Fisher, E.; Heathcote, L.; Palermo, T.M.; Williams, A.C.; Lau, J.; Ellert, U.; Neuhauser, H.; Roth-Isigkeit, A. Systematic review and meta-analysis of psychological therapies for children with chronic pain. *J. Pediatr. Psychol.* **2014**, *39*, 763–782. [CrossRef] [PubMed]
48. Huertas-Ceballos, A.A.; Logan, S.; Bennett, C.; Macarthur, C. Psychosocial interventions for recurrent abdominal pain (RAP) and irritable bowel syndrome (IBS) in childhood. *Cochrane Database Syst. Rev.* **2008**, CD003014. [CrossRef]
49. Sanders, M.R.; Shepherd, R.W.; Cleghorn, G.; Woolford, H. The treatment of recurrent abdominal pain in children: A controlled comparison of cognitive-behavioral family intervention and standard pediatric care. *J. Consult. Clin. Psychol.* **1994**, *62*, 306–314. [CrossRef] [PubMed]
50. Robins, P.M.; Smith, S.M.; Glutting, J.J.; Bishop, C.T. A randomized controlled trial of a cognitive-behavioral family intervention for pediatric recurrent abdominal pain. *J. Pediatr. Psychol.* **2005**, *30*, 397–408. [CrossRef] [PubMed]
51. Frerker, M.; Hechler, T.; Schmidt, P.; Zernikow, B. [Pain-related parental behavior: Maternal and paternal responses to chronic pain of their child and modifications following inpatient interdisciplinary pain treatment]. *Schmerz* **2016**, *30*, 241–247. [CrossRef] [PubMed]
52. Crushell, E.; Rowland, M.; Doherty, M.; Gormally, S.; Harty, S.; Bourke, B.; Drumm, B. Importance of parental conceptual model of illness in severe recurrent abdominal pain. *Pediatrics* **2003**, *112*, 1368–1372. [CrossRef] [PubMed]
53. Law, E.F.; Fisher, E.; Fales, J.; Noel, M.; Eccleston, C. Systematic review and meta-analysis of parent and family-based interventions for children and adolescents with chronic medical conditions. *J. Pediatr. Psychol.* **2014**, *39*, 866–886. [CrossRef] [PubMed]
54. Palermo, T.M.; Lewandowski Holley, A. The importance of the family environment in pediatric chronic pain. *JAMA Pediatr.* **2013**, *167*, 93–94. [CrossRef]

55. Levy, R.L.; Langer, S.L.; Romano, J.M.; Labus, J.; Walker, L.S.; Murphy, T.B.; van Tilburg, M.A.L.; Feld, L.D.; Christie, D.L.; Whitehead, W.E. Cognitive mediators of treatment outcomes in pediatric functional abdominal pain. *Clin. J. Pain* **2014**, *30*, 1033–1043. [CrossRef] [PubMed]
56. Hinz, A.; Schumacher, J.; Albani, C.; Schmid, G.; Brähler, E. Bevölkerungsrepräsentative Normierung der Skala zur Allgemeinen Selbstwirksamkeit. *Diagnostica* **2006**, *52*, 26–32. [CrossRef]
57. Romppel, M.; Herrmann-Lingen, C.; Wachter, R.; Edelmann, F.; Düngen, H.D.; Pieske, B.; Grande, G.A. Short form of the General Self-Efficacy Scale (GSE-6): Development, psychometric properties and validity in an intercultural non-clinical sample and a sample of patients at risk for heart failure. *GMS Psychosoc. Med.* **2013**, *10*, Doc01. [PubMed]
58. Lacasse, A.; Bourgault, P.; Tousignant-Laflamme, Y.; Courtemanche-Harel, R.; Choiniere, M. Development and validation of the French-Canadian Chronic Pain Self-efficacy Scale. *Pain Res. Manag.* **2015**, *20*, 75–83. [CrossRef] [PubMed]
59. McWilliams, L.A.; Kowal, J.; Wilson, K.G. Development and evaluation of short forms of the Pain Catastrophizing Scale and the Pain Self-efficacy Questionnaire. *Eur. J. Pain* **2015**, *19*, 1342–1349. [CrossRef] [PubMed]
60. Warschburger, P.; von Schwerin, A.D.; Buchholz, H.T.; Petermann, F. An educational program for parents of asthmatic preschool children: Short- and medium-term effects. *Patient Educ. Couns.* **2003**, *51*, 83–91. [CrossRef]
61. Goldbeck, L. The impact of newly diagnosed chronic paediatric conditions on parental quality of life. *Qual. Life Res.* **2006**, *15*, 1121–1131. [CrossRef] [PubMed]
62. West, C.A.; Besier, T.; Borth-Bruhns, T.; Goldbeck, L. Effectiveness of a family-oriented rehabilitation program on the quality of life of parents of chronically ill children. *Klin. Padiatr.* **2009**, *221*, 241–246. [CrossRef] [PubMed]
63. Greenley, R.N.; Cunningham, C. Parent quality of life in the context of pediatric inflammatory bowel disease. *J. Pediatr. Psychol.* **2009**, *34*, 129–136. [CrossRef] [PubMed]
64. Calvano, C.; Warschburger, P. Chronic abdominal pain in children and adolescents: Parental threat perception plays a major role in seeking medical consultations. *Pain Res. Manag.* **2016**, *2016*, 3183562. [CrossRef] [PubMed]
65. Warschburger, P.; Calvano, C.; Becker, S.; Friedt, M.; Hudert, C.; Posovszky, C.; Schier, M.; Wegscheider, K. Stop the pain: Study protocol for a randomized-controlled trial. *Trials* **2014**, *15*, 357. [CrossRef]

13

Can the Mindful Awareness and Resilience Skills for Adolescents (MARS-A) Program Be Provided Online? Voices from the Youth

Nicholas Chadi [1,*], Elli Weisbaum [2], Catherine Malboeuf-Hurtubise [3], Sara Ahola Kohut [4], Christine Viner [5], Miriam Kaufman [6], Jake Locke [7] and Dzung X. Vo [8]

1 Department of Pediatrics, Boston Children's Hospital, Harvard Medical School, 300 Longwood Avenue, Boston, MA 02115, USA
2 Institute of Medical Sciences, University of Toronto, 1 King's College Circle, Room 2374, Toronto, ON M5S 1A8, Canada; elliweisbaum@gmail.com
3 Department of Psychology, Bishop's University, 2600 College Street, Sherbrooke, QC J1M 1Z7, Canada; catherine.malboeuf.hurtubise@gmail.com
4 Department of Psychiatry, Hospital for Sick Children, University of Toronto, 555 University Avenue, Toronto, ON M5G 1X8, Canada; sara.aholakohut@sickkids.ca
5 Department of Pediatrics, Downstate Medical Center, State University of New York, 450 Clarkson Ave, Brooklyn, NY 11203, USA; christine.viner@gmail.com
6 Division of Adolescent Medicine, Department of Pediatrics, Hospital for Sick Children, University of Toronto, 555 University Avenue, Toronto, ON M5G 1X8, Canada; meejum1@icloud.com
7 Department of Child and Adolescent Psychiatry, British Columbia Children's Hospital, University of British Columbia, Vancouver, BCV6H 3N1, Canada; jlocke@cw.bc.ca
8 Division of Adolescent Health and Medicine, Department of Pediatrics, BC Children's Hospital, University of British Columbia, 4480 Oak St, Vancouver, BC V6H 3N1, Canada; dvo@cw.bc.ca
* Correspondence: nicholas.chadi@childrens.harvard.edu

Abstract: Mindfulness-based interventions (MBIs) have been shown to improve health and well-being in adolescents with chronic illnesses. Because they are most often delivered in person in a group setting, there are several barriers that limit access to MBIs for youth with limited mobility or who cannot access in-person MBIs in their communities. The objective of this study was to determine if eHealth is a viable platform to increase accessibility to MBIs for teens with chronic illnesses. This study reports the qualitative results of a mixed method randomized trial describing the experience of the Mindful Awareness and Resilience Skills for Adolescents (MARS-A) program, an eight-week MBI, delivered either in person or via eHealth. Participants were adolescents between the ages of 13 and 18 with a chronic illness recruited at a tertiary pediatric hospital in Toronto, Canada. Individual semi-structured post-participation audio-video interviews were conducted by a research assistant. A multiple-pass inductive process was used to review interview transcripts and interpret emergent themes from the participants' lived experiences. Fifteen participants (8 online and 7 in person) completed post-participation interviews. Four distinct themes emerged from participants in both groups: Creation of a safe space, fostering peer support and connection, integration of mindfulness skills into daily life, and improved well-being through the application of mindfulness. Direct quotations representative of those four themes are reported. Results from this study suggest that eHealth delivery of an adapted MBI for adolescents with chronic illnesses may be an acceptable and feasible mode of delivery for MBIs in this population. EHealth should be considered in future studies of MBIs for adolescents with chronic illnesses as a promising avenue to increase access to MBIs for youth who might not be able to access in-person programs.

Keywords: qualitative; mindfulness; meditation; chronic illness; adolescents; eHealth

1. Introduction

Adolescents with chronic illnesses face unique challenges that can have significant impacts on their development and well-being [1]. Adolescence is a period that typically involves the acquisition of independence and of a personal and social identity [2]. Managing a chronic illness and its associated appointments, procedures, and medications can disrupt this process [3]. Chronic health conditions (whether visible or not) can also cause emotional challenges and significant coping difficulties [4].

Mindfulness has been defined as "paying attention in a particular way: On purpose, in the present moment, and nonjudgmentally" [5]. Historically rooted in Eastern Buddhist and other contemplative traditions, mindfulness has recently gained popularity in both education and healthcare settings to promote health and well-being among adolescent populations [6]. In addition, mindfulness-based interventions (MBIs) for adolescents have been shown to have benefits on mood, stress, sleep, pain control, and concentration among many others in both clinical and non-clinical samples [7,8]. Emerging research has looked specifically at the feasibility and effectiveness of adapted MBIs for adolescents with chronic illnesses [9]. A randomized study conducted in 72 youth HIV-infected youth aged 14–22 who received an MBI or an active control intervention showed that mindfulness improved life satisfaction and cognitive accuracy in the context of negative emotion stimuli [10]. Another study conducted in 18 adolescents with functional somatic syndromes showed the high feasibility of an MBI and significant improvements in anxiety symptoms and level of functioning [11]. Finally, a number of small studies have shown that MBIs are well-received by adolescents with cancer and chronic pain conditions [12–16].

Despite these promising results, researchers have identified multiple barriers to implementation and dissemination of MBIs with adolescents with chronic illnesses. One barrier is that MBIs have traditionally been delivered in person in group settings [9]. This can pose a challenge for adolescents with mobility limitations, living in remote areas, or with limited access to transportation. Research conducted in adults has shown promise in the eHealth delivery of MBIs via online apps, web-based platforms, or hybrid modes of delivery [17–20]. To our knowledge, in-person and eHealth real-time group moderated MBIs have not been compared head-to-head in teens with chronic illnesses. Demonstrating the effectiveness of this new mode of delivery could have important implications to increase access to MBIs and potentially save costs of delivering this type of programming.

Studies conducted with adolescents have described the experience of participating in an MBI adapted for youth [21,22]. Qualitative data have revealed a number of benefits, including reduction of daily stressors and transformational shifts in life orientation and well-being [23]. It has been suggested that the incorporation of mindfulness practice in daily life demonstrates effective transmission of mindfulness skills to adolescents [24]. In this paper, we aim to describe the experience of adolescents with chronic illnesses receiving an MBI either in person or online. The overarching research question for this study was to determine if eHealth is a viable platform for teens with chronic illnesses. We hypothesized that eHealth would be an acceptable and feasible modality for the delivery of an adapted MBI in this population.

2. Materials and Methods

This paper will focus on the qualitative portion of a randomized mixed methods trial comparing the in-person and eHealth delivery of an adapted MBI for adolescents with chronic illnesses. All participants were included in both qualitative and quantitative analyses. Quantitative analyses sought to compare the acquisition of mindfulness skills and changes in mental health scores using standardized research questionnaires, changes in pre- and post-mindfulness salivary cortisol levels, and tracking of individual home practice between groups. The full description of the study protocol, including both qualitative and quantitative methods, has been published previously [25], and quantitative data will be reported separately. This study was a registered trial (ClinicalTrials.org: NCT03067207). All subjects gave their informed consent for inclusion before they participated in the study. The study was conducted in accordance with the Declaration of Helsinki, and the protocol was approved by the Ethics Committee of the Hospital for Sick Children in Toronto (project identification number: 1000053600).

Given our study's mixed methods design and to allow more flexibility in interpretation of the data, we decided to use a generic qualitative approach, combining elements of qualitative description [26] and interpretive description [27], rather than being guided by an explicit set of philosophical assumptions from an established qualitative methodology [28,29]. For our analysis of the in-depth interviews, we were guided by an interpretive lens, allowing concepts to emerge from the lived experiences of the participants, rather than from our own preconceived notions [30].

Participants were adolescents aged between 13 and 18 recruited from different subspecialty clinics in a tertiary pediatric hospital in Toronto, Canada. Participants were eligible to participate if they lived close enough to attend weekly in-person sessions. They needed to have a diagnosis of a medical or mental health condition requiring ongoing medical care, which included at least one physical symptom, such as chronic pain or headaches. Potential participants were referred by one of their health providers and later contacted by a research assistant (CV) who invited them to a recruitment meeting where the details of the study were explained and written informed consent was obtained from the teen and parent/guardian. Interested participants were then randomized and allocated to an in-person or eHealth group. In total, 58 participants were assessed for eligibility, 40 were excluded for not meeting inclusion criteria, for declining to participate, or for other reasons, including living too far and only being interested in the eHealth arm of the study. Eighteen participants were randomized (9 per group) and 14 (7 in each group) completed the MBI and post-participation interview. Two participants who had not completed the MBI, but had attended at least two mindfulness sessions (both in the eHealth group), were invited to participate in a post-participation interview, and one of them accepted.

Both groups received an eight-week evidence-informed MBI, the Mindful Awareness and Resilience Skills for Adolescents [31] (MARS-A) program, delivered either via eHealth, through a secure online platform allowing audio-visual group interactions in real time (Zoom Video Conferencing—Zoom Video Communications Inc., San Jose, CA, USA), or in person at the hospital. MARS-A sessions are 90 min in length, and the curriculum and facilitation are adapted for adolescents from eight-week evidence-based adult MBI's, including Mindfulness-Based Stress Reduction [32,33] and Mindfulness-Based Cognitive Therapy [34,35]. Each week, a different theme is explored, including introduction to mindfulness, informal mindfulness practice and gratitude, handling difficult emotions, and how best to take care of oneself. A more detailed thematic overview of the program can be found elsewhere [25,36]. Adaptations from adult MBIs include shorter sessions (90 min instead of 150 min), discussions focused on the challenges of coping with mental and physical illness in adolescence, and shorter group and home mindfulness practices. In-session activities included interactive group discussions related to weekly themes, mindfulness practices (i.e., sitting/breathing meditation, mindful movement, body scan, mindful eating, mindful listening), and review/inquiry of individual home practice. In-person and online groups were facilitated by co-authors, NC and EW, who both had extensive experience in MBIs for youth, were formally trained in teaching MARS-A, and had a long-standing personal mindfulness practice.

All participants took part in individual post-participation interviews through the same password-protected video conferencing platform used for the delivery of the MBI to the participants of the eHealth group. The video conferencing platform was chosen over phone or in-person interviews, since all participants, even participants in the in-person group, had been introduced to the platform at the time of enrollment. It was felt that this platform would allow a deeper connection with the interviewer than a phone interview and avoided the need for transportation for participants in the eHealth group. Interviews (average length 14 min, range 10–28 min) were conducted by a female research assistant with a medical degree (co-author, CV) who had received prior training in conducting semi-structured interviews and had met with participants at the moment of enrollment in the study. The interview template utilized was inspired by previous qualitative work with adolescents by co-authors, SAK [37] and NC [12]. Open-ended and semi-structured questions followed by specific probes were used to foster personal reflections about participants' lived experience of the MARS-A program (see Appendix A). The interviews were approached as an opportunity for data to be co-created, with space given for participants to elaborate on each question. Participants completed the interviews from a quiet room at home and were made aware that all interviews were audio-recorded and de-identified prior to transcription and analysis.

Data was analyzed manually through a multiple-pass inductive process [38]. In a first pass, co-authors, CV, NC, and EW, independently read through all the transcripts and coded them to identify emergent themes. Codes were generated using participants' own words whenever possible to minimize subjectivity. Co-authors, CV, NC, and EW, then met in person with the co-author, CMH, a child psychologist with extensive mindfulness facilitation experience who had reviewed the video-recordings of the MARS-A sessions to ensure facilitator quality and uniformity, and to review the themes that had been identified from the participants' semi-structured interviews. From this analysis, four key themes emerged, and a common coding scheme was developed. In a second pass, transcripts were recoded by NC and EW using the common coding scheme. In a third pass, codes were compared by EW and placed into corresponding theme categories. A final review of the transcripts was conducted by NC and EW to discuss classification until consensus was reached and to ensure that the language of participants, and not that of the investigators, guided the theme names and descriptions.

3. Results

The average number of sessions attended among participants who completed the MBI was 6.7 in the in-person group and 7 in the eHealth group. The average participant age was 15.3 years. There were two male participants in each group and all four of them completed post-participation interviews. Participants who did not complete the intervention mentioned lack of time (online group) and difficulty with transportation (in-person group) as reasons for non-completion. Table 1 details participant characteristics at baseline.

Four prominent themes emerged from the interview data: (1) Creating a safe space; (2) fostering peer support and connection; (3) integration of mindfulness skills into daily life; and (4) improved well-being through the application of mindfulness. These themes were similar, with only subtle differences between the in-person and eHealth groups and reflected the lived experience of the MARS-A participants. For brevity and clarity, we have used ellipses, (. . .), to indicate pauses and square brackets, ([. . .]), to indicate edits/omitted material when reporting supporting excerpts from interviews [39].

3.1. Creating a Safe Space

During their interviews, participants in both groups used the word, "safe", to describe their experience or environment. The use of the word, "safe", or concept of "safe space" arose most frequently in relation to the question, "What did you like the most about the program?" For both in-person and eHealth participants, the non-judgmental attitude of other group members who were experiencing similar challenges related to their chronic health condition allowed them to feel at ease during the MBI.

- In-person participant (IPP): [. . .] *it felt like a really safe space. Like it felt like you could really say whatever was on your mind.*
- IPP: [. . .] *you could say what you need to say, so like, afterwards if you're like stressed out about something then no one will like, judge you or make a comment . . .*
- EHealth participant (EHP): *I felt like it was a very safe environment . . . I felt like they were very welcoming, and it was comforting.*
- EHP: [. . .] *they made you feel like whatever you were feeling was like OK [. . .] Like, anytime I thought of something, I shared.*

Table 1. Participant characteristics at baseline.

Parameters	In-Person Group (n = 9)	Online Group (n = 9)
Average age (range)	15.2 (13–17)	15.4 (13–18)
Gender (%)		
Female	78	78
Male	22	22
Ethnicity (%)		
White/Caucasian	67	78
Asian	22	11
African-American	11	11
Primary diagnosis (%)		
Epilepsy	22	11
Anxiety	22	11
Somatic symptom disorder	11	11
Anorexia nervosa	11	11
Thalassemia	11	11
Diabetes	0	11
Obsessive-compulsive disorder	11	0
Juvenile idiopathic arthritis	0	11
Lupus	11	0
Cystic fibrosis	0	11
Asthma	0	11
Chronic pain (%)	44	44
Sleep difficulties (%)	67	78
Mental health (%)		
Any mental health diagnosis	89	78
Anxiety	78	67
Mood disorder	56	44
History of suicidal ideation	33	33
Other mental health diagnosis	33	22
Currently taking medication (%)	67	89
Substance use (past month) (%)		
Smoking/vaping (last month)	0	11
Alcohol (last month)	0	33
Other drugs	0	11
Past yoga/tai chi experience (%)	78	67
Previous meditation/mindfulness experience	44	44

3.2. Fostering Peer Support and Connection

Peer support and connection was reported in participants from both the in-person and online groups, with a focus on interaction with others either in person or through the audio-visual platform. These interactions were described as useful and allowed participants to compare their own challenges to those faced by their peers.

- IPP: *[. . .] you get to see like, other teens—what they're going through and stuff [...] I thought it was really useful.*
- IPP: *[. . .] then we started to get to know each other and like before the sessions started, or like when it ended we would talk to each other afterwards.*
- EHP: *[. . .] it was really interesting to hear the other kids and what they were saying [. . .] because I could relate to it, and I just didn't expect other people to be going through the same thing as me . . .*
- EHP: *I liked how I was able to interact with other people . . . other people who are in similar situations as me*

3.3. Integration of Mindfulness Skills into Daily Life

Implementing mindfulness practices outside of the formal sessions was a theme that emerged from both groups. Participants in both groups reported several concrete examples of how they were able to use the skills learned during the MBI to help them in their everyday life.

- IPP: *I liked how we could always learn new practices every week. And I feel like being able to try the practices out at school really helped.*
- IPP: *I liked the eating [practice] one too, because I could fit that into my daily life.*
- EHP: *I'm working and in the process of forgiving a bunch of people in my life, [...] so I definitely think that's going to be a helpful thing.*
- EHP: *I liked the techniques that I learned, the different kind of mindfulness things we went through because I use them throughout the day all the time.*

3.4. Improved Well-Being through the Application of Mindfulness

Reports from participants in the in-person and online groups suggested a positive impact of the intervention on well-being. Some of the benefits mentioned included: A reduction of anxiety and mood symptoms, an improvement in sleep, and the acquisition of new coping skills.

- IPP: *I feel like I'm less anxious about stuff and I feel a little bit happier about stuff now.*
- IPP: *I know that a couple times my stress level was a little bit lower which was helpful [...] like my sleeping patterns were consistent.*
- EHP: *I think the most useful part was how the program helps you cope with a lot of different things [...] it just helps you cope all around.*
- EHP: *I don't know what it is with the body scan, but it helps me go to sleep.*

4. Discussion

This article presents the qualitative results of a randomized study of an MBI for adolescents with chronic illnesses delivered in-person or via eHealth. The parallel emergence of four key themes—the creation of a safe space, the fostering of peer support and connections, the integration of mindfulness skills into daily life, and improved well-being through the application of mindfulness—in both the in-person and online groups suggests that an eHealth platform could present a viable alternative for the delivery of MBIs in this population.

Creating a safe space for learning, listening, and inquiry in which each participant feels comfortable and relaxed is an integral component of the MARS-A program and other eight-week mindfulness programs for adolescents [7,40]. This concept of creation of a safe space has been described in previous studies of adolescent MBIs [41] and was reported on several occasions by participants in both groups, yet, interestingly, was not included in any of the interview questions. Participants from the in-person group suggested that the lived experience of safe space allowed them to feel comfortable sharing their thoughts and emotions with the rest of the group. EHealth group participants' reflections mirrored the experience of safe space described by the in-person group, also describing an ease to share with others. An important question that remains unanswered is whether the creation of a safe space was the result of a non-specific group effect (unrelated to the mindfulness intervention) or, rather, was related to the facilitators' embodied mindfulness, which is considered to be integral to the pedagogy of mindfulness [42,43].

Although online participants' interactions, unlike in-person participants, were limited to viewing one another on screen during the formal session, with no designated time for informal social interactions before, after, or during sessions, the theme of fostering peer support and connection was reported in both groups. There was a slight difference in the nature of the connection described by each group, with the word, "friendship", used only by the in-person group and descriptors, like "similar", used more frequently by the online group. Nevertheless, both groups reported benefiting from meeting others with whom they had a shared lived experience, which is frequently reported in in-person studies of MBIs in pediatric populations [11,16].

A primary research question was whether the feeling of support and mutual learning could be fostered within the confines of online interaction. Online facilitation comes with its own novel set of challenges [44]. One of these challenges is having less physical cues to the emotional state of participants. During in-person sessions, facilitators have the chance to observe participants in informal interactions before and after the session and during the break. These informal interactions are removed in the online setting, which did not appear to limit participants' reports of group connectedness or the effectiveness of the intervention, as described in adult studies of MBIs delivered remotely [45].

One particularly striking finding regarding the group dynamic was seen in the reflection, "I got the sense that I wasn't alone", which was voiced by several participants. For individuals in the online group to feel this level of connection to their peers described in qualitative studies of in-person MBIs [15] speaks strongly to the viability of eHealth as a delivery platform for MBIs with adolescent populations. It also shows that a sense of community was fostered amongst participants, even though their description of their relationship to their peers—"friendship" vs. "support"—had a different quality between the in-person and online groups.

The question of whether the reported peer connectedness was attributed to the mindfulness intervention itself, or to a non-specific group effect, is challenging to answer without the presence of an active control group (e.g., non-mindfulness group therapy) [46,47]. It is worth noting that the intention of MBIs is usually not focused on fostering friendships per se, but rather on creating a sense of mindful peer connection and support [48], which was clearly reported by both groups. One could add that participants were part of a generation that has been exposed to technology and social media from an early age, which might have facilitated peer connection through the online platform [49].

Studies have indicated that pediatric participants in eight-week MBIs acquire the skillsets needed to apply mindfulness practices in their daily lives [11,15]. This integration of mindfulness skills can be assessed in different ways, including patient report and validated measurement scales [50], and is often used as a proxy to measure the effectiveness of MBIs [12,51]. In our study, participants were able to identify several real-life situations where the acquisition of new mindfulness skills would be useful for them (e.g., when eating, increased forgiveness). Both groups' willingness and ability to apply diverse mindful practices outside of the sessions suggests a successful adoption of the practices via in-person and online modalities.

Pediatric in-person studies have shown that the application of mindfulness can improve participants' well-being, specifically in relation to anxiety, pain, and sleep [14,16]. Both the in-person and online groups reported positive impacts in these three areas. In addition, participants explained that mindfulness had benefits on their happiness, body awareness, and reactions to difficult situations. On multiple occasions, participants went beyond simply describing foundational practices, such as sitting meditation, and were able to share high-level concepts, such as insight that their pain is connected to stress. This specific association has been described in previous in-person MBI studies, and is considered an indicator of increased mindfulness [16].

Qualitative data from post-participation interviews were meant to complement quantitative data from validated scales, logging of individual home practice, and measures of salivary cortisol levels also gathered during this study [52]. In brief, quantitative analyses from measurement scales and saliva samples were limited due to the small size of the sample, but there were similar levels of self-reported home practice between groups: In-person group: 6.5 times per participant/week (range = 1.4–13.4) and 28.8 min per participant/week (range = 4.3–154.7); and eHealth group: 6.0 times per participant/week (range = 2.9–9.7) and 30.6 min per participant/week (range = 6.6–107.8). Reported practices included all nine types of practices taught during MARS-A sessions (i.e., breathing meditation, body scan, mindful movement, eating meditation). These levels of individual practice, although much lower than those recommended (45 min per day) and observed (approximately 30 min per day) in adult MBIs [53], and lower than those reported in a recent in-person adolescent MBI study (median of 54 min per week) [11], provide some support that a number of different mindfulness practices were successfully integrated in participants' everyday life.

None of the participants recruited for this study (including potential participants that ultimately were not enrolled in the study) identified access to the technology required to participate in the eHealth group (computer/tablet, web camera, microphone, internet connection) as a barrier to participation. While there were some technical issues that impacted individuals and the entire group, such as mild delays (3–5 min) in establishing a stable internet connection for all members at the beginning of five of the eight eHealth sessions, loss of connection for a 30 s to 8 min on a total of 12 occasions for four of the eHealth participants, and a defective microphone requiring reliance on instant messaging functions for one of the participants during two of the sessions, along with some distractions from their own space (e.g., family talking loudly or a pet coming into the room), most online participants reported that the online platform was convenient and easy to use and shared that being at home, versus commuting, resulted in more ease for them before, during, and after the session. Although this was not reported by study participants, studies of MBIs provided remotely suggest that learning mindfulness skills in one's usual environment facilitates implementation of mindfulness skills and generalization to everyday life [54], with the added benefit of not having to plan additional time for transportation.

Study limitations: Due to a slower recruitment than anticipated, the sample size was small, and it is unclear if data saturation was reached. In addition, semi-structured interviews were short (less than thirty minutes), which could have limited the depth of participant reflections, and interviews took place immediately after the end of the MBI, which did not allow the capturing of any long-term effects of the intervention. In addition, interviews were conducted remotely through the same audio-video platform that was used for the delivery of the MBI in the eHealth group and was being trialed for feasibility. Finally, our study population was highly heterogeneous, limiting the possibility of applying findings to specific medical conditions.

5. Conclusions

Qualitative results from this study suggest that eHealth may be an acceptable and feasible mode of delivery for MBIs for adolescents with chronic illnesses. Given the small size and preliminary nature of our study, more research is needed to confirm these findings. Nonetheless, eHealth should be considered as an alternative option in future studies of MBIs for adolescents, and as a promising avenue to increase access to MBIs for youth who might not be able to access in-person programs.

Author Contributions: Conceptualization, N.C., M.K. and D.X.V.; Data curation, C.V.; Formal analysis, N.C., E.W., C.M.-H.and C.V.; Funding acquisition, N.C. and M.K.; Investigation, N.C. and C.V.; Methodology, N.C. and E.W.; Project administration, N.C. and C.V.; Supervision, S.A.K., M.K. and D.X.V.; Validation, C.M.-H. and C.V.; Visualization, N.C. and E.W.; Writing-original draft, N.C. and E.W.; Writing-review & editing, N.C., E.W., C.M.-H., S.A.K., C.V., M.K., J.L. and D.X.V.

Acknowledgments: The authors of this paper wish to acknowledge the contributions of Blathnaid McCoy, Abhaya Kulkarni, Nades Palaniyar, Danielle Ruskin, and Claire De Souza in drafting and submitting the initial study proposal.

Appendix A

Post-Intervention Semi-Structured Interview Guide

Participant ID: ________

Interviewer:

____

Date:

____

Start Time: ________ AM/PM End Time: ________ AM/PM

Hello, my name is (insert research assistant's name). I am one of the research assistants for the Mindfulness research project you are participating in at SickKids Hospital. First, I would like to thank you for participating in the research project. Now that you have completed the eight-week mindfulness program, I would like to ask you a few questions about the program. Our research team is interested in hearing your opinion about things that went well or were helpful for you and things that could be changed to improve the program in the future. This conversation should not take more than 15 to 20 min of your time. Is this still a good time for you to conduct this interview? [If no: Can I call you back at another time? What is the best time to reach you?]

1. **What did you like the most about the program?** *Probe: What were some of the good things that came out of the mindfulness sessions?*
2. **What did you like the least about the program?** *Probes: Were there some parts of the program that you didn't like? Why? What ways could we improve on those parts?*
3. **What was the most useful part of the program for you?** *Probes: Are there some things that you learned the program that you think you will use in the future?*
4. **What did you think of the teens in your group?** *Probes: Did you enjoy being part of a group? If so, how or in what way? Was the size of the group too large/small? Did you find that you had enough/too much time to share your experience?*
5. (For participants in the eHealth arm) **What did you think of the iMeet platform?** *Probes: What issues, if any, did you have with the iMeet platform? What did you like/dislike about doing the program at home? Online/remotely?*
6. **How did you find your instructors?** *Probes: Is there something that your instructors could have done differently? What did you like/dislike about your instructors?*
7. **Did you practice mindfulness between the sessions? If yes, approximately how many times a week did you practice and for how long? If no, why not?** *Probe: What made it easy/difficult to practice at home? What were the barriers to home practice?*
8. (If yes at the previous question) **Which mindfulness practices did you do at home? Why did you choose this/these practice(s)?**
9. **What changes, if any, did you see in yourself after finishing the mindfulness program?** *Probes: Better sleep, feeling happier, more energy, less anxious/stressed, less pain, increased school/social event attendance*
10. **Would you recommend the mindfulness program to a friend or to another young person with a health condition?** *Probes: If no, why not? If yes, why would you recommend it?*
11. **Do you think that you will continue to practice mindfulness? Why or Why not?**
12. **Do you have any other comments that you would like to share with us about the program?** *Probes: positive/negative experiences? General thoughts and feelings about program?*

Thanks again for your time and your participation in the program.

References

1. Pinquart, M.; Teubert, D. Academic, physical, and social functioning of children and adolescents with chronic physical illness: A meta-analysis. *J. Pediatr. Psychol.* **2012**, *37*, 376–389. [CrossRef] [PubMed]
2. Christie, D.; Viner, R. Adolescent development. *BMJ* **2005**, *330*, 301–304. [CrossRef] [PubMed]
3. Chadi, N.; Amaria, K.; Kaufman, M. Expand your HEADS, follow the THRxEADS! *Paediatr. Child Health* **2017**, *22*, 23–25. [CrossRef] [PubMed]
4. Warschburger, P.; Hanig, J.; Friedt, M.; Posovszky, C.; Schier, M.; Calvano, C. Health-related quality of life in children with abdominal pain due to functional or organic gastrointestinal disorders. *J. Pediatr. Psychol.* **2014**, *39*, 45–54. [CrossRef] [PubMed]
5. Kabat-Zinn, J. *Wherever You Go, There You Are: Mindfulness Meditation in Everyday Life*, 10th ed.; Hachette Books: New York, NY, USA, 2005; ISBN 978-1401307783.
6. Zenner, C.; Herrnleben-Kurz, S.; Walach, H. Mindfulness-based interventions in schools-A systematic review and meta-analysis. *Front. Psychol.* **2014**, *5*, 603. [CrossRef] [PubMed]
7. Vo, D.X.; Doyle, J.; Christie, D. Mindfulness and Adolescence: A Clinical Review of Recent Mindfulness-Based Studies in Clinical and Nonclinical Adolescent Populations. *Adolesc. Med. State Art Rev.* **2014**, *25*, 455–472. [PubMed]
8. Zoogman, S.; Goldberg, S.B.; Hoyt, W.T.; Miller, L. Mindfulness Interventions with Youth: A Meta-Analysis. *Mindfulness* **2015**, *6*, 290–302. [CrossRef]
9. Ahola Kohut, S.; Stinson, J.; Davies-Chalmers, C.; Ruskin, D.; van Wyk, M. Mindfulness-Based Interventions in Clinical Samples of Adolescents with Chronic Illness: A Systematic Review. *J. Altern. Complement. Med.* **2017**. [CrossRef] [PubMed]
10. Webb, L.; Perry-Parrish, C.; Ellen, J.; Sibinga, E. Mindfulness instruction for HIV-infected youth: A randomized controlled trial. *AIDS Care* **2018**, *30*, 688–695. [CrossRef] [PubMed]
11. Ali, A.; Weiss, T.R.; Dutton, A.; McKee, D.; Jones, K.D.; Kashikar-Zuck, S.; Silverman, W.K.; Shapiro, E.D. Mindfulness-Based Stress Reduction for Adolescents with Functional Somatic Syndromes: A Pilot Cohort Study. *J. Pediatr.* **2017**, *183*, 184–190. [CrossRef] [PubMed]
12. Chadi, N.; McMahon, A.; Vadnais, M.; Malboeuf-Hurtubise, C.; Djemli, A.; Dobkin, P.L.; Lacroix, J.; Luu, T.M.; Haley, N. Mindfulness-based intervention for female adolescents with chronic pain: A pilot randomized trial. *J. Can. Acad. Child Adolesc. Psychiatry* **2016**, *25*, 159–168. [PubMed]
13. Malboeuf-Hurtubise, C.; Achille, M.; Hardouin, M.; Vadnais, M. Impact of a mindfulness-based randomized, wait-list controlled clinical trial intervention on mood, sleep and quality of life in teenagers with cancer. *Psychosom. Med.* **2014**, *76*, A30.
14. Ruskin, D.A.; Gagnon, M.M.; Kohut, S.A.; Stinson, J.N.; Walker, K.S. A Mindfulness Program Adapted for Adolescents With Chronic Pain: Feasibility, Acceptability, and Initial Outcomes. *Clin. J. Pain.* **2017**. [CrossRef] [PubMed]
15. Ruskin, D.; Harris, L.; Stinson, J.; Kohut, S.A.; Walker, K.; McCarthy, E. "I Learned to Let Go of My Pain". The Effects of Mindfulness Meditation on Adolescents with Chronic Pain: An Analysis of Participants' Treatment Experience. *Children* **2017**, *4*, 110. [CrossRef] [PubMed]
16. Waelde, L.; Feinstein, A.; Bhandari, R.; Griffin, A.; Yoon, I.; Golianu, B. A Pilot Study of Mindfulness Meditation for Pediatric Chronic Pain. *Children* **2017**, *4*, 32. [CrossRef] [PubMed]
17. Murray, G.; Leitan, N.D.; Berk, M.; Thomas, N.; Michalak, E.; Berk, L.; Johnson, S.L.; Jones, S.; Perich, T.; Allen, N.B.; et al. Online mindfulness-based intervention for late-stage bipolar disorder: Pilot evidence for feasibility and effectiveness. *J. Affect. Disord.* **2015**, *178*, 46–51. [CrossRef] [PubMed]
18. Boggs, J.M.; Beck, A.; Felder, J.N.; Dimidjian, S.; Metcalf, C.A.; Segal, Z.V. Web-based intervention in mindfulness meditation for reducing residual depressive symptoms and relapse prophylaxis: A qualitative study. *J. Med. Internet Res.* **2014**, *16*, e87. [CrossRef] [PubMed]
19. Cavalera, C.; Pagnini, F.; Rovaris, M.; Mendozzi, L.; Pugnetti, L.; Garegnani, M.; Molinari, E. A telemedicine meditation intervention for people with multiple sclerosis and their caregivers: Study protocol for a randomized controlled trial. *Trials* **2016**, *17*, 4. [CrossRef] [PubMed]
20. Mikolasek, M.; Berg, J.; Witt, C.M.; Barth, J. Effectiveness of Mindfulness- and Relaxation-Based eHealth Interventions for Patients with Medical Conditions: A Systematic Review and Synthesis. *Int. J. Behav. Med.* **2018**, *25*, 1–16. [CrossRef] [PubMed]

21. Sibinga, E.M.S.; Perry-Parrish, C.; Thorpe, K.; Mika, M.; Ellen, J.M. A Small Mixed-Method RCT of Mindfulness Instruction for Urban Youth. *Explore J. Sci. Heal.* **2014**, *10*, 180–186. [CrossRef] [PubMed]
22. Monshat, K.; Khong, B.; Hassed, C.; Vella-Brodrick, D.; Norrish, J.; Burns, J.; Herrman, H. A conscious control over life and my emotions: Mindfulness practice and healthy young people. A qualitative study. *J. Adolesc. Health* **2013**, *52*, 572–577. [CrossRef] [PubMed]
23. Kerrigan, D.; Johnson, K.; Stewart, M.; Magyari, T.; Hutton, N.; Ellen, J.M.; Sibinga, E.M.S. Perceptions, experiences, and shifts in perspective occurring among urban youth participating in a mindfulness-based stress reduction program. *Complement. Ther. Clin. Pract.* **2011**, *17*, 96–101. [CrossRef] [PubMed]
24. Caldwell, C. Mindfulness & Bodyfulness: A New Paradigm. *J. Contempl. Inq.* **2014**, *1*, 77–96.
25. Chadi, N.; Kaufman, M.; Weisbaum, E.; Malboeuf-Hurtubise, C.; Kohut, S.A.; Viner, C.; Locke, J.; Vo, D.X. In-Person Versus eHealth Mindfulness-Based Intervention for Adolescents With Chronic Illness: Protocol for a Randomized Controlled Trial. *JMIR Res. Protoc.* **2017**, *6*, e241. [CrossRef] [PubMed]
26. Sandelowski, M. Whatever happened to qualitative description? *Res. Nurs. Health* **2000**, *23*, 334–340. [CrossRef]
27. Thorne, S.; Kirkham, S.R.; MacDonald-Emes, J. Interpretive description: A noncategorical qualitative alternative for developing nursing knowledge. *Res. Nurs. Health* **1997**, *20*, 169–177. [CrossRef]
28. Caelli, K.; Ray, L.; Mill, J. 'Clear as Mud': Toward Greater Clarity in Generic Qualitative Research. *Int. J. Qual. Methods* **2003**, *2*, 1–13. [CrossRef]
29. Kahlke, R.M. Generic Qualitative Approaches: Pitfalls and Benefits of Methodological Mixology. *Int. J. Qual. Methods* **2014**, *13*, 37–52. [CrossRef]
30. Schwartz-Shea, P.; Yanow, D. *Interpretive Research Design: Concepts and Processes*; Routhledge: New York, NY, USA, 2012.
31. Vo, D.X.; Locke, J.J.; Johnson, A.; Marshall, S.K. The Effectiveness of the Mindful Awareness and Resilience Skills for Adolescents (MARS-A) Intervention on Adolescent Mental Health: A Pilot Clinical Trial. *J. Adolesc. Health* **2015**, *56*, S27. [CrossRef]
32. Biegel, G.M.; Brown, K.W.; Shapiro, S.L.; Schubert, C.M. Mindfulness-based stress reduction for the treatment of adolescent psychiatric outpatients: A randomized clinical trial. *J. Consult. Clin. Psychol.* **2009**, *77*, 855–866. [CrossRef] [PubMed]
33. Kabat-Zinn, J. *Full Catastrophe Living: Using the Wisdom of Your Body and Mind to Face Stress, Pain, and Illness*; Delta Trade Paperbacks: New York, NY, USA, 1991.
34. Teasdale, J.D.; Segal, Z.V.; Williams, J.M.; Ridgeway, V.A.; Soulsby, J.M.; Lau, M.A. Prevention of relapse/recurrence in major depression by mindfulness-based cognitive therapy. *J. Consult. Clin. Psychol.* **2000**, *68*, 615–623. [CrossRef] [PubMed]
35. Segal Williams, J.M.G.; Teasdale, J.D.; Segal, Z. *Mindfulness-Based Cognitive Therapy for Depression*; Guilford Press: New York, NY, USA, 2013.
36. Vo, D. *The Mindful Teen. Powerful Skill to Help You Handle Stress One Moment At a Time*; New Harbinger Publications: Vancouver, BC, Canada, 2015.
37. Ahola Kohut, S.; Stinson, J.; Forgeron, P.; van Wyk, M.; Harris, L.; Luca, S. A qualitative content analysis of peer mentoring video calls in adolescents with chronic illness. *J. Health Psychol.* **2016**, *23*, 788–799. [CrossRef] [PubMed]
38. Dierckx de Casterlé, B.; Gastmans, C.; Bryon, E.; Denier, Y. QUAGOL: A guide for qualitative data analysis. *Int. J. Nurs. Stud.* **2012**, *49*, 360–371. [CrossRef] [PubMed]
39. De Zoysa, N.; Ruths, F.A.; Walsh, J.; Hutton, J. Mindfulness Based Cognitive Therapy for Mental Health Professionals: A Long-Term Qualitative Follow-up Study. *Mindfulness* **2014**, *5*, 10–17. [CrossRef]
40. Bluth, K.; Campo, R.A.; Pruteanu-Malinici, S.; Reams, A.; Mullarkey, M.; Broderick, P.C. A School-Based Mindfulness Pilot Study for Ethnically Diverse At-Risk Adolescents. *Mindfulness* **2016**, *7*, 90–104. [CrossRef] [PubMed]
41. Dariotis, J.K.; Mirabal-Beltran, R.; Cluxton-Keller, F.; Gould, L.F.; Greenberg, M.T.; Mendelson, T. A Qualitative Evaluation of Student Learning and Skills Use in a School-Based Mindfulness and Yoga Program. *Mindfulness* **2016**, *7*, 76–89. [CrossRef] [PubMed]
42. McCown, D.; Reibel, D.; Micozzi, M.S. *Teaching Mindfulness: A Practical Guide for Clinicians and Educators*; Springer: Berlin, Germany, 2010; ISBN 9780387094830.

43. Crane, R.S.; Kuyken, W.; Hastings, R.P.; Rothwell, N.; Williams, J.M.G. Training Teachers to Deliver Mindfulness-Based Interventions: Learning from the UK Experience. *Mindfulness* **2010**, *1*, 74–86. [CrossRef] [PubMed]
44. Sansom-Daly, U.M.; Wakefield, C.E.; McGill, B.C.; Patterson, P. Ethical and Clinical Challenges Delivering Group-based Cognitive-Behavioural Therapy to Adolescents and Young Adults with Cancer Using Videoconferencing Technology. *Aust. Psychol.* **2015**, *50*, 271–278. [CrossRef]
45. Colgan, D.D.; Wahbeh, H.; Pleet, M.; Besler, K.; Christopher, M. A Qualitative Study of Mindfulness Among Veterans With Posttraumatic Stress Disorder: Practices Differentially Affect Symptoms, Aspects of Well-Being, and Potential Mechanisms of Action. *J. Evid.-Based Complement. Altern. Med.* **2017**, *22*, 482–493. [CrossRef]
46. Hyland, T. The Limits of Mindfulness: Emerging Issues for Education. *Br. J. Educ. Stud.* **2016**, *64*, 97–117. [CrossRef]
47. Van Dam, N.T.; van Vugt, M.K.; Vago, D.R.; Schmalzl, L.; Saron, C.D.; Olendzki, A.; Meissner, T.; Lazar, S.W.; Kerr, C.E.; Gorchov, J.; et al. Mind the Hype: A Critical Evaluation and Prescriptive Agenda for Research on Mindfulness and Meditation. *Perspect. Psychol. Sci.* **2018**, *13*, 36–61. [CrossRef] [PubMed]
48. Bluth, K.; Gaylord, S.A.; Campo, R.A.; Mullarkey, M.C.; Hobbs, L. Making Friends with Yourself: A Mixed Methods Pilot Study of a Mindful Self-Compassion Program for Adolescents. *Mindfulness* **2016**, *7*, 479–492. [CrossRef] [PubMed]
49. Lenhart, A. *Teens, Social Media and Technology Overview*; Pew Research Center: Washington, DC, USA, 2015.
50. Brown, K.W.; West, A.M.; Loverich, T.M.; Biegel, G.M. Assessing adolescent mindfulness: Validation of an adapted Mindful Attention Awareness Scale in adolescent normative and psychiatric populations. *Psychol. Assess.* **2011**, *23*, 1023–1033. [CrossRef] [PubMed]
51. Ramasubramanian, S. Mindfulness, stress coping and everyday resilience among emerging youth in a university setting: A mixed methods approach. *Int. J. Adolesc. Youth* **2017**, *22*, 308–321. [CrossRef]
52. Chadi, N.; Kaufman, M.; Weisbaum, E.; Malboeuf-Hurtubise, C.; Kohut, S.A.; Locke, J.; Vo, D.X. Comparison of an in-Person vs. Ehealth Mindfulness Meditation-Based Intervention for Adolescents with Chronic Medical Conditions: A Mixed Methods Study. *J. Adolesc. Health* **2018**, *62*, S12. [CrossRef]
53. Parsons, C.E.; Crane, C.; Parsons, L.J.; Fjorback, L.O.; Kuyken, W. Home practice in Mindfulness-Based Cognitive Therapy and Mindfulness-Based Stress Reduction: A systematic review and meta-analysis of participants' mindfulness practice and its association with outcomes. *Behav. Res. Ther.* **2017**, *95*, 29–41. [CrossRef] [PubMed]
54. Bazarko, D.; Cate, R.A.; Azocar, F.; Kreitzer, M.J. The Impact of an Innovative Mindfulness-Based Stress Reduction Program on the Health and Well-Being of Nurses Employed in a Corporate Setting. *J. Workplace Behav. Health* **2013**, *28*, 107–133. [CrossRef] [PubMed]

14

Integrating Pediatric Hypnosis with Complementary Modalities: Clinical Perspectives on Personalized Treatment

Pamela Kaiser [1,*], Daniel P. Kohen [1,2,3], Melanie L. Brown [3,4], Rebecca L. Kajander [1] and Andrew J. Barnes [1,3]

[1] National Pediatric Hypnosis Training Institute (NPHTI), 29 Western Terrace, Minneapolis, MN 55426, USA; dpkohen@umn.edu (D.P.K.); rebeccakajander@gmail.com (R.L.K.); drbarnes@umn.edu (A.J.B.)

[2] Partners-in-Healing, 10505 Wayzata Blvd #200, Minnetonka, MN 55305, USA

[3] Department of Pediatrics, University of Minnesota, 717 Delaware St SE #353, Minneapolis, MN 55414, USA; melanie.brown@childrensmn.org

[4] Children's Hospitals and Clinics of Minnesota, 2525 Chicago Ave, Minneapolis, MN 55404, USA

* Correspondence: drpkaiser@gmail.com

Abstract: While pediatric integrative medicine (PIM) emphasizes an "evidence-based practice using multiple therapeutic modalities"; paradoxically, literature reviews examining the prevalence and/or efficacy of such mind–body approaches often address PIM modalities separately. Such contributions are relevant, yet documentation of how to deliver combined complementary approaches in children and youth are scarce. Nevertheless, integrative practitioners in clinical practice routinely mix approaches to meet the individual needs of each patient. Best practices are flexible, and include blending and augmenting services within the same session, and/or connecting modalities sequentially for an incremental effect, and/or referring to outside resources for additional interventions. Resonating with integrative medicine's definition, this article's goal is to demonstrate paradigms that "bring together complementary approaches in a coordinated way within clinical practice" by linking clinical hypnosis, the trail-blazer modality in PIM's history, with mindfulness, biofeedback, acupuncture, and yoga. Following the consideration of the overlap of guided imagery with hypnosis and an abridged literature report, this clinical perspective considers the selection of modalities within a collaborative relationship with the child/teen and parents, emphasizing goodness-of-fit with patients' contexts, e.g., symptoms, resources, interests, goals, and developmental stage. Case vignettes illustrate practical strategies for mixing approaches.

Keywords: integrative medicine; hypnosis; mindfulness; biofeedback; acupuncture; yoga; guided imagery; self-regulation; complementary; education

---

1. Introduction

1.1. Clinical Hypnosis: The Roots of Pediatric Integrative Medicine (PIM)

The cornerstone of pediatric mind–body approaches is clinical hypnosis—i.e., positive, mastery-oriented suggestions coupled with imagery to optimize individualized goals related to health, well-being, self-regulation, and resilience [1,2]—which supports a family [3] and preventative [4] perspective [5]. This approach is unified by utilization of the child's internal resources, interests, context, and capacity for healthy dissociation and imaginative involvement [6,7].

Although pediatric integrative medicine (PIM) is one of the newest recognized academic subspecialties [8], the clinical utility of hypnosis has long been recognized as an approach complementary to conventional medicine and has been cited in the medical literature within the past two centuries [9]. Fundamental to PIM's growth and credibility, the field of pediatric hypnosis (see overviews of research [5] and training [10]) began to distinguish itself as a mind–body modality in the 1960s–1980s.

Clinical hypnosis helped set the standard for the broad applications of pediatric integrative health. Groundbreaking publications addressed its efficacy in combination with or in lieu of conventional medical approaches for a remarkable range of pediatric health issues. These have included hypnosis for pediatric learning problems [11–13], anesthesia [14], asthma [15], drug abuse [16], burns [17], enuresis [18–20], functional megacolon [21], warts [22], sleep disorders [23,24], habit disorders [1], autism [25], pelvic exams [26], cancer [2], pain and procedure-related anxiety [27], psychoneuroimmunology [28,29], healing [30], refractory irritable bowel syndrome [31], hemophilia [32], chronic illness [33], hospitalization [34], emergencies [35], aphasia [36], Tourette's syndrome [37–39], migraine [40,41], sickle cell disease [42], chemotherapy-related nausea and vomiting [43], and behavioral issues [44].

Current reviews highlight further evidence- and empirically-based incorporation of hypnosis for children's health care [5,45–48]. Applications to specific behavioral and physical concerns and contexts include anxiety [49,50], asthma [51], cystic fibrosis [52], dental issues [53], enuresis [54], habits [55], headaches [56], vocal cord dysfunction [57], pain [58,59], palliative care [60], primary care [61], psychoneuroimmunology [62], and the potential value in pediatric inflammatory bowel disease [63].

One particularly exciting area of research is the work of Vlieger's team in the Netherlands showing strong efficacy of pediatric hypnosis as the sole treatment for gut disorders. For example, in double-blind study gut-directed hypnotherapy (HT) was shown to be highly effective for pain frequency and intensity in pediatric patients (ages 8–18) with diagnoses of functional abdominal pain or irritable bowel syndrome compared to standard medical therapy (SMT), with continued efficacy at one year follow-up (85% for HT group compared to 25% for SMT group) [64]. Subsequent studies by the same group showed similar results [65–67].

Going forward, hypnosis' cutting-edge research includes the work of Amir Raz, Ph.D., Canada Research Chair in the Cognitive Neuroscience of Attention at the Department of Psychiatry at McGill University. The thrust of his team's and colleagues' cognitive neuroscience and neuroimaging studies is to expand the understanding of hypnosis' underlying mechanisms related to attention, self-regulation, expectation, and consciousness [68].

1.2. Guided Imagery vs. Hypnosis

Definitive conclusions about the value of pediatric guided imagery (GI) are obscured by a muddle of inaccurate and contradictory differentiations from clinical hypnosis [69,70], the overlap of the two approaches, and GI's low methodological quality of research to date [71–73]. It is difficult to find a clear definition of GI distinguishing it from clinical hypnosis, given mistaken assertions—e.g., that pediatric hypnosis does not involve imagery [73–75]. Even professional organizations (and many GI websites) struggle with accurate differentiation [76,77].

While there is some evidence for the efficacy of GI scripts [71], the literature suggests that this modality—infused with hypnotic elements—could be analogous to the clinician-designed hypnotic experience. Congruence between hypnosis and GI include the involvement of the child's senses, incorporation of their imagination, focus on attention, and enhancement of well-being and self-regulation. Like GI, combining imagery while tapping the child's senses is routinely used in pediatric hypnosis [78] and both often incorporate relaxation. Further support for this hypothesis is the literature's repeated recognition of these overlapping elements. Martin Rossman, MD (a student of hypnosis and early advocate of GI) borrowed from Ericksonian hypnosis and other popular modalities to delineate key GI steps for 'healing' various health conditions. In point of fact, all but one are hypnotic elements [69]. We can only speculate that perhaps the 1970s origins of this modality stem, even if only in part, from a purposeful disengagement from the myths and other negative preconceived notions associated with the term 'hypnosis'. The inter-relation between the two continues: a current review of high-quality studies of gut-directed hypnotherapy for children included guided imagery with the rationale that GI "is a technique that is highly comparable to hypnotherapy, because both are using relaxation and imageries and both aim to change mental and physical experiences with the use of suggestions" (p. 223) [79]. Beyond this blended/overlapping view, some authors explicitly consider the two modalities as completely equivalent [80–82].

It is important to clarify the mistaken assumption of some authors that hypnosis does not include imagery. Experts from the 1800s to recent times note "the importance of imagery and its integral role in hypnosis, particularly in children" (p. 21) [44]. In a 1984 seminal article entitled "Use of Relaxation-Mental Imagery (Self-Hypnosis) in the Management of 505 Pediatric Behavioral Encounters", the protocol included the "cultivation of natural imaginative skills" (p. 22) [44]. Another key paper described hypnosis "as a process of 'cultivation of imagination' for the patient's own benefit" [44].

One clear disparity between hypnosis and GI is the required intensive training in pediatric hypnosis for licensed clinicians with advanced degrees to design tailor-made, individualized sessions vs. the abundant, ready-made GI scripts available to clinicians and lay people. The non-profit National Pediatric Hypnosis Training Institute (www.NPHTI.org) offers the only recurring pediatric-specific clinical hypnosis skills training workshops in North America. NPHTI provides extensive, supervised experiential learning practice of skills as well as to become adept with careful monitoring of each patient's psychophysiological phenomena and responses; checking in as needed and adjusting the pacing, content, delivery, and prosody (voice speed, cadence, etc.) of the thoughtfully planned, goal-related suggestions, rich imagery, and metaphoric stories.

By contrast, the author of GI scripts imposes his/her own imagery onto the child/teen which could be inferred incorrectly that children prefer that sensory modality and type of imagery. Such scripts written for "every patient" are read-aloud by the clinician or lay people who must look at their paper rather than attending to the content's impact on their patient. A recent study found that the use of a home-based CD-script vs. a therapist-read script (followed by the same home-based CD) for students with IBS, FAP, or FAPS had comparably very favorable results [67]. Based on the article's description of the delivery of these approaches, it appears that this was a comparison of *two ways of delivering an identical GI script*. Furthermore, there were a number of qualified subjects dropped due to insufficient motivation, either due to preference for a therapist-led intervention or lack of interest in protocol requirements. Clearly, the researchers are to be commended for an otherwise exquisitely designed study, including controlling for relevant confounders (e.g., anxiety and depression) in this demonstration of a cost-effective intervention for a large group of children. Because it is our opinion that a personalized approach optimizes the potential for a meaningful therapeutic outcome, hopefully, future studies will contrast the individually designed intervention of pediatric hypnosis with these two different modes of script delivery.

1.3. Integrating Hypnosis with PIM

Other pediatric mind–body approaches also share some elements with hypnosis: mindfulness, biofeedback, yoga (and perhaps to a lesser degree) acupuncture also utilize the child/teen's unfolding curiosity for novelty and learning; overall motivation for mastery; capacity for focused, narrowed attention; openness to positive suggestions and expanding internal resources; and willingness to practice emerging skills. Breath is often incorporated and patients learn the easily accessible value of slowed, diaphragmatic ('belly') breathing to activate the parasympathetic nervous system (aka the 'calming control center'). It may be safe to say that the over-arching intent of mind–body modalities is to offer these "gifts" to maximize one's own health, well-being, self-regulation, self-confidence, and self-efficacy.

Following a brief synopsis of the literature, the following sections offer clinical perspectives from clinicians on *how* to interlink hypnosis with four distinct complementary mind–body approaches (mindfulness, biofeedback, acupuncture, and yoga). The additional case vignettes illustrate ways to blend PIM approaches, highlighting the importance of context for goodness-of-fit as well as practical points and considerations when personalizing PIM treatment.

2. Integrating Mindfulness and Hypnosis

2.1. Background

A specific form of meditative practice called "mindfulness" was popularized by Jon Kabat-Zinn [83,84] who defined mindfulness as "the awareness that emerges through paying attention on purpose, in the present moment, and non-judgmentally to the unfolding of experience moment by moment" [85]. Early works by Kabat-Zinn summarized the history of mindfulness as well as its emergence into clinical contexts as a broadened approach to mind–body interventions.

Mindfulness continues to gain popularity, with an increasing presence in school curricula, workplace wellbeing initiatives, and health care settings. In clinics and hospitals, mindfulness-based stress reduction is prototypical of such practices in health care, first developed as a program to relieve suffering among adults with chronic conditions [86]. Similar practices have been used in other therapies (albeit not necessarily called 'mindfulness') including acceptance and commitment therapy, dialectical-behavioral therapy, and mindfulness-based cognitive therapy [87].

Experience-based practice with formal meditative approaches (such as the body scan, moving meditation, and sitting meditation) and informal meditation during everyday activities (such as eating) are called "guided mindfulness meditations" because they use in-person or recorded instructions. Collectively, these guided experiences and self-directed practices are called mindfulness-based practices (MBPs) [87]. Some MBPs are delivered in a group format, others individually, and others a combination. A number of apps, recordings, and lay-press books detail mindfulness activities for children and adolescents, and these very frequently include developmentally-tailored exercises and therapeutic metaphors (e.g., Sitting Still Like a Frog [88] and Breathe, Think, Do with Sesame [89]).

Guided mindfulness and other MBPs differ from clinical hypnosis in that the former is rooted within a contemplative philosophy with historical roots that did not include therapeutic goals. The hallmark of hypnosis is the use of specific therapeutic suggestions oriented towards one or more health-related goals. However, as therapist Michael Yapko, Ph.D. points out in his seminal book, *Mindfulness and Hypnosis: The Power of Suggestion to Transform Experience* [90], mindfulness applied in a clinical context always implies goal-oriented changes in one's health or experience of health (as opposed to mindfulness practiced for spiritual contemplation). Thus, both mindfulness and hypnosis training done with a health professional require some level of interactional suggestions that, at the very least, facilitate a patient's focus, absorption, and awareness to achieve therapeutic outcomes. For these reasons, Yapko advocates for clinicians using MBPs to develop a deep understanding of hypnotic suggestion, verbal and nonverbal communication, and inter- and intra-personal processes. Furthermore, the precise terminology used in clinical practice (mindfulness, hypnosis, et al.) is perhaps less important than gaining an appreciation for both hypnosis and mindfulness as processes that lead to self-regulation and associated neurobiological changes.

In fact, therapeutic goals are now a common component of mindfulness and simple MBPs as part of an integrative approach for children with psychological and mind–body issues, including those with chronic worries; rumination or being too 'in their heads'; many 'what-ifs' who seek frequent reassurance; frequent over-estimation of the potential for negatives such as risk, threat, or danger; generalized anxiety disorder; major depression; and/or sleep-onset or sleep-maintenance insomnia. This modality is perfect to help these children and youth quiet their minds and be more fully present in the current moment (instead of being 'stuck' in the imagined negative future). This can be practiced and summarized with children and adolescents briefly with these simple steps developed by the first author (P.K.):

- Focus your attention on being present, in this very moment . . . now THIS very moment . . . now THIS very moment . . .

- Amplify this moment-to-moment awareness by focusing on your five senses: be aware of what you hear NOW, what you see NOW, what you feel NOW, what you smell NOW, and what you taste NOW . . . and integrate that to being just present in this very moment . . .
- NOW, the final of the three steps: Create a feeling of deep Appreciation . . . it could be for your pet, your friend or another wonderful person, the shower, your favorite food, the sunset, your bed, or anything else that you really truly are grateful for.

Pediatric well-being can be improved through guided mindfulness and other MBPs in other contexts. A recent meta-analysis of MBPs in children and adolescents showed positive effects on academic achievement, school functioning, negative emotionality, subjective distress, internalizing symptoms, and a number of physical health indicators [91]. For example, in a randomized controlled trial, African-American teens with elevated blood pressure were taught to sit "upright in a comfortable position with eyes closed . . . focus on diaphragm movements while breathing . . . acknowledge and accept [unwanted thoughts, ideas or images] without making judgments about them and shift attention back to diaphragmatic breathing", and encouraged to practice this for 10 min before and after school for three months. The MBP group had significant reductions in systolic blood pressure during the school day and at night, as well as decreased urinary excretion of sodium and resting heart rate [92]. MBPs are also being investigated to help reverse the impact of trauma and adversity during childhood [93] and to help parents of children with intellectual and developmental differences to decrease parenting stress and indirectly promote behavioral competence in their children [94]. Some of the MBPs studied in children have shown benefits with just one session of guided mindfulness, whereas others have used multiple guided sessions with active home practice.

Other elements now thought to be important to such mindfulness-based programs that strikingly overlap with the inherent phenomena, process, and purposes of hypnosis include (a) dissociating from, and letting go of reactive or distressing thoughts and feelings and (b) cultivating absorbed attention, intention, and evoking curiosity to foster emotional-behavioral self-regulation [87]. Further, mental imagery a mainstay of clinical hypnosis, is now commonly used within various MBPs, e.g., by suggesting that feelings or thoughts are like moving ants on a log floating down a river in order to help shift from ruminative or perseverative thinking to more flexible thinking or positive alterative thoughts.

Ongoing research aims to better specify the ways in which mindfulness and hypnosis work, including the extent to which they affect the central nervous system [95,96]. One example of the practical overlap between hypnosis and mindfulness can be seen in a series of studies in which four-to-six-year-olds were instructed to pretend to be "an exemplar other [such as Batman]". These young children performed better on tasks of executive function and perseverance than did their peers who were instructed to take either a first-person or third-person perspective on themselves [97,98]. The utilization of the hero as a figure in play is also a classic developmental marker of preschool- and early-school-aged children's beneficial use of imagination. Thus, the imaginative suggestions to embody a powerful hero are commonly employed in self-hypnosis with children at this developmental stage, and the resulting 'self-distancing' is often part of mindfulness-based approaches. The outcome of this hero-role-play—improved executive function—demonstrates how self-regulation can be promoted in children, tailored to their developmental level, through the integration of mindfulness and hypnosis.

In a similar way, "jettison" techniques [5] blend mindful awareness with hypnotic phenomena, and are particular well-suited to school-age and adolescent patients—these strategies use self-generated imagery (e.g., picturing a distressful emotion as a shape, color, or other metaphor such as a liquid in the body) and focused sensorimotor action (e.g., to allow the pictured emotion to 'flow' or 'move' gradually down an arm into a fist that clenches to hold the emotional imagery until it is 'released' as the fisted fingers release and relax as if a faucet opening) to 'externalize' and self-regulate emotions—clearly blending mindfulness with hypnosis.

To further underline the commonalities between pediatric clinical hypnosis and MBPs, children and adolescents who learn self-hypnosis in clinical settings will frequently and spontaneously refer to their home practice as 'meditation'. Indeed, when invited to demonstrate their self-hypnosis to the clinician or parent, some young people will adopt a stereotypical meditative posture such as the index fingers touching the thumbs while the dorsum of each hand rests upon each knee (which is itself a yogic pose called 'gyan mudra', symbolizing attunement with higher power, wisdom, and knowledge).

Regardless of whether it is called mindfulness, meditation, hypnosis, or something else made up like "that thing the doctor showed me how to do", such child-generated language is to be encouraged and built upon, not only as hypnotic ego-strengthening and utilization of a child's individual strengths and talents, but also as post-hypnotic suggestions that empower children to apply therapeutic strategies across contexts. Because of the powerful self-regulation that can result from mindfulness-based hypnotic approaches as summarized above, clinical applications can include decreasing ruminative cognitions among vulnerable children [99], and preventive care and general health promotion from infancy through adolescence [9].

Best practices for mindfulness-based hypnosis [100] in pediatrics include a strong relationship (rapport and therapeutic resonance) with the patient and family, in addition to a thorough understanding of the patient's developmental level, history, and temperament. For children with a cognitive level of 8–10 years or less, it is often helpful to help parents learn these approaches for themselves and also how to best incorporate them into their daily routine with their child (either as something each person does individually or as a collective experience). For older children and adolescents, having a recording with which to practice can also be useful, especially for children who are just learning. At times, mindfulness-based approaches can be taught first, and hypnotic approaches added to this later—this can work especially well for children with shorter attention spans or who do not enjoy or have facility with mental imagery, because such children can benefit from brief mindfully-oriented strategies to re-orient their awareness (i.e., 1-to-5-min practices). With practice, these children can utilize more complex and longer hypnotic strategies with or without imagery (e g., with cognitively-behaviorally oriented suggestions). For children with longer attention spans, or who enjoy physical activity or more kinesthetic experiences, active/alert hypnosis can be taught first (e.g., with eyes open, standing/moving) and mindfulness added over time through activity-based practices (such as moving a hula hoop gradually up the body as a 'body scan' to engage somatic awareness). For children who are very imaginative, imagery-oriented, and/or have average-to-high executive function or attention spans, hypnosis and mindfulness can be seamlessly woven together from the outset for sessions of 5–20 min in length—some children will make their preferences for various approaches known over time, so longitudinal dialogue and debriefing with each individual patient and family about how they do their ongoing practice is essential for the clinician to learn how and when to blend approaches or lean more heavily on one approach.

2.2. *Case Example*

M. was first referred to the developmental-behavioral pediatrician at age 10 by his psychiatrist for recurrent abdominal pain. The psychiatrist had previously diagnosed M. with attention-deficit/hyperactivity disorder, inattentive type, co-occurring with generalized anxiety disorder, each treated with appropriate medications that had somewhat improved his ability to manage the symptoms of these conditions. These medications did not seem to affect his abdominal pain for better or worse, and a thorough medical evaluation by his primary care physician had confirmed the diagnosis of recurrent abdominal pain. His mother said that at home he would often cry in the morning due to the pain, and many nights he would "work himself up" worrying about the pain recurring the next day. His mother also indicated in private that he had experienced high levels of family dysfunction and maltreatment in early childhood. He presented as a thin, somewhat disheveled-appearing boy who was distracted, inattentive, and behaviorally inhibited. He spoke tentatively and with much elaboration about the characteristics of the pain, saying only "it hurts a lot sometimes" in the periumbilical region and could be "dull", occurring most often before school.

The first visit's goals were to establish therapeutic resonance and to help M develop new ways of discriminating various levels of comfort. To do so, after acknowledging the reality of M.'s physical pain, the clinician reframed it as "discomfort" and affirming his "strength . . . shown so well already . . . because that's what it means to get to school every morning even if we're feeling uncomfortable". The clinician 'wondered' with M. about "what else (he) might notice between today and the next visit about how the body feels or what the brain is thinking right before, or during, or even after, the discomfort shows up" to evoke M.'s curiosity and enlist his ability to be mindful, i.e., "pay attention on purpose", of his experiences. At the following visit, M. said he had noticed that his "heart beat differently, like not faster but weird" right before an episode of abdominal discomfort. The clinician affirmed this new awareness, then began to teach M. about mindfulness: being aware of bodily sensations and perceptions when "the heart started to beat differently, and if the breathing changed or the chest changed in other ways, and when that abdomen began to feel any change in its level of comfort, and when any other parts had other differences in how they felt" (this language was also chosen to help him learn to distance himself from his bodily sensations when in pain, also known as hypnotic dissociation).

The clinician then got out his stethoscope and offered to teach M. how to use it, and M. responded with interest. As M. began to listen to his heartbeat, the clinician suggested that he "just notice the little or big differences" in his heart rate when inhaling vs. exhaling vs. holding his breath vs. hyperventilating. As he did so, he became very attentionally absorbed, and gradually began to smile. When he took off the stethoscope, the clinician asked him what else he noticed physically at that moment, and he responded that his entire body felt "relaxed" and that his abdominal area felt "calm and cool". He was instructed to become more and more aware of sensory changes, in the tradition of a mindful body scan, i.e., "just take a few moments, or a few minutes, one or two or more times every day for the next two week, to check in with your body and notice how every part is feeling . . . like changes in temperature, or changes in how heavy or light a part feels, or tingly, or bigger or smaller, or differences between one side or area and another, or even colors that might look different on the skin if any part needs calming or cooling or comfort, then you can make that happen, because you discovered how to do that just now." He was instructed to do this practice in the manner of alert hypnosis (i.e., eyes open with focused attention) although no specific name was given to him for this practice.

Several visits later, M. reported that he had been regularly practicing his "noticing" (his word for the body scan) and his abdominal pain had completely abated. Over the next five years, his abdominal pain remained in full remission. He had transient, intermittent episodes of milder somatic complaints as well as mood difficulties, usually during times of life transition such as starting at a new school. Over time, with the clinician's guidance, he discussed the traumatic events and adversity he had faced earlier in his childhood and connected these experiences to "stress . . . and stress makes me have more (aches and pains) and be crabby".

At this time (a bit more than five years after the initial visit) the clinician invited him to learn self-hypnosis to address the long-term goal of handling stress more effectively, and he said he was motivated to do so. To begin, he was simply asked to do the "noticing" body scan that he had previously found helpful; as he did so, he spontaneously closed his eyes and the clinician suggested he talk aloud to himself as he noticed each part of his body felt. The clinician then suggested he could "change any of those (sensations) now if they're not yet comfortable, or just allow them to be how they are until they change themselves to be more comfortable". Suggestions for self-paced stress reduction were then permissively offered, included metaphoric imagery such as letting go of one or more balloons filled with stress and watching them slowly rise, the stress getting smaller and smaller as the balloons went higher and higher into the sky, as well as imagery for strength such as pulling a heavy load of stress and watching it get smaller and eventually fade away to nothing as he got stronger and pulled it further. It was further suggested that by pulling that heavy load so far, he had become so strong that most stressors would bounce off of him and the few that did not bounce off would be easy for him to move around or transform into something harmless. He was then offered post-hypnotic suggestions, i.e., suggestions given during the hypnotic experience to be recalled and used with automaticity within the context of the patient's everyday life, for a "power word" of M's choosing, that he could use every time he would be practicing self-hypnosis at home which would then allow him to quickly and easily engage this "inner-strength stress-relief system" during times of distress or recovery from stressors. M. continues to do this self-hypnosis practice several times per week and uses his "power word" to deal effectively with life's ups and downs, including interpersonal relationships, family transitions, and school.

2.3. Summary

In the case of M., the session with the stethoscope integrated a mindfulness-based approach (i.e., body scan and nonjudgmental awareness of, and ability to distance himself from (dissociate), unpleasant physical sensations) to promote M. orienting towards (instead of avoiding) his somatic experiences in a neutral manner, and as a hypnotic and post-hypnotic suggestion for self-regulation of neurophysiology (e.g., pain perception and stress reactivity). His subsequent use of these strategies on his own demonstrates the enduring value of mindfulness-oriented self-hypnotic approaches that empower young people who have faced chronic 'toxic' stress.

3. Integrating Biofeedback and Hypnosis

3.1. Background

Similar to hypnosis—and hypnosis with children [9,101–103]—biofeedback has had fluctuating definitions in its extensive literature [104–106]. Most theorists would agree that biofeedback utilizes technology typically with computer-based equipment) to monitor a patient's various physiologic functions and in real time relay this to the patient, i.e., feed these measurements back to the patient for their use in acknowledging and then manipulating/altering the physiologic variable in the direction of a pre-determined, agreed-upon therapeutic direction and outcome [104,107,108]. Modern advances in computer technology commonly display the feedback in sophisticated, colorful, and engaging visual and/or auditory modes. This feedback is also used by the clinician to assess and monitor the patient's responses to events during the session (e.g., to specific suggestions for relaxation and/or mental imagery).

It is common, appropriate, and effective to invite children to consider and learn computerized biofeedback by presenting it as a "video game for your body". With the everyday, even constant availability and prevalence of videogames, high tech formats are relevant and syntonic with popular culture, so much so that 'apps' on smart-phones and 'smart watches' and other portable devices now can and do provide multiple biofeedback options to children and adults alike, not to mention comparable resources on social media. Indeed, they are even promoted as therapeutic devices (e.g., Inner Balance from Heartmath [109], Elvira Lang's "My Comfort Talk" [110], Ben Furman's "KIDS SKILLS" [111]). Types of feedback modalities commonly and typically utilized are heart rate variability for children with anxiety, stress, positional orthostatic tachycardia syndrome (POTS), and a host of other conditions (www.heartmath.com); or EMG (electromyography) and peripheral skin temperature for migraine headaches [112,113].

It has been our experience that most, if not all, biofeedback with children includes hypnotic suggestions whether or not 'named' and/or intended as such. Increasingly, even more extensive hypnotherapeutic procedures are commonly and often elegantly integrated with the electronic feedback information and re-structuring of that information in the direction of the collaboratively agreed upon (between children, parents, and clinician) therapeutic outcomes. In clinical as well as research studies, reference to, or identification of, the hypnotic elements are barely mentioned in passing if at all. For example, in most scientific paper describing biofeedback research, several paragraphs are often devoted to a description of the electronic monitoring equipment and the nature of the electrodes and operating systems, before a one- or two-line statement almost blithely states something like "and the child was instructed to relax and imagine a favorite activity". This obvious hypnotic invitation/suggestion is rarely characterized as such though it seems it is integral to the clinical experience and, we believe, to the success of the therapeutic intervention. To our knowledge, no one has sought to discriminate the differential influence of the biofeedback process vs. the hypnotic suggestions per se.

As the biofeedback experience proceeds, and particularly as the clinician observes the 'results' of improving physiologic regulation, the clinician commonly offers 'ego-strengthening' suggestions including compliments and verbal feedback that the subject is 'doing well', doing it 'right', and 'the more you do it the better you get'. These reinforcing hypnotic suggestions are often used to provide future-oriented (i.e., 'post-hypnotic') suggestions for continued practice/rehearsal of the hypnotic-biofeedback strategy at home as a self-empowerment approach. Because anxious children typically experience exaggerated psychophysiological stress reactivity, they benefit from learning relaxation skills and self-regulation strategies to reduce over-arousal [5]. Examples include "as you notice on the computer how well you have slowed your breathing ... "; or "while your skin temperature is going up in your fingertips, it's great to notice how much your headache is going away"; or "the more you notice how relaxed your muscles are, just realize and notice how happy and proud you feel, and how those worries are disappearing ... and the more you do this every day for 5 or 10 min, the more and sooner you'll be successful (in resolving that (problem) or eliminating that (pain, anxiety, worry)".

We have come to understand that biofeedback is a form of self-hypnosis and self-hypnosis is the ultimate form of biofeedback [108]. More than 40 years ago, the late Psychologist, Beata Jencks, Ph.D. published Your Body-Biofeedback at its Best [114] reflecting her initial training in the art of J.H. Schultz's "Standard Autogenic Training" and her emphasis on Mind–body integration. Jencks' work had substantial influence in a study applying hypnosis and pulmonary function biofeedback in a preschool family asthma education program [15].

Writing in the first textbook on Integrative Pediatrics in the chapter "A Pediatric Perspective on Mind–body Medicine" Kohen wrote about the hypnosis/biofeedback interface:

> Hypnosis and biofeedback are strategies directed at evoking innate experiential resources to alter psycho-physiologic responses which have become maladaptive. Hypnosis relies on the resonance and rapport of a therapeutic relationship and the language of positive expectancy to (help the child to) cultivate the imagination. Biofeedback provides an external somatic focus as a proxy for internal psycho-physiological change. BOTH involve narrowly focused, intensified attention and heightened responsiveness to new ideas and associations. This 'trance' state can be reinforced by the clinician's therapeutic language AND by the nature of the electronic/computerized information being received in the feedback. [115] (p. 287)

3.2. Case Example

A 12-year-old boy, F., was referred to the developmental-behavioral pediatrician by his primary care pediatrician for the presenting complaint of school phobia. Though his school refusal had begun soon after the beginning of his first semester in 6th grade in his first year at the Junior High School, most of his elementary school peers were in the same school and as a good student he did not find the classes difficult or the teachers challenging, intimidating, or otherwise problematic. In fact, as is often the case, academic or peer-related anxiety was not the concern.

He reportedly had "difficulty falling asleep" though this too was a function of underlying separation anxiety and not insomnia or other sleep disorder. He spoke of being afraid of the dark, not liking it, and being upset that his parents and siblings were asleep before he was, i.e., that he was the one awake and, "What if something happens?!" His mother noted that even when he told his parents he was "feeling fine now" and would "baby-sit" his younger six-year-old sister when the parents were going out for dinner for 2 h before dark, as soon as they would begin to back the car down the driveway, he would run after the moving car, crying and not wanting to be left alone. On occasion when they would go out and he and his sister stayed with a "baby-sitter" he frequently called his parents every 5–10 min at the restaurant to find out when they would come home.

After developing rapport during the initial visit, F. was willing to acknowledge that he had a lot of "worry" and "nervousness"; and that this made him afraid to go to school, to be away from his parents, and to do stuff. When he thought about this he said he said he thought it was "dumb" and that he wished it would go away. He was especially embarrassed about having hyperventilation and crying "so easily, like a baby" when he was anxious.

He was intrigued by the idea that with self-hypnosis he could learn to use his mind to be "the boss of his body". He quickly learned the self-hypnotic technique of "three and six" [116], focusing on his own body's biofeedback by paying careful attention to his respiratory cycle, i.e., slowly breathing in to a slow count to three, then slowly breathing out to a slow count to six. A "second" three and six would be identical along with eye closure. The next breath (also three and six) would keep eyes closed and begin to imagine favorite place imagery, and the next three and six would begin to add progressive relaxation linked to each successive out-breath.

Though F.'s anxiety improved, and he was able to more easily make it to school, he continued to call his mother frequently from school, with varying complaints that he "didn't feel well" or "needed to come home", and frequent visits to the nurse's office. Despite his mother's effectiveness in being sensitive in listening to F., she followed guidance to not pick him up early from school, and the School Nurse was equally collaborative in offering comfort and reassurance while dispatching F. back to class. As this continued, and in the context of knowing that F. also found comfort in successfully immersing himself in video games he could WIN, it was decided to introduce him to biofeedback by offering to show him "a computer-game for your body". He was immediately intrigued by the graphics and the easy-to-understand process of the Emwave PRO computerized biofeedback (Heartmath Inc., Boulder Creek, CA). As children commonly do, as he became focused and absorbed in attending to the images on the computer screen (monitoring and measuring his heart rate variability), he spontaneously moved into a hypnotic state, evidenced by his body stillness in his chair, fixed gaze stare at the computer screen (with infrequent blinking), and spontaneous slowing of respirations, along with slowing of heart rate, without any verbal hypnotic suggestion to do any of those behaviors.

He quickly became proficient at 'winning' the various games available in this program through control of his heart rate variability (HRV); and his pride and confidence in his growing competence were natural by-products of the process. As he enjoyed these biofeedback sessions, hypnotic suggestions were brief and focused upon suggestions directed at strengthening inner resources such as self-confidence (such as "you're doing this exactly right!" or "wonderful!") and post-hypnotic suggestions to foster competence and control over target symptoms (such as "the more you do this, the better you get", and "pretty soon you'll be so good at this that you'll hardly notice any of that anxiety or worry or nervous feelings that used to be there before ... "). After two biofeedback sessions he and his family were encouraged to consider obtaining a personalized, portable version of the Emwave program, the Emwave PSR (Personal Stress Reliever), which monitors and gives visual and auditory feedback of pacing and slowing of breathing, signaling when HRV is in a positive 'coherence' state.

F. continued to improve. One day he came in for an appointment after school and was eager to report, "You won't believe what happened today!" He said that at lunchtime he was on the playground and three older boys began bullying him. He said he did not know why, but they were pushing him around and he was getting sad and nervous and he began to cry and ran away. Luckily, they did not follow him. He ran to his locker, planning to get his Emwave PSR from his backpack and find a private place he could practice his Emwave and calm himself ("I didn't want to cry more or call my Mom or go to the Nurse."). He got his backpack, found a place in a corner where he could be in private. All set to practice his Emwave he discovered that it was not in his backpack! Hearing this, the clinician said "Oh, no! What did you DO to SOLVE this?" (Note the suggestions of the clinician regarding their confidence to help himself). F. said "Well, I decided all that I could do was "just pretend and imagine that I did have the Emwave, so I pretended to attach it (the HRV monitoring electrode) to my earlobe, and then I imagined I was holding it in my hand, and I closed my eyes and was doing the imagination and my breathing got slower and I was fine and didn't feel like crying any more. I realized then that actually I am the Emwave, and the Emwave is me!" Beyond complimenting F., the clinician asked if it was okay to tell that story to other students, of course without mentioning his name . . . and he too was thrilled that his experience could be of help to others in that way.

It was clearly a combination of self-hypnosis and biofeedback that allowed F. to develop mastery over his symptoms, and to cope with parental separation and stressful situations at school.

3.3. Summary

In the foregoing, it was critical to identify a biofeedback system and modalities within that system that would be concordant with the abilities, interests, and maturation and cognitive developmental style of the child, 12-year-old F. Rapport with F. and knowledge of his facility and interest in videogames were identified as key resources that made this easy to accomplish, in part because the HRV biofeedback system selected has games that appeal to various ages and interests in childhood and adolescence. Just as we emphasize the importance of tailoring hypnotic approaches to the developmental level and capacity of the young [9,102], so it is essential that biofeedback approaches be selected that appeal to the interests and developmental capacity of the patient.

As reflected in the described case of F, hypnosis and biofeedback share similar (if not identical) characteristics, including:

- positive expectations for therapeutic outcomes;
- absorption/concentration/focused, narrowed attention;
- spontaneous relaxation in association with vigilant attention;
- concurrent psychophysiological changes (used to give feedback to the subject that they are "doing this 'exactly right'"—biofeedback clinicians may simply refer to these as encouragement or positive verbal feedback).

4. Integrating Acupuncture and Hypnosis

4.1. Background

Acupuncture is a form of eastern medicine that originated in China over 2000 years ago. The traditional concept of acupuncture is that Qi, the basic life force, travels along channels, i.e., meridians, which can be accessed by fine instruments (traditionally acupuncture needles) to balance and remove obstructions to its flow in order to treat mental and physical ailments and improve health. Acupuncture is one of the most popular complementary medicine modalities in the US [117] according to a 2008 survey [118], with 20% of children in the US having used it. Acupuncture has been used to treat several conditions [119] and is gaining particular attention for its usefulness in treating pain. The mechanism of acupuncture is not completely known, but acupuncture can cause an endogenous opioid response that is blunted by naloxone in a dose dependent fashion [120].

The unity between mind and body, i.e., an interactive relationship between the two, is an important component of Eastern medicine. As a result of this interaction, hypnosis and acupuncture may be uniquely suited to complement each other as therapies [121]. Numerous studies have supported the use of hypnosis for both procedural and chronic pain. Kemper [122] previously reported that acupuncture is well tolerated in pediatrics with many patients identifying it as "helpful and pleasant". Others note that acupuncture is safe and well tolerated in the pediatric population when carried out by appropriately trained individuals [123,124]. Zeltzer et al.'s [125] study provided further support for the feasibility and acceptability of acupuncture in the pediatric population and illustrated its utility in combination with hypnosis. In this study of over 31 children with chronic pain at the UCLA pain center, acupuncture was combined with a standardized hypnosis program using a pain dial technique in which the children imagined being in a plane cockpit with a dial connected to the area of pain. Rather than using the word pain, but they suggested using the phrase "altering the feeling as needed". The 28 children completing the study reported decreased symptoms [125,126].

Acupuncture is well tolerated in patients from infancy to adulthood [127]. The management of commons symptoms such as pain, nausea, and other GI distress are particularly good fits for a combination of hypnosis and acupuncture. Recommended ages for the combination of the two include any child who is of appropriate age for hypnosis. Hypnosis may help in the tolerability of painful acupoints and augment the response to acupuncture in painful conditions such as headache [128]. Acupuncture may be useful in facilitating and augmenting hypnotic suggestion in patients who are preparing for dental and surgical procedures and have a history of phobias and panic attacks [129]. In a study of 108 adults with history of panic attacks and dental/surgical phobias, the acupuncture point GV-24 (the "third eye" point on the forehead) was found to enhance hypnotic induction [129]. GV-20 (the "governing vessel" point on the scalp vertex) and surrounding points have been used to decrease anxiety associated with dental procedures [130]. Though more research is needed, the combined use of hypnosis with acupuncture appears to be beneficial for pediatric patients.

4.2. Case Example

J. is a 14-year-old adolescent with sickle cell disease who was referred to an outpatient integrative medicine clinic by her hematologist for assistance with pain management. J.'s sickle cell symptoms had been relatively well controlled until about a year ago when she began to present with painful crises requiring hospitalization every two months. She was receiving a number of medications for pain as needed including: acetaminophen, ibuprofen, gabapentin, and oxycodone. The hematologist had recommended hydroxyurea. The family was considering the addition of hydroxyurea but had some concerns about side effects.

The initial integrative medicine visit was 90 min. Considerable time was spent listening to J's story and how her sickle cell disease affected her life including her relationships and interactions with friends and family. We also discussed her goals for this session and for management of her pain in general, including the potential benefits of adding hydroxyurea as recommended by her hematologist. After development of rapport, J. was able to recognize that her fear of the pain, or of pain coming, was interfering with the enjoyment of her daily life. J.'s main goal was to be able to fully participate in the activities that she enjoyed with her friends. Her parents were concerned that she was beginning to isolate herself and hoped that when her pain was controlled that she would be able to continue to participate in the afterschool activities that she used to enjoy. Though she did continue to attend school despite the pain, she was worried about being too active—that doing so would cause the pain to return and that she would need to go back to the hospital for pain management. J. and her parents were very interested in acupuncture for pain management, but J. said that she was afraid of needles and too scared to have acupuncture.

The clinician and J. discussed using her imagination to help her relax and explained that when she was in a more relaxed state she might be surprised to find that she does not mind having acupuncture at all and that she may find the experience to be pleasant and helpful (all of these were alert hypnotic suggestions to enlist her cooperation). It was explained that some people also call this way of using your imagination hypnosis and that hypnosis is about using the mind and imagination to give her the power to be able to do the things that she wants such as having acupuncture and spending time with her friends without worry. She was curious about the process and agreed to proceed with reassurance that she was in control and could stop whenever she liked. This provided the safe space to allow her to more fully experience the trance state.

The clinician proceeded with hypnosis using favorite place imagery for calming and relaxation during the acupuncture session. The clinician began with a conversational induction, speaking to J. in a calm and soothing voice about what we were planning to do. Reassurance was provided that she would remain in control and the discussion centered around 'wondering' what this experience would be like for her. It was also suggested that she would be able to speak and interact while maintaining a calm and relaxed state. Her gaze became fixed and her breath elongated as she began to deepen into trance, she then was invited her to close her eyes. Her eyelids closed. A few moments later rapid movement of her eyes beneath her closed lids was noted. Then, she was invited to imagine a door beyond which was her favorite place with all of her senses. As she explored her favorite place, she was able to report that her favorite place was her grandmother's house. She was encouraged her to fully imagine being there, including paying particular attention to the look, the feel, sounds, and the smells. As she explored her favorite place, she became comfortable enough to accept the acupuncture needles. Encouragement and praise were provided for her continuing to fully experience her favorite place during acupuncture. She was able to share that in her favorite place she felt, "warm", "safe", and "loved". It was suggested that she could continue to maintain those feelings.

At that time, it was asked if she was ready to proceed with the treatment. She nodded that she was. With her permission, a needle was placed in GV-20 for deeper relaxation and then auricular acupuncture was performed using the battlefield technique for pain management [131]. J. did not appear to notice when the needles were placed. After the needles were placed, she was invited to bring her awareness back to the room. As she brought her awareness back to the room, she maintained a calm and relaxed state and was pleasantly surprised to find that in her experience, "the needles don't hurt at all!" We completed the acupuncture treatment and the needles were removed. There were no complications. She tolerated the procedure well and requested to continue acupuncture and hypnosis at future visits. Weekly acupuncture was recommended for six weeks and she tolerated all future treatments well. The family decided to start hydroxyurea. J. continued to use self-hypnosis with favorite place imagery at home for pain and anxiety and her hospital admissions decreased. The combination of acupuncture and hypnosis allowed J. to fully explore treatment options that she initially feared. Had it not been for the combination of acupuncture and hypnosis, J. would not have been relaxed and comfortable enough to allow the needles. It is also likely that needling at GV-20 allowed for deeper relaxation and deepening of the trance state. In addition, J. also developed the skill of self-hypnosis which provided another tool in her toolbox to help her better manage her pain.

4.3. Summary

Acupuncture and hypnosis are useful tools on their own, but when used in combination can work synergistically. In the case presented above, hypnosis allowed for relaxed state that provided an opening for the acceptance of the acupuncture needles. Acupuncture to GV-20 likely assisted with deepening which may have augmented the hypnotic state and experience.

5. Integrating Yoga and Hypnosis

5.1. Background

The practice of yoga, an ancient mind–body, "moving meditation" modality originating from India, traditionally involved a set of beliefs and rituals with an over-arching goal of a person's union with Supreme Reality or the Universal Self [132]. Various yoga systems emphasized different paths toward that goal. By contrast, the version used by adults in the United States primarily focuses on combining various exercises involving postures ('asanas'), regulation of breathing ('pranayama'), and, at times, meditation to achieve emotional balance [133].

Moving beyond the one-on-one tradition, group instruction became the norm. In recent years a plethora of yoga programs for children and teens has propagated across the U.S. In 2012, 3.1% of U.S. children (1.7 million) used some form of yoga [118]. Parents, teachers, professionals and others with no yoga experience can become certified to teach youth in groups by completing an online (webinars and home-study) or live program. Some may pursue an optional registration as a registered children's yoga teacher (RCYT) with Yoga Alliance, a non-profit organization with a mission to foster "integrity and diversity of teaching yoga" [134]. The RCYT designation is accomplished by fulfilling their requirements, i.e., the equivalent of over 40 days of training acquired over time, and an annual fee. YogaKids, a registered children's yoga school offers such training through a sequence of levels [135].

Of note, YogaKids describes that future teachers of YogaKids learn how to combine yoga with other activities involving music, books, games, art, reading, writing, and science for a group of children. Thus, perhaps not surprisingly, yoga has found its way into the classroom [136]. On the one hand, this combination seems developmentally on target to facilitate children's learning and enjoyment; on the other, it begs the research question whether such confounders are controlled or measured in studies. One would be hard pressed to conclude that benefits of yoga group classes of this nature are solely due to learning yoga poses, postures, and breathing. Clearly, learning yoga in a more narrowed sense (postures, breathing, with or without meditation) or on a one-on-one basis would offer a very different learning environment.

Yoga Calm is another child- and family-oriented yoga program that incorporates "mindfulness" and "relaxation and reflection activities" with a goal of "self-regulation" and "social-emotional learning" [137]. Parents and professionals seeking certification and instructor training must complete the required 40 h of online courses and 40 h of practicum. This training is distinguished by providing graduate level college credits and continuing education units from many colleges and organizations. Further, efforts to ground their program with science is evident by their listing of research in these related domains (i.e., self-regulation, etc.) and their active engagement in research projects in collaboration with the University of Minnesota, a public-school system, and a children's hospital.

Early reviews of yoga focusing on the physical and mental health for children and teens expressed caution in making conclusions, citing only preliminary benefits due to methodological limitations [133,138,139]. More recently, some clinicians writing about yoga vary in their interpretation about potential benefits for children/teens' physical [140,141] and mental health [142,143]. Further, randomly chosen websites and blogs about this topic frequently reveal far-reaching conclusions, with minimal mention of the still preliminary conclusions. Hopefully correcting this trend is a 2017 Clinical Report by the AAP about pediatric integrative medicine that noted that while recent studies suggest benefits of yoga for children, the committee advocated for more systematic studies to ferret out this inquiry [144].

While PIM research has progressed remarkably, to date, research reviews of yoga focusing on outcomes of physical and mental health for children/teens have not yet examined differences based on many variables that complicate the comparison and contrast of findings and obscure conclusions about efficacy. As this area of study continues to unfold, investigators surely will begin to examine such variables as content (yoga type, elements, exercises, and other activities); format (e.g., session number, frequency, and time frame); context (individual vs. group (and size) vs. home); age range; home practice expectations and adherence; teacher's expertise; and long-term outcomes.

Exciting, fresh lines of research about the neuroscience underpinnings of therapeutic yoga are very promising and adds credibility to this PIM modality. Similarly, sound exploration of theoretical models for potential self-regulatory mechanisms of yoga for psychological and physical health is expanding. An article by researchers from Harvard and other institutions [145] provide evidence of yoga's top-down (cognitive) and bottom-up (emotions generated by the limbic system) pathways for self-regulation of cognition, emotions, behavior, and physiology. They also propose an intriguing model whereby these yoga-based processes may influence self-regulation of physical and emotional stress.

A complementary article by a group of University of California researchers offers a comprehensive, scholarly literature review, including a unique, methodical deconstruction of yoga's main components, i.e., "posture or movement sequences, conscious regulation of the breath, and techniques to improve attentional focus" [146]. Cogent hypotheses are laid out regarding how the neurocircuitry and physiological processes promoted by yoga may explain the mechanisms for change. They propose that yoga's main components may directly activate the vagal afferent system and other circuits, possibly resulting in enhanced autonomic, emotional, and cognitive regulation. Building on these neurophysiological frameworks, a recent paper connects therapeutic yoga to polyvagal theory (PVT), developed by Porges in 2011, to further explain the patterns of autonomic regulation related to emotional expression and social behavior and relationships [147].

Information about combining traditional yoga with hypnosis is scarce. Dalal and Barber's 2008 chapter (a modestly revised version of a 1969 paper) on this topic is the notable exception with its discussion and challenge of the purported similarities, i.e., an altered state of consciousness (trance states) with associated unusual phenomena [148]. Like some of the other PIM modalities, the shared elements of pediatric hypnosis and westernized yoga include the pre-requisite building of trust and alliance or rapport; goals toward self-regulation, health, well-being, and emotional balance; narrowed attention and inner absorption; frequent use of the breath; reduced psychophysiological reactivity via activation of the parasympathetic nervous system with vagal tone to evoke calmness; and varying degrees of dissociation. The latest theories on hypnosis emphasize its top-down neurophysiological components [68,95].

5.2. Case Example

S. is a 14-year-old female referred for integrative therapies to help her manage physical symptoms of headache and body aches, difficulty with sleep onset, and a history of generalized anxiety disorder. S.'s anxiety problems began at eight years of age with separation anxiety and specific phobia symptoms. On the first day of ninth grade, she had a panic episode with multiple symptoms including racing heartbeat, shaking, sweating, cold extremities, and fear of "losing it". Subsequently, she developed recurrent headaches due to clenching her teeth and general increased muscle tension of her neck, shoulders and back. In addition to being an excellent student, she was also an accomplished dancer but had become unable to participate in recitals due to performance anxiety.

At her first appointment, considerable time was spent developing rapport by listening closely to her story, learning about her family, her interests, and her goals for this intervention. She specifically said she wished to learn skills to avoid taking more "anti-anxiety pills", feel more comfortable in the classroom, and be able to dance in recitals with her friends. The clinician discussed with S. how she might learn to help herself achieve these goals by learning about the brain/body connections, combining yoga and hypnosis.

Yoga was defined for S. as "uniting the mind, body and spirit." It includes using the breath ('pranayama'), physical poses ('asanas'), and conscious awareness to create balance. She had done a little of this in a physical education class. She was more unsure of hypnosis, so the clinician talked about how it is "using your imagination on purpose", which she already knew how to do since she practiced her dance routines in her mind. S. also described how she occasionally reminds herself (to reframe worries) that she "can do it!" The clinician suggested she might reframe her worries and fears to experiencing herself as strong, competent and successful. Hypnosis was further defined as beginning with focused attention on the breath, the body, or an image and may be intensified with greater sensory, or imagery awareness. The process then shifts to using specific goal-oriented suggestions to change one's symptoms, perceptions, or behavior. The clinician emphasized that it is important to be certain that the use of hypnosis is appropriate for the desired outcome. S. and the clinician collaboratively planned for S. to spend time before the next visit simply noticing how she felt physically and emotionally when she was doing something she really enjoyed.

At the second visit, S. could more easily describe how her heart raced, her muscles tightened, her hands got sweaty and she forgot what she wanted to say when anxious, in contrast to how she felt when she was calm. The clinician again reviewed the possibilities of S. learning to help herself by using interventions such as yoga and hypnosis to help her become more aware of her ability to be in control in healthy, positive ways. The clinician invited S. to begin with heart/belly breathing because all these modalities use breathing as a means of inducing calmness, relaxation, increasing body awareness, and being in the present moment. The clinician then gently put one hand over her own heart and the other hand over her own abdomen. The clinician further suggested that S focus her attention on her breath as it moved through her body and simply say to herself, "I breathe in (in breath) and I breathe out (out breath)". As she did this she naturally elongated the exhalation and commented on feeling relaxed. After this invitation of narrowed attention to induce the hypnotic experience, the clinician then suggested that S. continue breathing in this easy and natural way while she imagined herself in her favorite place—laying in a hammock in her back yard. Utilizing this classic imagery technique to intensify the hypnotic experience, she visualized her mother's colorful flower garden, felt the warm sun on her arms and legs and the gentle sway of the hammock. The clinician suggested that S allow herself to be absorbed inside her mind by these images and sensations and say to herself, "I am safe and calm" while doing so. Her assignment following this visit was to practice her self-hypnosis (i.e., breathing, favorite place imagery, and positive suggestions to herself) daily for approximately 10 min as well as any time she began to feel anxious.

At the next visit she wanted to learn more about yoga. The clinician invited her to stand in "mountain pose" with her feet about hip width apart, imagining her feet reaching deep into the roots of the earth. During this heightened focus on her body's position and posture, S. was then offered hypnotic suggestions of self-efficacy and self-regulation, to repeat phrases in her mind, such as "I am strong" and "I can do this". She then brought her hands to her heart and energetically pushed her hands and arms above her head—like an exploding volcano releasing worries, fears, negative self-talk, and anything that she no longer needed. This hypnotic metaphor, imagery, and suggestions were combined with the "releasing" process (movement and pose) in yoga that needs to occur before someone can calm down. Using her love of dance, she then created a routine that included using her breath to calmly sustain her while she gracefully moved her body—stretching forward/backward, and side to side releasing tension while imagining strength and courage to move further out into her world with confidence and success.

After this introduction to combining hypnosis with yoga, S. found a class in her community where she could practice yoga with the support of others. She continued to interweave the practice the hypnotic phenomena of intentional breathing, focused attention, and absorption in mental imagery of favorite activities and rehearsal of future successes (as post-hypnotic suggestions).

5.3. Summary

This case illustrates that hypnosis and yoga can work well together to manage physical symptoms, anxious thoughts and negative self-perceptions and are readily accepted by children and teens as a means of improving self-care and resilience. They can easily build on patients' knowledge and experiences.

6. Discussion

PIM touts a growing array of approaches that initially were considered to be solely adjunctive interventions. For several years now, diligent efforts have preliminarily documented the efficacy and safety of separate integrative strategies that improve quality of care in order to recognize PIM as credible and viable by mainstream pediatrics. In spite of the epic history and groundwork of hypnosis as a common root of mind–body PIM, hypnosis may be overlooked as an integrative approach. There is confusion in the PIM literature where hypnosis 'belongs', as it has variably been considered a conventional [149], complementary [118,150], or cast-aside [8] approach. Yet a 2016 article published on the website of the National Center for Complementary and Integrative Health (NCCIH) includes hypnosis as a complementary approach [151]. Might this diminished inclusion be partially due to the recognition that some other PIM modalities (e.g., aromatherapy (essential oils) and nutritional supplements) perhaps sound more acceptable, are simpler to teach, are quicker to grasp, or are easier to incorporate—thus, hypnosis has become out of sight and out of mind?

A related question concerns guided imagery (GI): despite both its heritage and oft-revealed overlapping ingredients with hypnosis as discussed above in this article, might this more neutral name (guided imagery) and its scripts similarly be preferred by some institutions, journals, and clinicians?

It is our reasoning that GI bypasses the investment of time, effort, and cost needed to acquire skills that characterize the uniquely therapeutic communication of hypnosis.

Beyond these two thorny questions, we have highlighted three key themes throughout this paper: (1) common components shared by pediatric hypnosis with GI as well as other mind–body techniques form the core of PIM, i.e., mindfulness, biofeedback, acupuncture, and yoga; and (2) permutations of combined PIM modalities reveal that individual PIM modalities are actually evolving by 'borrowing' elements from one another. Just like the 'blending trend' of integrative approaches with CBT, e.g., "cognitive hypnotherapy" [152,153] and "mindfulness-based cognitive therapy" [154], emerging new terms in integrative health publications further illustrate this trajectory, such as "mindful self-hypnosis" [155]. Research is needed to document the efficacy of combining these multi-modal approaches [156].

A third key theme of this paper is the value and importance of designing personalized treatments in PIM. Health professionals new to PIM modalities quickly discover the range of responses among children/teens, driven by underlying developmental, learning, experiential, and other individual differences. While some clinicians choose to deliver the same 'procedure' to every patient, others are embracing the critical importance of establishing rapport and solidifying trust and attunement in order to maximize each patient's receptivity, cooperation, and adherence to acquiring new skills. As clinicians become more seasoned and secure in their use of PIM modalities, they invite and incorporate the child/teen's own specific goals while contemplating goodness-of-fit between each patient and the potpourri of PIM approaches. The case vignettes we chose for this paper illustrated the additive value of incorporating hypnosis as well as numerous practical strategies and clinical acumen as guidelines for integrating PIM modalities to achieve this goal of individualized care. Honing one's sensitivity to and flexibility in the selection, timing, and presentation of integrative approaches completes the criteria toward a new PIM benchmark for designing personalized treatment with each patient. Beyond the *sequential* use of integrative approaches, future research may find that a more refined delivery model [156], of 'mingling modalities' as illustrated in the case vignettes, could potentially offer a synergistic effect that might become PIM's new norm.

Acquiring expertise in such a practice model takes time, mentoring, and ongoing training. PIM approaches vary widely in terms of effort, time, and cost to achieve competence or mastery, and differ in terms of complex skill development (e.g., hypnosis, biofeedback, and acupuncture) vs. knowledge attainment (e.g., nutritional supplements, essential oils). Obviously, such variations differentially lend themselves to hands-on learning, intensive supervised practice, and ongoing mentoring [10] vs. online webinars and lectures. The phenomenal launches of the online pediatric integrative medicine in residency (PIMR) curriculum [157] and the first pediatric integrative medicine fellowship (under the direction of Ann Ming Yeh, M.D., at Stanford) are ground-breaking contributions to medical education. While the PIMR curriculum includes some on-site activities, hopefully residency program directors (and future iterations of PIMR) will include opportunities for clinicians-in-training to have access to skills training in hypnosis as a fundamental principle and core construct underlying many PIM modalities that prioritize goals relating to children's self-regulation.

While the current integrative medicine board-certification exam in the US includes hypnosis as an area of core content [158], more work remains to incorporate hypnosis into formal curricula. For the thematic reasons outlined in this paper, we recommend that clinical hypnosis be more deeply and broadly promoted as a fundamental root of PIM. Basically, pediatric hypnosis combines imagery with nuanced verbal and nonverbal suggestions to promote therapeutic change from within. As such, curricula in PIM will be strengthened by specific, detailed training in hypnosis in order to develop the nuanced capacities of creating a design (in collaboration with the child/teen) of multi-sensorial imagery and of formulating therapeutic suggestions including an awareness and use of voice prosody, including the speaker's word selection, phrasing, rate, stress, loudness, pitch, and quality [159]. Further, research on clinicians' training in purposeful word choice to design positive suggestions shows substantial evidence of the positive benefits for patients undergoing surgery and procedures, as well as for those experiencing chronic pain, somatization, warts, etc. [160,161]. Creating 'therapeutic presence' via prosodic vocalizations, facial expressions, and gestures has shown to enhance a child and parent's sense of safety within the clinician–patient encounter [162]. Thus, learning such refined details in delivering suggestions speaks to the pragmatic utility of including hypnosis in training for all pediatric professionals to better address physical, mental, and behavioral health issues in an integrative manner.

Author Contributions: Conceptualization, P.K.; Methodology, P.K. and A.J.B.; Writing—Original Draft Preparation, P.K., D.P.K., M.L.B., R.L.K., and A.J.B.; Writing—Review & Editing, P.K. and A.J.B.

References

1. Olness, K.; Gardner, G.G. Some guidelines for uses of hypnotherapy in pediatrics. *Pediatrics* **1978**, *62*, 228–233. [PubMed]
2. Olness, K. Hypnosis in pediatric practice. *Curr. Probl. Pediatr.* **1981**, *12*, 1–47. [CrossRef]
3. Gardner, G.G. Hypnosis with children. *Int. J. Clin. Exp. Hypn.* **1974**, *22*, 20–38. [CrossRef] [PubMed]
4. Olness, K.N.; Conroy, M.M. A Pilot Study of Voluntary Control of Transcutaneous PO_2 by Children: A Brief Communication. *Int. J. Clin. Exp. Hypn.* **1985**, *33*, 1–5. [CrossRef] [PubMed]
5. Kohen, D.P.; Kaiser, P. Clinical hypnosis with children and adolescents—What? Why? How?: Origins, applications, and efficacy. *Children* **2014**, *1*, 74–98. [CrossRef] [PubMed]
6. Erickson, M.H. Pediatric hypnotherapy. *Am. J. Clin. Hypn.* **1958**, *1*, 25–29. [CrossRef]
7. Hilgard, J.R. *Personality and Hypnosis: A Study of Imaginative Involvement*, 2nd ed.; University of Chicago Press: Chicago, IL, USA, 1979.
8. Vohra, S.; Surette, S.; Mittra, D.; Rosen, L.D.; Gardiner, P.; Kemper, K.J. Pediatric integrative medicine: Pediatrics' newest subspecialty? *BMC Pediatr.* **2012**, *12*, 123. [CrossRef] [PubMed]
9. Kohen, D.P.; Olness, K.O. *Hypnosis and Hypnotherapy with Children*, 4th ed.; Routledge, Taylor & Francis Group: New York, NY, USA, 2011.
10. Kohen, D.P.; Kaiser, P.; Olness, K. State-of-the-art pediatric hypnosis training: Remodeling curriculum and refining faculty development. *Am. J. Clin. Hypn.* **2017**, *59*, 292–310. [CrossRef] [PubMed]
11. Krippner, S. The use of hypnosis with elementary and secondary school children in a summer reading clinic. *Am. J. Clin. Hypn.* **1966**, *8*, 261–266. [CrossRef] [PubMed]
12. Jampolsky, G.; Haight, M. Hypnosis and sensory motor stimulation to aid children with learning problems. *J. Learn. Disabil.* **1970**, *3*, 570–575. [CrossRef]
13. Johnson, L.S.; Johnson, D.L.; Olson, M.R.; Newman, J.P. The uses of hypnotherapy with learning disabled children. *J. Clin. Psychol.* **1981**, *37*, 291–299. [CrossRef]
14. Antitch, J.L. The use of hypnosis in pediatric anesthesia. *J. Am. Soc. Psychosom. Dent. Med.* **1967**, *14*, 70–75. [PubMed]
15. Kohen, D.P.; Wynne, E. Applying hypnosis in a preschool family asthma education program: Uses of storytelling, imagery, and relaxation. *Am. J. Clin. Hypn.* **1997**, *39*, 169–181. [CrossRef] [PubMed]
16. Baumann, F. Hypnosis and the adolescent drug abuser. *Am. J. Clin. Hypn.* **1970**, *13*, 17–21. [CrossRef] [PubMed]
17. Labaw, W.L. Adjunctive trance therapy with severely burned children. *Int. J. Child Psychother.* **1973**, *2*, 89–92.
18. Olness, K. The use of self-hypnosis in the treatment of childhood nocturnal enuresis. A report on forty patients. *Clin. Pediatr.* **1975**, *14*. [CrossRef] [PubMed]
19. Edwards, S.D.; Van der Spuy, H.I. Hypnotherapy as a treatment for enuresis. *J. Child Psychol. Psychiatry.* **1985**, *26*, 161–170. [CrossRef] [PubMed]
20. Friman, P.C.; Handwerk, M.L.; Swearer, S.M.; McGinnis, J.C.; Warzak, W.J. Do children with primary nocturnal enuresis have clinically significant behavior problems? *Arch. Pediatr. Adolesc. Med.* **1998**, *152*, 537–539. [CrossRef] [PubMed]
21. Olness, K. Autohypnosis in functional megacolon in children. *Am. J. Clin. Hypn.* **1976**, *19*, 28–32. [CrossRef] [PubMed]

22. Clawson, T.A.; Swade, R.H. The hypnotic control of blood flow and pain: The cure of warts and the potential for the use of hypnosis in the treatment of cancer. *Am. J. Clin. Hypn.* **1975**, *17*, 160–169. [CrossRef] [PubMed]
23. Porter, J. Guided fantasy as a treatment for childhood insomnia. *Aust. N. Z. J. Psychiatry* **1975**, *9*, 169–172. [CrossRef] [PubMed]
24. Kohen, D.P.; Mahowald, M.W.; Rosen, G.M. Sleep-terror disorder in children: The role of self-hypnosis in management. *Am. J. Clin. Hypn.* **1992**, *34*, 233–244. [CrossRef] [PubMed]
25. Gardner, G.G.; Tarnow, J.D. Adjunctive hypnotherapy with an autistic boy. *Am. J. Clin. Hypn.* **1980**, *22*, 173–179. [CrossRef] [PubMed]
26. Kohen, D.P. Relaxation/mental imagery (self-hypnosis) and pelvic examinations in adolescents. *J. Dev. Behav. Pediatr.* **1980**, *1*, 180–186. [CrossRef] [PubMed]
27. Zeltzer, L.; LeBaron, S. Hypnosis and nonhypnotic techniques for reduction of pain and anxiety during painful procedures in children and adolescents with cancer. *J. Pediatr.* **1982**, *101*, 1032–1035. [PubMed]
28. Hall, H.R. Hypnosis and the immune system: A review with implications for cancer and the psychology of healing. *Am. J. Clin. Hypn.* **1982**, *25*, 92–103. [CrossRef] [PubMed]
29. Olness, K.; Culbert, T.; Uden, D. Self-regulation of salivary immunoglobulin A by children. *Pediatrics* **1989**, *83*, 66–71. [PubMed]
30. Hall, H.R. Hypnosis, suggestion, and the psychology of healing: A historical perspective. *Adv. Inst. Adv. Heal.* **1986**, *3*, 29–37.
31. Whorwell, P.J.; Prior, A.; Faragher, E.B. Controlled trial of hypnotherapy in the treatment of severe refractory irritable-bowel syndrome. *Lancet* **1984**, *2*, 1232–1234. [CrossRef]
32. Swirsky-Sacchetti, T.; Margolis, C.G. The effects of a comprehensive self-hypnosis training program on the use of factor VIII in severe hemophilia. *Int. J. Clin. Exp. Hypn.* **1986**, *34*, 71–83. [CrossRef] [PubMed]
33. Zeltzer, L.K.; LeBaron, S. Fantasy in children and adolescents with chronic illness. *J. Dev. Behav. Pediatr.* **1986**, *7*, 195–198. [CrossRef] [PubMed]
34. Barnes, A.J.; Kohen, D.P. Clinical hypnosis as an effective adjunct in the care of pediatric inpatients. *J. Pediatr.* **2006**, *149*, 563–565. [CrossRef] [PubMed]
35. Kohen, D.P. Applications of relaxation/mental imagery (self-hypnosis) in pediatric emergencies. *Int. J. Clin. Exp. Hypn.* **1986**, *34*, 283–294. [CrossRef] [PubMed]
36. Thompson, C.K.; Hall, H.R.; Sison, C.E. Effects of hypnosis and imagery training on naming behavior in aphasia. *Brain Lang.* **1986**, *28*, 141–153. [CrossRef]
37. Kohen, D.P.; Botts, P. Relaxation-imagery (self-hypnosis) in Tourette syndrome: Experience with four children. *Am. J. Clin. Hypn.* **1987**, *29*, 227–237. [CrossRef] [PubMed]
38. Young, M.H.; Montano, R.J. A new hypnobehavioral method for the treatment of children with Tourette's disorder. *Am. J. Clin. Hypn.* **1988**, *31*, 97–106. [CrossRef] [PubMed]
39. Culbertson, F.M. A four-step hypnotherapy model for Gilles de la Tourette's syndrome. *Am. J. Clin. Hypn.* **1989**, *31*, 252–256. [CrossRef] [PubMed]
40. Olness, K.; MacDonald, J.T.; Uden, D.L. Comparison of self-hypnosis and propranolol in the treatment of juvenile classic migraine. *Pediatrics* **1987**, *79*, 593–597. [PubMed]
41. McGrath, P.J.; Humphreys, P.; Goodman, J.T.; Keene, D.; Firestone, P.; Jacob, P.; Cunningham, S.J. Relaxation prophylaxis for childhood migraine: a randomized placebo-controlled trial. *Dev. Med. Child Neurol.* **1988**, *30*, 626–631. [CrossRef] [PubMed]
42. Dinges, D.F.; Whitehouse, W.G.; Orne, E.C.; Bloom, P.B.; Carlin, M.M.; Bauer, N.K.; Gillen, K.A.; Shapiro, B.S.; Ohene-Frempong, K.; Dampier, C.; et al. Self-hypnosis training as an adjunctive treatment in the management of pain associated with sickle cell disease. *Int. J. Clin. Exp. Hypn.* **1997**, *45*, 417–432. [CrossRef] [PubMed]
43. Jacknow, D.S.; Tschann, J.M.; Link, M.P.; Boyce, W.T. Hypnosis in the prevention of chemotherapy-related nausea and vomiting in children: a prospective study. *J. Dev. Behav. Pediatr.* **1994**, *15*, 258–264. [CrossRef] [PubMed]
44. Kohen, D.P.; Olness, K.N.; Colwell, S.O.; Heimel, A. The use of relaxation-mental imagery (self-hypnosis) in the management of 505 pediatric behavioral encounters. *J. Dev. Behav. Pediatr.* **1984**, *5*, 21–25. [CrossRef] [PubMed]
45. Wingert, A.; Ali, S. The Cochrane Library and procedural pain in children: an overview of reviews. *Evidence-Based Child Heal. A Cochrane Rev. J.* **2012**, *7*, 1363–1399.

46. Uman, L.S.; Birnie, K.A.; Noel, M.; Parker, J.A.; Chambers, C.T.; McGrath, P.J.; Kisely, S.R. Psychological interventions for needle-related procedural pain and distress in children and adolescents. *Cochrane Database Syst. Rev.* **2013**, *10*, CD005179. [CrossRef] [PubMed]
47. Olness, K.O. Pediatrics. In *Handbook of Medical and Psychological Hypnosis: Foundations, Applications, and Professional Issues*; Elkins, G.R., Ed.; Springer Publishing Company, LLC: New York, NY, USA, 2017; pp. 371–378.
48. Sawni, A.; Breuner, C.C. Clinical hypnosis, an effective mind-body modality for adolescents with behavioral and physical complaints. *Children* **2017**, *4*, 19. [CrossRef] [PubMed]
49. Kaiser, P. Childhood anxiety, worry, and fear: individualizing hypnosis goals and suggestions for self-regulation. *Am. J. Clin. Hypn.* **2011**, *54*, 16–31. [CrossRef] [PubMed]
50. Kaiser, P. Anxiety in Children and Teens. In *Handbook of Medical and Psychological Hypnosis: Foundations, Applications, and Professional Issues*; Elkins, G.R., Ed.; Springer Publishing Company, LLC: New York, NY, USA, 2017; pp. 477–484.
51. Anbar, R.D. Asthma. In *Handbook of Medical and Psychological Hypnosis: Foundations, Applications, and Professional Issues*; Elkins, G.R., Ed.; Springer Publishing Company, LLC: New York, NY, USA, 2017; pp. 161–168.
52. Anbar, R.D. Cystic Fibrosis. In *Handbook of Medical and Psychological Hypnosis: Foundations, Applications, and Professional Issues*; Elkins, G.R., Ed.; Springer Publishing Company, LLC: New York, NY, USA, 2017; pp. 199–204.
53. Hogg, F. Hypnosis. In *Dental Fear and Anxiety in Pediatric Patients*; Campbell, C., Ed.; Springer International Publishing: Basel, Switzerland, 2017; pp. 153–172.
54. Lazarus, J.E. Enuresis. In *Handbook of Medical and Psychological Hypnosis: Foundations, Applications, and Professional Issues*; Elkins, G.R., Ed.; Springer Publishing Company, LLC: New York, NY, USA, 2017; pp. 225–234.
55. Kohen, D.P. Nail Biting. In *Handbook of Medical and Psychological Hypnosis: Foundations, Applications, and Professional Issues*; Elkins, G.R., Ed.; Springer Publishing Company, LLC: New York, NY, USA, 2017; pp. 321–325.
56. Kohen, D.P. Headaches—Children. In *Handbook of Medical and Psychological Hypnosis: Foundations, Applications, and Professional Issues*; Elkins, G.R., Ed.; Springer Publishing Company, LLC: New York, NY, USA, 2017; pp. 259–271.
57. Anbar, R.D.; Fernandez, B.A. Vocal Cord Dysfunction. In *Handbook of Medical and Psychological Hypnosis: Foundations, Applications, and Professional Issues*; Elkins, G.R., Ed.; Springer Publishing Company, LLC: New York, NY, USA, 2017; pp. 429–434.
58. Kuttner, L. *A Child in Pain: What Health Professionals Can Do to Help*; Crown House Publishing: Camarthen, UK, 2010.
59. Saadat, H. Clinical Hypnosis in Children. In *Handbook of Pediatric Chronic Pain: Current Science and Integrative Practice (Perspectives on Pain in Psychology)*; McClain, B.C., Suresh, S., Eds.; Springer-Verlag: New York, NY, USA, 2011.
60. Friedrichsdorf, S.J.; Kohen, D.P. Integration of hypnosis into pediatric palliative care. *Ann. Palliat. Med.* **2018**, *7*, 136–150. [CrossRef] [PubMed]
61. Pendergrast, R.A. Incorporating hypnosis into pediatric clinical encounters. *Children* **2017**, *4*, 18. [CrossRef] [PubMed]
62. Hall, H.R.; Olness, K.O. Hypnosis, imagery, self-regulation and immune activity. In *Psychoneuroimmunology and Psychotherapy*; Schubert, C., Ed.; Schattauer-Verlag: Stuttgart, Germany, 2014.
63. Yeh, A.M.; Wren, A.; Golianu, B. Mind-body interventions for pediatric inflammatory bowel disease. *Children* **2017**, *4*, 22. [CrossRef] [PubMed]
64. Vlieger, A.M.; Menko-Frankenhuis, C.; Wolfkamp, S.C.; Tromp, E.; Benninga, M.A. Hypnotherapy for children with functional abdominal pain or irritable bowel syndrome: A randomized controlled trial. *Gastroenterology* **2007**, *133*, 1430–1436. [CrossRef] [PubMed]
65. Vlieger, A.M.; Rutten, J.M.T.M.; Govers, A.M.A.P.; Frankenhuis, C.; Benninga, M.A. Long-term follow-up of gut-directed hypnotherapy vs. standard care in children with functional abdominal pain or irritable bowel syndrome. *Am. J. Gastroenterol.* **2012**, *107*, 627–631. [CrossRef] [PubMed]

66. Rutten, J.M.; Vlieger, A.M.; Frankenhuis, C.; George, E.K.; Groeneweg, M.; Norbruis, O.F.; Tjon a Ten, W.; Van Wering, H.; Dijkgraaf, M.G.; Merkus, M.P.; et al. Gut-directed hypnotherapy in children with irritable bowel syndrome or functional abdominal pain (syndrome): a randomized controlled trial on self exercises at home using CD versus individual therapy by qualified therapists. *BMC Pediatr.* **2014**, *14*, 140. [CrossRef] [PubMed]
67. Rutten, J.M.T.M.; Vlieger, A.M.; Frankenhuis, C.; George, E.K.; Groeneweg, M.; Norbruis, O.F.; Tjon a Ten, W.; van Wering, H.M.; Dijkgraaf, M.G.W.; Merkus, M.P.; et al. Home-based hypnotherapy self-exercises vs individual hypnotherapy with a therapist for treatment of pediatric irritable bowel syndrome, functional abdominal pain, or functional abdominal pain syndrome. *JAMA Pediatr.* **2017**, *171*, 470. [CrossRef] [PubMed]
68. Terhune, D.B.; Cleeremans, A.; Raz, A.; Lynn, S.J. Hypnosis and top-down regulation of consciousness. *Neurosci. Biobehav. Rev.* **2017**, *81*, 59–74. [CrossRef] [PubMed]
69. Rossman, M. *Guided Imagery for Self-Healing: An Essential Resource for Anyone Seeking Wellness*; H.J. Kramer, Inc.: Tiburon, CA, USA, 2000.
70. Fung, E. Relaxation, guided imagery and hypnosis training not just for the Olympic athletes. In *NASW Child Welfare, Section Connection*; National Association of Social Workers: Chicago, IL, USA, 2008; Issue 2.
71. Roffe, L.; Schmidt, K.; Ernst, E. A systematic review of guided imagery as an adjuvant cancer therapy. *Psychooncology.* **2005**, *14*, 607–617. [CrossRef] [PubMed]
72. Hadjibalassi, M.; Lambrinou, E.; Papastavrou, E.; Papathanassoglou, E. The effect of guided imagery on physiological and psychological outcomes of adult ICU patients: A systematic literature review and methodological implications. *Aust. Crit. Care* **2018**, *31*, 73–86. [CrossRef] [PubMed]
73. Weydert, J.A.; Shapiro, D.E.; Acra, S.A.; Monheim, C.J.; Chambers, A.S.; Ball, T.M. Evaluation of guided imagery as treatment for recurrent abdominal pain in children: A randomized controlled trial. *BMC Pediatr.* **2006**, *6*, 29. [CrossRef] [PubMed]
74. Gruzelier, J.H. A review of the impact of hypnosis, relaxation, guided imagery and individual differences on aspects of immunity and health. *Stress* **2002**, *5*, 147–163. [CrossRef] [PubMed]
75. Dormoy, M. *Imagery Work with Kids: Essential Practices to Help Them Manage Stress, Reduce Anxiety & Build Self-Esteem*; W.W. Norton & Company: New York, NY, USA, 2016.
76. American Psychological Association. Want Better Health? Use Your Head! Available online: http://www.apa.org/research/action/head.aspx (accessed on 24 July 2018).
77. Vohra, S.; McClafferty, H.; Becker, D.; Bethell, C.; Culbert, T.; King-Jones, S.; Rosen, L.; Sibinga, E.; Bailey, M.; Weydert, J.; et al. Mind-body therapies in children and youth. *Pediatrics* **2016**, *138*, e20161896.
78. Huynh, M.E.; Vandvik, I.H.; Diseth, T.H. Hypnotherapy in child psychiatry: The state of the art. *Clin. Child Psychol. Psychiatry* **2008**, *13*, 377–393. [CrossRef] [PubMed]
79. Rutten, J.M.; Reitsma, J.B.; Vlieger, A.M.; Benninga, M.A. Gut-directed hypnotherapy for functional abdominal pain or irritable bowel syndrome in children: A systematic review. *Arch. Dis. Child.* **2013**, *98*, 252–257. [CrossRef] [PubMed]
80. Lambert, S.A. The effects of hypnosis/guided imagery on the postoperative course of children. *J. Dev. Behav. Pediatr.* **1996**, *17*, 307–310. [CrossRef] [PubMed]
81. Brown, J.L. Imagination training: A tool with many uses. *Contemp. Pediatr.* **1995**, *12*, 22–26, 29–30. [PubMed]
82. Van Tilburg, M.A.; Chitkara, D.K.; Palsson, O.S.; Turner, M.; Blois-Martin, N.; Ulshen, M.; Whitehead, W.E. Audio-recorded guided imagery treatment reduces functional abdominal pain in children: a pilot study. *Pediatrics* **2009**, *124*, e890–e897. [CrossRef] [PubMed]
83. Kabat-Zinn, J. *Full Catastophe Living*; Delacorte Press: New York, NY, USA, 1990.
84. Kabat-Zinn, J. *Full Catastrophe Liviing: Using the Wisdom of Your Body and Mind to Face Stress, Pain, and Illness*; Bantam Dell: New York, NY, USA, 2013.
85. Kabat-Zinn, J. Mindfulness-based interventions in context: Past, present, and future. *Clin. Psychol. Sci. Pract.* **2003**, *10*, 144–156. [CrossRef]
86. Kabat-Zinn, J.; Lipworth, L.; Burncy, R.; Sellers, W. Four-year follow-up of a meditation-based program for the self-regulation of chronic pain: Treatment outcomes and compliance. *Clin. J. Pain* **1986**, *3*, 60. [CrossRef]
87. Crane, R.S.; Brewer, J.; Feldman, C.; Kabat-Zinn, J.; Santorelli, S.; Williams, J.M.G.; Kuyken, W. What defines mindfulness-based programs? The warp and the weft. *Psychol. Med.* **2017**, *47*, 990–999. [CrossRef] [PubMed]
88. Snel, E. *Sitting Still Like a Frog: Mindfulness Exercises for Kids (and Their Parents)*; Shambhala Publication: Boulder, CO, USA, 2013.

89. Breathe, Think, Do with Sesame. Available online: https://sesamestreetincommunities.org/activities/breathe-think-do/ (accessed on 3 August 2018).
90. Yapko, M. *Mindfulness and Hypnosis: The Power of Suggestion to Transform Experience*; W.W. Norton & Company: New York, NY, USA, 2011.
91. Klingbeil, D.A.; Renshaw, T.L.; Willenbrink, J.B.; Copek, R.A.; Chan, K.T.; Haddock, A.; Yassine, J.; Clifton, J. Mindfulness-based interventions with youth: A comprehensive meta-analysis of group-design studies. *J. Sch. Psychol.* **2017**, *63*, 77–103. [CrossRef] [PubMed]
92. Barnes, V.A.; Pendergrast, R.A.; Harshfield, G.A.; Treiber, F.A. Impact of breathing awareness meditation on ambulatory blood pressure and sodium handling in prehypertensive African American adolescents. *Ethn. Dis.* **2008**, *18*, 1–5. [PubMed]
93. Ortiz, R.; Sibinga, E. The role of mindfulness in reducing the adverse effects of childhood stress and trauma. *Children* **2017**, *4*, 16. [CrossRef] [PubMed]
94. Crnic, K.A.; Neece, C.L.; McIntyre, L.L.; Blacher, J.; Baker, B.L. Intellectual disability and developmental risk: Promoting intervention to improve child and family well-being. *Child Dev.* **2017**, *88*, 436–445. [CrossRef] [PubMed]
95. Wark, D.M. Traditional and alert hypnotic phenomena: Development through anteriorization. *Am. J. Clin. Hypn.* **2015**, *57*, 254–266. [CrossRef] [PubMed]
96. Tang, Y.Y.; Hölzel, B.K.; Posner, M.I. The neuroscience of mindfulness meditation. *Nat. Rev. Neurosci.* **2015**, *16*, 213–225. [CrossRef] [PubMed]
97. White, R.E.; Carlson, S.M. What would Batman do? Self-distancing improves executive function in young children. *Dev. Sci.* **2016**, *19*, 419–426. [CrossRef] [PubMed]
98. White, R.E.; Prager, E.O.; Schaefer, C.; Kross, E.; Duckworth, A.L.; Carlson, S.M. The "Batman Effect": Improving perseverance in young children. *Child Dev.* **2017**, *88*, 1563–1571. [CrossRef] [PubMed]
99. Lyons, L. *Using Hypnosis with Children: Creating and Delivering Effective Interventions*; W.W. Norton & Company: New York, NY, USA, 2015.
100. Alladin, A. Mindfulness-based hypnosis: Blending science, beliefs, and wisdoms to catalyze healing. *Am. J. Clin. Hypn.* **2014**, *56*, 285–302. [CrossRef] [PubMed]
101. Lynn, S.J.; Rhue, J.W. (Eds.) *Theories of Hypnosis: Current Models and Perspectives*; Guilford Press Inc.: New York, NY, USA, 1988.
102. Sugarman, L.I.; Wester, W.C., II (Eds.) *Therapeutic Hypnosis with Children and Adolescents*; Crown House: Carmarthen, UK, 2013; Volume 2.
103. Yapko, M.D. *Trancework: An Introduction to the Practice of Clinical Hypnosis*, 5th ed.; Guilford Press Inc.: New York, NY, USA, 2018.
104. Schwartz, M. *Biofeedback: A Practitioner's Guide*; Guilford Press Inc.: New York, NY, USA, 1987.
105. Sugarman, L.I. Hypnosis and Biofeedback. In *Pediatric Primary Care*; Hoekelman, R.A., Friedman, S.R., Nelson, N.M., Seidel, H.M., Weitzman, M.L., Eds.; Mosby: St Louis, MO, USA, 2000.
106. Shaffer, F.; Moss, D. Biofeedback. In *Textbook of Complementary and Alternative Medicine*; Yuan, C.S., Bieber, E.J., Bauer, B.A., Eds.; Taylor & Francis Group: New York, NY, USA, 2005.
107. Barowsky, E. The use of biofeedback in the treatment of disorders of childhood. *Ann. N. Y. Acad. Sci.* **1990**, *602*, 221–233. [CrossRef] [PubMed]
108. Culbert, T.P.; Reaney, J.B.; Kohen, D.P. "Cyberphysiologic" strategies for children: The clinical hypnosis/biofeedback interface. *Int. J. Clin. Exp. Hypn.* **1994**, *42*, 97–117. [CrossRef] [PubMed]
109. Heartmath Inner Balance. Available online: www.heartmath.com (accessed on 3 August 2018).
110. Lang, E.V. My Comfort Talk. Available online: www.comforttalk.com (accessed on 3 August 2018).
111. Furman, B. Kids' Skills App. Available online: http://www.kidsskillsapp.com (accessed on 3 August 2018).
112. Dikel, W.; Olness, K. Self-hypnosis, biofeedback, and voluntary peripheral temperature control in children. *Pediatrics* **1980**, *66*, 335–340. [PubMed]
113. Culbert, T.P.; Banez, G. Pediatric Applications of Biofeedback Other than Headache. In *Biofeedback: A Practitioner's Guide*; Schwartz, M., Andrasik, F., Eds.; Guilford Press Inc.: New York, NY, USA, 2003.
114. Jencks, B. *Your Body—Biofeedback at Its Best*; Nelson-Hall Company: Chicago, IL, USA, 1977.
115. Kohen, D.P. Pediatric Perspective on Mind-Body Medicine. In *Integrative Pediatrics*; Culbert, T.P., Olness, K.O., Eds.; Oxford University Press: New York, NY, USA, 2010; pp. 267–301.

116. Kohen, D.P. The "3 and 6" Hypnotic Induction Technique for Children and Adolescents. In *The Art and Practice of Hypnotic Induction: Favorite Methods of Master Clinicians*; Jensen, M.P., Ed.; Denny Creek Press: Kirkland, WA, USA, 2017.
117. Lu, D.P.; Lu, G.P. A Historical Review and Perspective on the Impact of Acupuncture on US Medicine and Society. *Med. Acupunct.* **2013**, *25*, 311–316. [CrossRef] [PubMed]
118. Black, L.I.; Clarke, T.C.; Barnes, P.M.; Stussman, B.J.; Nahin, R.L. Use of complementary health approaches among children aged 4-17 years in the United States: National Health Interview Survey, 2007–2012. *Natl. Health Stat. Report.* **2015**, *78*, 1–19.
119. Lee, M.S.; Ernst, E. Acupuncture for pain: An overview of Cochrane reviews. *Chin. J. Integr. Med.* **2011**, *17*, 187–189. [CrossRef] [PubMed]
120. Pomeranz, B.; Chiu, D. Naloxone blockade of acupuncture analgesia: Endorphin implicated. *Life Sci.* **1976**, *19*, 1757–1762. [CrossRef]
121. Schiff, E.; Gurgevich, S.; Caspi, O. Potential synergism between hypnosis and acupuncture—Is the whole more than the sum of its parts? *Evid. Based. Complement. Alternat. Med.* **2007**, *4*, 233–240. [CrossRef] [PubMed]
122. Kemper, K.J.; Sarah, R.; Silver-Highfield, E.; Xiarhos, E.; Barnes, L.; Berde, C. On pins and needles? Pediatric pain patients' experience with acupuncture. *Pediatrics* **2000**, *105*, 941–947. [PubMed]
123. Jindal, V.; Ge, A.; Mansky, P.J. Safety and efficacy of acupuncture in children. *J. Pediatr. Hematol. Oncol.* **2008**, *30*, 431–442. [CrossRef] [PubMed]
124. Slover, R.; Neuenkirchen, G.L.; Olamikan, S.; Kent, S. Chronic pediatric pain. *Adv. Pediatr.* **2010**, *57*, 141–162. [CrossRef] [PubMed]
125. Waterhouse, M.; Stelling, C.; Powers, M.; Levy, S.; Zeltzer, L.K. Acupuncture and hypotherapy in the treatment of chronic pain in children. *Clin. Acupunct. Orient. Med.* **2000**, *1*, 139–150. [CrossRef]
126. Zeltzer, L.K.; Tsao, J.C.I.; Stelling, C.; Powers, M.; Levy, S.; Waterhouse, M. A phase I study on the feasibility and acceptability of an acupuncture/hypnosis intervention for chronic pediatric pain. *J. Pain Symptom Manage.* **2002**, *24*, 437–446. [CrossRef]
127. Golianu, B.; Krane, E.; Seybold, J.; Almgren, C.; Anand, K.J.S. Non-pharmacological techniques for pain management in neonates. *Semin. Perinatol.* **2007**, *31*, 318–322. [CrossRef] [PubMed]
128. Samuels, N. Integration of hypnosis with acupuncture: Possible benefits and case examples. *Am. J. Clin. Hypn.* **2005**, *47*, 243–248. [CrossRef] [PubMed]
129. Lu, D.P.; Lu, G.P. A comparison of the clinical effectiveness of various acupuncture points in reducing anxiety to facilitate hypnotic induction. *Int. J. Clin. Exp. Hypn.* **2013**, *61*, 271–281. [CrossRef] [PubMed]
130. Rosted, P.; Bundgaard, M.; Gordon, S.; Pedersen, A.M.L. Acupuncture in the management of anxiety related to dental treatment: A case series. *Acupunct. Med.* **2010**, *28*, 3–5. [CrossRef] [PubMed]
131. Tsai, S.-L.; Fox, L.M.; Murakami, M.; Tsung, J.W. Auricular acupuncture in emergency department treatment of acute pain. *Ann. Emerg. Med.* **2016**, *68*, 583–585. [CrossRef] [PubMed]
132. Barber, T.X. *LSD, Marijuana, Yoga and Hypnosis*; Aldine Transaction Publishing: New Brunswick, NJ, USA, 2008.
133. Sibinga, E.M.S.; Kemper, K.J. Complementary, holistic, and integrative medicine: Meditation practices for pediatric health. *Pediatr. Rev.* **2010**, *31*, e91–e103. [CrossRef] [PubMed]
134. Yoga Alliance. Yoga Alliance Home Page. Available online: www.yogaalliance.org (accessed on 3 August 2018).
135. Yoga Kids. Yoga Kids Training and Certificiation. Available online: www.yogakids.com/training-and-certification (accessed on 3 August 2018).
136. Butzer, B.; Ebert, M.; Telles, S.; Khalsa, S.B.S. School-based yoga programs in the United States: A survey. *Adv. Mind. Body. Med.* **2015**, *29*, 18–26. [PubMed]
137. Yoga Calm. Yoga Calm Home Page. Available online: https://www.yogacalm.org/ (accessed on 3 August 2018).
138. Birdee, G.S.; Yeh, G.Y.; Wayne, P.M.; Phillips, R.S.; Davis, R.B.; Gardiner, P. Clinical applications of yoga for the pediatric population: A systematic review. *Acad. Pediatr.* **2009**, *9*, 212–220. [CrossRef] [PubMed]
139. Kaley-Isley, L.C.; Peterson, J.; Fischer, C.; Peterson, E. Yoga as a complementary therapy for children and adolescents: A guide for clinicians. *Psychiatry* **2010**, *7*, 20–32. [PubMed]

140. Telles, S. Iyengar Yoga for Adolescents and Young Adults with Irritable Bowel Syndrome. In *Child and Adolescent Mental Health*; Nayar, U., Ed.; SAGE Publications: Thousand Oaks, CA, USA, 2012; pp. 219–227.
141. Evans, S.; Lung, K.C.; Seidman, L.C.; Sternlieb, B.; Zeltzer, L.K.; Tsao, J.C.I. Iyengar yoga for adolescents and young adults with irritable bowel syndrome. *J. Pediatr. Gastroenterol. Nutr.* **2014**, *59*, 244–253. [CrossRef] [PubMed]
142. Noggle, J.J.; Steiner, N.J.; Minami, T.; Khalsa, S.B. Benefits of yoga for psychosocial well-being in a US high school curriculum: A preliminary randomized controlled trial. *J. Dev. Behav. Pediatr.* **2012**, *33*, 193–201. [CrossRef] [PubMed]
143. Khalsa, S.B. Yoga in schools research: Improving mental and emotional health. In Proceedings of the Second International Conference on Yoga for Health and Social Transformation, Haridwar, India, 7–10 January 2013.
144. McClafferty, H.; Vohra, S.; Bailey, M.; Brown, M.; Esparham, A.; Gerstbacher, D.; Golianu, B.; Niemi, A.-K.; Sibinga, E.; Weydert, J.; et al. Section on Integrative Medicine. Pediatric Integrative Medicine. *Pediatrics* **2017**, *140*, e20171961. [CrossRef] [PubMed]
145. Gard, T.; Noggle, J.J.; Park, C.L.; Vago, D.R.; Wilson, A. Potential self-regulatory mechanisms of yoga for psychological health. *Front. Hum. Neurosci.* **2014**, *8*, 770. [CrossRef] [PubMed]
146. Schmalzl, L.; Powers, C.; Henje Blom, E. Neurophysiological and neurocognitive mechanisms underlying the effects of yoga-based practices: towards a comprehensive theoretical framework. *Front. Hum. Neurosci.* **2015**, *9*, 235. [CrossRef] [PubMed]
147. Sullivan, M.B.; Erb, M.; Schmalzl, L.; Moonaz, S.; Noggle Taylor, J.; Porges, S.W. Yoga therapy and polyvagal theory: The convergence of traditional wisdom and contemporary neuroscience for self-regulation and resilience. *Front. Hum. Neurosci.* **2018**, *12*, 67. [CrossRef] [PubMed]
148. Dalal, A.; Barber, T.X. Yoga and Hypnotism. In *LSD, Marijuana, Yoga, and Hypnosis*; Aldine Transaction Publishing: New Brunswick, NJ, USA, 2008; pp. 117–132.
149. Landier, W.; Tse, A.M. Use of complementary and alternative medical interventions for the management of procedure-related pain, anxiety, and distress in pediatric oncology: an integrative review. *J. Pediatr. Nurs.* **2010**, *25*, 566–579. [CrossRef] [PubMed]
150. Bethell, C.; Kemper, K.J.; Gombojav, N.; Koch, T.K. Complementary and conventional medicine use among youth with recurrent headaches. *Pediatrics* **2013**, *132*, e1173–e1183. [CrossRef] [PubMed]
151. National Institutes of Health/National Center for Complementary and Integrative Health. Complementary, Alternative, or Integrative Health: What's In a Name? NCCIH. Available online: https://nccih.nih.gov/health/integrative-health (accessed on 12 June 2018).
152. Robertson, D. *Cognitive Hypnotherapy: An Integrated Approach to the Treatment of Emotional Disorders*; Karnac: London, UK, 2012.
153. Alladin, A. Cognitive hypnotherapy for accessing and healing emotional injuries for anxiety disorders. *Am. J. Clin. Hypn.* **2016**, *59*, 24–46. [CrossRef] [PubMed]
154. Semple, R.J.; Lee, J. Mindfulness-based cognitive therapy for children. In *Mindfulness-Based Treatment Approaches: Clinician's Guide to Evidence Base and Applications*; Baer, R., Ed.; Elsevier: Amsterdam, The Netherlands, 2014; pp. 161–188.
155. Elkins, G.R.; Roberts, R.L.; Simicich, L. Mindful self-hypnosis for self-care: An integrative model and illustrative case example. *Am. J. Clin. Hypn.* **2018**, *61*, 45–56. [CrossRef] [PubMed]
156. Kemper, K.J. Integrative medicine is becoming mainstream: Research on multimodal interventions needs to catch up. *Complement. Ther. Med.* **2018**, in press. [CrossRef] [PubMed]
157. McClafferty, H.; Dodds, S.; Brooks, A.; Brenner, M.; Brown, M.; Frazer, P.; Mark, J.; Weydert, J.; Wilcox, G.; Lebensohn, P.; et al. Pediatric Integrative Medicine in Residency (PIMR): Description of a new online educational curriculum. *Children* **2015**, *2*, 98–107. [CrossRef] [PubMed]
158. American Board of Physician Subspecialties Integrative Medicine Exam Description. Available online: http://www.abpsus.org/integrative-medicine-description (accessed on 15 June 2018).
159. Shriberg, L.D.; Kwiatkowski, J. Developmental phonological disorders. I: A clinical profile. *J. Speech Hear. Res.* **1994**, *37*, 1100–1126. [CrossRef] [PubMed]
160. Kekecs, Z.; Varga, K. Positive suggestion techniques in somatic medicine: A review of the empirical studies. *Interv. Med. Appl. Sci.* **2013**, *5*, 101–111. [CrossRef] [PubMed]

161. Lang, E.V.; Hatsiopoulou, O.; Koch, T.; Berbaum, K.; Lutgendorf, S.; Kettenmann, E.; Logan, H.; Kaptchuk, T.J. Can words hurt? Patient-provider interactions during invasive procedures. *Pain* **2005**, *114*, 303–309. [CrossRef] [PubMed]
162. Geller, S.M.; Porges, S.W. Therapeutic presence: Neurophysiological mechanisms mediating feeling safe in therapeutic relationships. *J. Psychother. Integr.* **2014**, *24*, 178–192. [CrossRef]

15

Perspectives on Technology-Assisted Relaxation Approaches to Support Mind-Body Skills Practice in Children and Teens: Clinical Experience and Commentary

Timothy Culbert

PrairieCare Medical Group, Chaska, MN 55419, USA; tculbert@prairie-care.com; Tel.: +1-952-903-1380

Abstract: It has been well-established that a variety of mind-body (MB) techniques, including yoga, mental imagery, hypnosis, biofeedback, and meditation, are effective at addressing symptoms such as pain, anxiety, nausea, and insomnia, as well as helping with a wide variety of medical, emotional, and behavioral issues in pediatric populations. In addition, MB skills can also be health-promoting in the long-term, and with regular practice, could potentially contribute to longer attention spans, social skills, emotional regulation, and enhanced immune system functioning. Importantly, the benefits accrued from MB skills are largely dose-dependent, meaning that individuals who practice with some consistency tend to benefit the most, both in the short- and long-term. However, clinical experience suggests that for busy patients, the regular practice of MB skills can be challenging and treatment adherence commonly becomes an issue. This commentary reviews the concept of technology-assisted relaxation as an engaging and effective option to enhance treatment adherence (i.e., daily practice) for pediatric patients, for whom MB skills have been recommended to address physical and mental health challenges.

Keywords: technology; mind-body skills; biofeedback; mobile applications; meditation; multimedia; computer games; children; relaxation; stress; video games

---

1. Introduction

Interactive electronic devices can play a positive role in healthcare [1–17]. Technology-assisted relaxation is currently a very popular topic for healthcare consumers, including products which are available in the form of multimedia mobile applications for smartphones or tablets. Devices can be used in a variety of situations and are available in numerous formats, such as teaching relaxation techniques, providing interactive electronic physiological monitoring (biofeedback) which facilitates self-regulation, or stand-alone electrotherapeutic technologies, which can influence brainwave frequencies. Therapeutic technologies are rapidly emerging as a unique and effective way to provide health information and as a source for patient self-management tools. Recently, a number of new options for mind-body (MB) skills training have been developed, including technologies that support stress management approaches, emotional regulation strategies, and self-calming techniques. Although many healthcare providers are aware of the need for effective stress management strategies for patients of all ages, busy clinicians may not have the time to stay up-to-date with these new technological offerings. However, in many cases, companies are launching direct-to-consumer advertising of their product benefits, which allows patients and families direct access to, and use of, these approaches, as they seek attractive options for treating stress-mediated mental and physical challenges.

It is well-known that children are regularly utilizing interactive electronic media, such as smartphones or tablets, at home and school [18]. In a 2015 article in *Pediatrics* by Kabali et al. [19], the following was discovered about the use of mobile devices by children and families: "[a] cross-sectional study [was performed including] 350 children aged 6 months to 4 years, seen October to November 2014, at a pediatric clinic in an urban, low-income, minority community. The survey was adapted from Common Sense Media's 2013 nationwide survey...[and it was found that] most households had television (97%), tablets (83%), and smartphones (77%). At age 4, half the children had their own television and three-fourths [had] their own mobile device. Almost all children (96.6%) used mobile devices, and most started using before one years of age. Parents gave children devices when doing house chores (70%), to keep them calm (65%), and at bedtime (29%)." This study suggests that, even if not explicitly stated, many parents are currently utilizing technology with their children as a non-pharmacological option for purposes of calming and distraction.

After over twenty years working in the clinical practice of developmental/behavioral and integrative pediatrics, the author has witnessed the many benefits of teaching children a variety of MB skills, as an important therapeutic element in a comprehensive treatment plan. This commentary offers his opinions and perspectives on the way in which technology can enhance the process of learning and practicing MB skills for children and teens. Therefore, this paper is not intended to provide an exhaustive review of the literature on this subject, but instead is meant to reflect the author's clinical experience and what he has found to be useful in his own clinical practice.

One important goal of this commentary is to raise awareness of these technologies among clinicians, so that healthcare providers might better understand alternative therapeutic options and consequently discuss these options with their patients. An additional hope is that healthcare providers may creatively integrate these newer technology-assisted relaxation approaches, when indicated, into appealing treatment strategies for pediatric patients for whom MB skills are indicated.

1.1. *Complementary Approaches and Pediatric Practice*

Complementary and alternative medicine (CAM) is quite popular for children and teenagers seeking natural approaches [20–22] for a variety of medical and mental health issues, partly because families are now seeking out more natural and less invasive therapies. Many children and parents prefer non-pharmacological therapies, if available, for common complaints such as headaches, abdominal pain, insomnia, anxiety, stress, inattention, anger, or emotional dysregulation. Within the CAM domain, MB and self-regulation skills are particularly effective in managing a number of common symptoms of childhood with a very positive risk/benefit ratio in a safe, cost-effective, and time-efficient manner [23]. The attractiveness of these options can be seen in a recent review by Vohra and McClafferty et al., who note that MB therapies "are popular and ranked among the top ten complementary and integrative medicine practices reportedly used by adults and children" [1].

1.2. *Chronic Over-Arousal*

It is also reasonable to argue that, for most children and teenagers, the demands and exposures of modern life are increasingly leading to chronic autonomic nervous system (ANS) over-arousal, in a way that is often unrecognized by the majority of individuals, who commonly accept it as their normal baseline reference mode of experience. However, this constant over-arousal can cause physical and emotional regulation problems [24–26]. In fact, since this state of ANS imbalance (stress) is so often recognized as a normal baseline mood, individuals may feel uncomfortable with calmer, quieter states of mind and body, as these can feel unfamiliar or uncomfortable. Evidence suggests that this heightened baseline and continuous state of chronic stress may be depleting for the mind, body, and spirit, and when left unchecked, can lead to many physical and mental health problems [27]. For example, stress may serve as an epigenetic modifier [28,29], while accessing a relaxation response achieved from practicing MB techniques (i.e., dialing up parasympathetic nervous system activity and reducing sympathetic arousal), may counterbalance this stress-effect and help to turn on health-promoting genes and processes.

A chronic state of nervous system over-arousal can also contribute to the etiology and/or maintenance of a number of physical issues (inflammation, pain, immune dysregulation, insomnia) and mental health symptoms (anxiety, depression, inattention), for which medications are commonly prescribed [24–27]. For these reasons, it is important that all children and teenagers learn MB balancing skills early on, so that they might also have the option to utilize non-pharmacological alternatives that can facilitate the MB's natural healing capacity and perhaps address the causative issue at a more foundational level. It has also been well-established that the regular practice of a variety of MB techniques, including yoga, mental imagery, hypnosis, biofeedback, and meditation, are effective for re-balancing the ANS in pediatric populations and for addressing physical and emotional symptoms, such as pain, anxiety, insomnia, and gastrointestinal complaints [1,30–32]. Additionally, with regular practice, MB skills can be health-promoting in the long-term, contributing to better attention spans, social skills, emotional regulation, enhanced immune system function, and decreased inflammation [6,25,29,33].

1.3. Mind-Body Skills for Autonomic Nervous System Re-Balancing

Currently, there are no definitive studies detailing the exact amount of practice of MB skills required for optimal success, in terms of short-term symptom control (e.g., to reduce acute pain or anxiety), or long-term health and wellness improvements (e.g., baseline levels of stress, happiness, attention, inflammation). In clinical settings, some individuals do appear to achieve benefits—at least acutely—with only a single practice or a few experiences, but mastery and sustained change likely requires consistent practice of the skill, in order to use these skills effectively for the re-patterning of neurobiological processes and consequently create a new baseline. Therefore, it can be reasonably assumed that the benefits accrued from MB skills are likely dose-dependent. Despite the recognition that cost-efficient, safe, and effective MB techniques are readily available and can be used to address a variety of the aforementioned issues, children and teenagers often don't practice MB skills, and certainly not to an optimal level to be able to achieve the best possible therapeutic benefit.

Clinical experience suggests that: (1) although many kids are familiar with the concept of relaxation, few have learned any formal MB skills; (2) many kids, when asked how they relax, suggest alternative methods, such as to read a book, do an art project, play a video game, or watch TV, which may or may not be objectively relaxing in terms of ANS arousal; (3) kids that have learned MB skills don't practice them consistently in the appropriate situations; (4) kids that practice MB skills often get bored with that practice; (5) kids that understand and have practiced some form of MB skills are not necessarily applying them in a way that could be effective in-the moment; and (6) kids often don't believe that a change in their thinking and feeling can really result in a physical change in the body.

1.4. Technology for Healing

The selective use of technology, although problematic in many ways, can be quite useful for children and teenagers to learn and practice MB skills, especially for those who have been reluctant to do so because it is perceived as another boring, non-preferred task, such as homework or household chores. Most individuals would prefer to interact with electronic media in the age of cellphones, computers, video game systems, or TV sets. This preference can be used to the advantage of healthcare providers, by becoming familiar with new "healing technologies", that can be harnessed to provide technology-assisted relaxation training and can make the process of learning and practicing effective MB skills much more engaging, playful, and user-friendly for kids.

Many studies have focused on the potential downside of technology, suggesting that too much exposure to electronic media and/or exposure to certain types of inappropriate electronic media content, may have negative impacts on the developing child, such as contributing to a short attention span, sedentary behavior, over-arousal, aggressive behavior, depression, insomnia, and unhealthy food choices related to advertisements. However, not enough attention has been paid to the concept of utilizing these interactive electronic multimedia devices in order to engage children and teenagers in constructive, health-promoting, self-care skill development and symptom management. In this commentary, concepts such as play, therapeutic play, self-regulation, and MB skills, and their relationship to new electronic media, are reviewed. This commentary also reviews some of the most helpful software and devices currently used in the field of technology-assisted relaxation.

2. Benefits of MB Skills

MB techniques typically focus on the interactions and connections between the brain, the body, and the subsequent behaviors. There are many ways in which emotional, spiritual, cognitive, and psychosocial phenomena can directly affect physical and mental health. A compilation of potential benefits of practicing MB skills is listed in Table 1.

Teaching self-regulation and/or MB skills of any kind often involves assisting individuals to achieve a state of improved MB health and healing by shifting the balance of: (1) the ANS (from sympathetic activity to parasympathetic activity); (2) emotions (from negative to positive); (3) thoughts (from unhelpful to helpful) and; (4) a sense of control over health status (from external to internal) [23,33].

Table 1. Potential benefits of mind-body (MB) skills training.

Eliciting the "Relaxation Response"
Autonomic Nervous System Balancing: decreasing sympathetic nervous system activity while dialing up parasympathetic nervous system activity
Enhanced Emotional Regulation
Training Attention and Cultivating Awareness
Stress Management
Modifying the central nervous system (CNS)
Performance Enhancement
Improved Social Interactions
Improved Decision Making
Increasing Peace and Happiness
Building Emotional and Physical Resilience
Pain and Symptom Management

3. The Interface of Video Games, Self-Regulation and Healing

Many healthcare providers know that, when teaching kids self-care skills, they are more effective and more likely to be practiced and operationalized, if the skills are customized to the child's interests and learning style, and delivered in a way that is playful, non-threatening, developmentally appropriate, and novel. Delivering treatments through "play" experiences or games, is an ideal, developmentally appropriate way to proceed in therapeutic interaction, and is often referred to as "therapeutic play." Over the past several years, playing video games, texting, and watching online videos have become popular activities for children and teens [34–36]. What exactly is it that seems to make video games so popular? One component of their appeal may involve the experience of "mastery" and being recognized as an expert. For a child with limited opportunities to experience success in activities such as sports, music, or theater, being talented at video games could have a positive impact on their self-esteem.

Additionally, video game designers also know what it takes to engage kids. In their 1983 book *Mind at Play: The Psychology of Video Games*, psychologists Loftus and Loftus describe the three elements that drive the design of successful, addictive video games and make them intrinsically motivating (i.e., curiosity, fantasy, and challenge) [37]. These concepts are still relevant and can therefore be used to inform the design of effective MB, self-care strategies for kids. In particular, children aged four to 13 years are developmentally driven towards mastery, have a rich fantasy life, move easily between real life and their imagination, and are engaged by experiences that are multimedia, interactive, and novel—thus evoking a strong sense of curiosity. The designers and marketers of computer games, mobile apps, and related software and gadgets have often exploited these elements in the design of popular multimedia entertainment that have become highly recognized brand names, such as *Final Fantasy*, *Angry Birds*, *Legend of Zelda*, and *Kingdom Hearts*, along with many games based on movies and cartoons, such as *Toy Story*, *Pokemon* and *Cars*. Interestingly, popular children's books are now among the top-sellers for mobile apps, but have also gone far beyond the book form—interactive elements have been added, such as gaming features and audio enhancements (i.e., entertaining sound effects).

Consequently, technology-assisted relaxation devices have been increasingly designed to harness the same power, absorption, and fun of these electronic games features and mobile applications, but for the service of health instead of strictly entertainment. Multimedia interactive game play can be utilized to connect with the imagistic, emotional, and sensory elements of the right brain for symptom management and healing. The following section will review the concept of MB skills, along with current electronics–based options for kids and teenagers that leverage the idea of "therapeutic play", in order to practice MB skills at home, at school, or in clinical settings. This listing is not complete, but has been gathered by the experience of the author, who has personally used the majority of these products in both inpatient and outpatient settings. Additionally, the paper will review common products that the author and his colleagues have found useful for supporting children in their regular, daily practice of MB skills. These products are organized by the type of technology involved: (1) mobile applications (for smart phones and tablet computers), which only involve software; (2) biofeedback devices (either stand-alone or computer-based), which involve hardware (a physiological sensor) and software; (3) other technology-assisted relaxation devices that are specialized portable technologies involving electrical stimulation.

4. Definitions of MB Skills

1. *Breathwork:* the conscious control of the rate, rhythm, and depth of breathing; a technique used in relaxation and meditative practices in order to reduce psychological stress and increase parasympathetic nervous system activity.
2. *Biofeedback*: a technique you can use to learn to control your body's functions, such as your heart rate, hand temperature, or muscle tension. With biofeedback, you're connected to electrical sensors or electromechanical devices that provide you with auditory and visual information about your body. This feedback helps you to then control a desired physiological function in a therapeutic direction, which provides the opportunity to more objectively observe the mind-body connection and understand how a change in thinking or feeling can directly correlate with a change in physiology.
3. *Guided and/or Mental Imagery/Self-hypnosis*: commonly invokes all of the five senses in journeys of imagination (and fantasy) and facilitates an intensification of focus, less attention to peripheral factors, more awareness of internal events/sensations, and enhanced suggestibility.
4. *Meditation and Mindfulness*: practices involving concentrated focus or intentional attention training, in order to increase awareness of the present moment or to reduce stress.
5. *Yoga*: a Hindu spiritual and ascetic discipline derived from the Sanskrit word *yuj*, meaning union. It includes body postures, breathwork, and meditative practices.

5. Electronic Mobile Applications for Smartphones and Tablet Computers

Mobile apps are often game-like in design and can include features of immersive, attention-maintaining properties of fantasy and imagery, offer interactivity and control, and can include useful behavioral change elements, such as symptom assessment, tailored messages, tracking progress, and goal setting.

5.1. Mobile Apps for Breathwork

5.1.1. Breathe2Relax

According to its website [38], "this (app) is a portable stress management tool which provides detailed information on the effects of stress on the body and instructions and practice exercises to help users learn the stress management skill called diaphragmatic breathing." This app also includes effective explanations and illustrations of the respiratory system.

5.1.2. Breathing Zone

This is a well-designed mobile app that basically serves as an interactive breath pacer. The user has the flexibility to pick the beginning breath pace, ending breath pace, and cueing audio for each breath (chime, water, voice, etc.), along with an optional timer.

5.1.3. Belly Bio Interactive Breathing

This is an interactive app for the iPhone that utilizes the phone's accelerometer to monitor proper diaphragmatic (belly) breathing techniques, by providing feedback about the movement of the user's stomach.

5.1.4. Breathing Bubbles

Breathing Bubbles is an app that helps kids to practice releasing worries and focus on pleasant feelings, while using a bubble as a visual representation for this release.

5.2. Mobile Apps for Meditation and Mindfulness

Meditation has been proven to be a helpful tool addressing medical and mental health issues, for both the pediatric and adult populations [2,31].

5.2.1. Take a Chill

According to the developers [39], "this mobile app offers mindfulness meditation exercises and texted practice reminders. As a teen, there are moments in your life when you're really stressed and just need to 'Take a Chill'." This app is full of tools to help manage that stress and incorporate mindful practices into a daily routine. Using quick mindful exercises and thoughtful activities, teenagers learn to begin to overcome those moments, whether it's studying for a test or preventing negative thoughts and patterns. Features in the app include:

1. Quick Exercises: two illustrated exercises for in-the-moment situations
2. Daily Dose: daily activities to help reinforce concepts and increase your mindful practice
3. Progress: see your progress and activity overtime
4. Reminders: keep yourself motivated with three types of Reminders
5. Motivational Quotes: receive a new motivational quote after each use

5.2.2. Stop, Breathe and Think

The creators [40] state that, "with this app, you can develop and apply awareness, kindness and compassion in your daily life through a meditative process called *Stop, Breathe and Think*: (1) Stop:

Stop what you are doing. Check in with what you are thinking, and how you are feeling; (2) Breathe: Practice mindful breathing to create space between your thoughts, emotions and reactions; (3) Think: Learn to broaden your perspective and strengthen your force field of peace and calm by practicing one of the meditations."

5.2.3. Smiling Mind

The creators of this app [41] state that, "*Smiling Mind* is a modern meditation approach, a unique web- and app-based program developed by psychologists and educators to help bring balance to people's lives by teaching meditation and related skills."

5.3. Mobile Apps for Yoga

Yoga can be used as another helpful tool to address a variety of psychological and physical conditions of childhood [30].

5.3.1. The Adventures of Superstretch

This is a mobile app [42] that teaches yoga with videos of real kids doing yoga postures, and animated narrators offering information, instructions, and insight. It is a helpful way to get sedentary kids moving in a fun, non-threatening process. The app's designers have declared that "kids don't have to be athletes, flexible or fit to do this. We've designed it to be non-competitive and even bring in partner activities to show we're all in this together. In yoga, there's no perfect. In each pose, the kids are just being kids—doing poses the best they can. No need to be perfect, to 'succeed' or do it 'right'. We are allowing ourselves to be present, in the moment. It's ok to fall out of poses. It's ok to laugh, to roar like a lion—in fact, that's the whole point. Be courageous, creative and just try."

5.3.2. Yoga by Teens

According to the developers [43], "within this app, kids can join yoga teens, Lauren, Emily and Jessica Parsons in a class that is designed and taught by teens. *Yoga by Teens* teaches basic hatha yoga poses that are fun, challenging and help to build strength and flexibility, as well as develop self-confidence and self-esteem. Its message is that yoga is for all ages and levels of ability, including people with special needs."

5.3.3. Kids Yogaverse: I Am Love

The website [44] claims, "this is a great app which allows kids to calm down and be ready for the day. It teaches individuals to always think about good things and always know that you are smart. It is beautifully hand-drawn and incorporates 13 yoga poses for children demonstrated by children. Get ready to open your heart, expand your mind and reveal that *you* are the real treasure to love. The yoga poses help you to stretch out and wake up your mind. The material on this app can be enjoyed by listening to the book, or reading the book." Additional interactive features include:

1. Animated Poses: follow the children as they do the real poses through the yoga journey
2. Breath Affirmations: press the Breath button on each page and you will hear a special message just for you
3. Guess What?: press the Guess What button and learn amazing new facts

5.4. Mobile Apps for Imagery, Movement and More

5.4.1. Healing Buddies Comfort Kit

The author has developed this free mobile app with the local children's hospital, called the *The Healing Buddies Comfort Kit,* for use in children's hospitals and clinical settings. It provides an interactive, game-like, colorful, multimedia way for kids and teens to learn a variety of integrative and holistic techniques in order to manage bothersome symptoms. It includes guided sessions of imagery, muscle relaxation, and breathing for a variety of symptoms that kids might experience at home, in hospitals, or anywhere, such as pain, nausea, fatigue, insomnia, and anxiety.

5.4.2. Me Moves

This app (now available as a digital download) is accessible on tablet computers, cellphones, and computers. The interaction involves using your arms and upper body to slowly follow and engage in graceful upper body movements, to the beat of a metronome and lovely background music. Kids with any kind of over-arousal or anxiety tendencies, including kids with autism and ADHD, can greatly benefit from this program. The developers [45] state that, "mirroring those on the screen, users are transformed by the music, images, movement, and the expressive features of emotion. This easy to use, interactive program has been widely praised by therapists, educators, and parents."

6. Biofeedback Devices (Stand-Alone, Computer-Based and Smartphone-Based)

Training MB self-regulation skills using biofeedback-based relaxation techniques and technologies can be quite engaging, interactive, and effective for treating a variety of conditions [1,3], which has been described by kids as "a videogame for your body". A therapist might use several different biofeedback methods. Determining the method that is right for your client depends on their specific health problems and goals. Biofeedback methods include:

1. *Brainwave*: also known as an electroencephalograph (EEG) and neurofeedback, this type of device uses head sensors to monitor brain wave frequencies.
2. *Heart rate*: this type of biofeedback uses an infrared finger or earlobe sensor, called a photoplethysmograph, to measure your heart rate and variability (HRV).
3. *Muscle*: electromyography (EMG) biofeedback, which involves placing sensors on skeletal muscles to measure the electrical activity that causes muscle contraction.
4. *Sweat glands*: sensors attached around your fingers or on your palm measure sweat gland activity (also called electrodermal activity; EDA).
5. *Temperature:* sensors read the temperature of your fingers/hands that is controlled by blood flow to the periphery (which is influenced by ANS balance).

6.1. HeartMath Products (Heart Rate Variability)

These products are available as a Mac- or PC-based program with game features (*emWave Pro* and *emWave Pro Plus*), as a mobile app for smartphones or tablet computers (called *Inner Balance*), or as a portable, handheld version (called *emWave2*, which features color changing LEDs that signal the user about ANS balance and an optimal state of psychophysiological harmony, termed "coherence".) The user receives information about the heart rate variability pattern as a proxy for ANS balance and emotional regulation. *HeartMath's emWave Pro* also contains video games, for example one game challenges the user to color in a picture that starts as black and white as they move into a more optimal ANS balance and shift to a positive emotional state. Another game format rewards the user with a hot air balloon ride over beautiful landscapes. With the newest game, dual drive, the user controls the speed and handling of a sports car by staying in optimal ANS balance. With the portable, handheld version (*emWave2*), the user can follow a breathing pacer and will then see a specific LED change from red (low coherence), to blue (medium coherence), to green (high coherence). Features of "Inner Balance" include the ability to customize screens with photographs and personally-selected music. This serves as a great tool for kids with any kind of chronic pain, anxiety, insomnia, tics, or anger management challenges.

6.2. Muse (Electrical Brain Activity)

The Muse is a brain-sensing headband that measures electrical brain signals using seven finely calibrated sensors—two on the forehead, two behind the ears, and three reference sensors. The headband uses information from these EEG sensors to measure whether your mind is calm and focused, or active and wandering, and translates that data into active sounds to guide you. There is a companion app for smartphones or tablets that provides audio and visual feedback to guide training.

6.3. The Pip (ElectroDermal Response)

The skin pores (sweat glands) on your fingertips are sensitive to changing levels of stress. *The Pip* accurately captures these changes, and through audio and visual feedback, allows you to be aware and change your response pattern. It achieves this by detecting variations in your EDA. This product comes with interactive software to provide audio and visual feedback and summary information about stress response patterns.

6.4. eSense (Peripheral Temperature Monitor)

According to its website [46], "*eSense* is a small sensor for measuring your skin temperature with the microphone input of your smartphone or tablet (Android or Apple iOS.). Hand warming training is an especially effective and common biofeedback method. The temperature of our hands is connected to our stress level: when we are stressed, we tend to have cold hands. Immediate feedback enables you to voluntarily increase the skin temperature in your fingers, thus increasing your peripheral blood circulation, leading to relaxation and stress reduction. *eSense* provides you, in various ways, with exact feedback about your momentary stress level (e.g., with measurement curves, video display and audio feedback features)."

6.5. Antense (Electromyography)

The developers [47] state that, "the *Antense* anti-tension device is a simple yet effective way to eliminate stress by helping you develop a greater sense of body awareness in the comfort and privacy of your home. A common cause of the discomfort associated with stress or tension is the contraction of your scalp, face and neck muscles. Learning how to relax these muscles is an essential step toward relief and prevention of this discomfort. Because these muscles are not normally under your conscious, direct control, a monitoring or guidance system is necessary to indicate or feedback to you their level of activity. EMG. The *Antense* biofeedback device provides this monitoring. The instrument continuously monitors and averages the EMG activity in the frontalis (forehead) muscle and converts it into a pleasant tone. Using patented technology, *Antense* measures these contractions and instantly converts the signal into a pleasant tone-pitch proportional to the level of muscle tension in your body. With the variations in the tone as a guide, you can quickly train your muscles to relax relieving the discomfort and preventing future problems related to tense facial muscles like headaches. By learning to feel how stress changes your body, you will quickly understand how to release that tension and stress and learn how to relax at will."

7. Other Technology-Assisted Relaxation Devices

As technology marches on, there are some additional, very promising gadgets that can assist individuals in achieving a deep relaxation response and decrease sympathetic nervous arousal, while enhancing parasympathetic nervous system activity. The available scientific literature regarding the use of these devices by children and teens is very limited, so they should be used with caution. However, these devices are generally safe and easy to use, and are available for anyone to purchase, without the prescription of a healthcare provider. Although there is still only limited research on the use of these technologies, they are worth considering and have shown promising preliminary results in adult populations [48–50].

7.1. *Cranial Electrotherapeutic Stimulation (CES)*

The concept of applying electrical stimulation for healing purposes has been in use for at least 2000 years. Machines that deliver a small, pulsed electric current across the head are now claiming efficacy for a variety of medical and mental health conditions. Cranial electrotherapeutic stimulation (CES) is a technology which applies small levels of electrical stimulation across the cranium, to benefit patients with issues such as anxiety, depression, insomnia, ADHD, and chronic pain [41,43,44].

One of the developers of a CES product called *alpha-stim* [51], states that, "our brain basically creates four different frequencies of brain waves each day: beta, alpha, theta and delta. Alpha waves are created when we are in a state of quiet, calm, focused contemplation, and are often associated with meditative states and practices. The CES device sends pulses of very low amperage (i.e., less than 1.0 milliampere) electricity through thin wires attached to electrodes clipped to the ear lobes or stuck to the skin over the bony prominences just to the front of, or behind each ear. The frequency of the electrical pulses can be adjusted—usually from 0.5 Hz to 100 Hz—depending on the treatment effect desired." You could think of these new gadgets that passively cultivate alpha waves as a passive form of meditation. Basically, you place small sensors on your earlobes, dial up the device (about the size of a thick cellphone), and passively enjoy the cultivation of alpha brain waves. Although the exact mechanisms of alpha wave stimulation are not known, some have claimed that these waves could promote the release of neurotransmitters, like serotonin, and the elicitation of alpha wave frequencies in the brain. In alpha wave states, people tend to feel calm, relaxed, and report an enhanced mental focus. Products include *alpha-stim*, *CES Ultra*, and *Fisher Wallace* (Table 2).

7.2. *Audio-Visual Entertainment (AVE)*

The brain is capable of being tuned in a remarkable variety of ways. For instance, certain music or light-pulsing colored sunglasses can significantly alter brain wave frequency, which affects different functions, depending upon the chosen frequency. Beta waves are associated with active problem solving, alpha waves with a calm, focused mind, theta with creative thinking, and delta waves with sleep. Brainwave entrainment refers to any practice intended to cause brain waves to fall into step—or certain frequencies—by using a periodic stimulus of some type. One potential desirable result of brainwave entrainment is to synchronize the two hemispheres of our brain with their brainwave frequency patterns. Potential benefits of hemisphere synchronization include promoting happiness, optimism, and contentment [52–54].

For simple audio entrainment, products include various music or nature sound CD's with embedded beats, vibration, and or therapeutic suggestions. Examples of this include CD's by Jeffrey Thompson, and holo-synch and hemi-synch recordings. When pulsing LED lights are added to audio entrainment, audio-visual entrainment is subsequently created: products include the *DAVID*, the *Dream Machine*, and *Proteus* (Table 2). Some of the benefits which have been seen from the use of brain entrainment include: healthier sleep patterns and more restful sleep each night; a greater ability to relax and meditate (some describe brain entrainment as the ultimate meditation tool); a lowering of situation-specific and overall stress levels; improvements in cognitive function and creativity; easing of negative emotions which affect health and happiness; and an overall sense of peace and well-being.

7.3. *Transcutaneous (tc) Vagal Nerve Stimulation (tc-VNS)*

The concept of influencing neurons with electricity has been used for over a century, when patients were treated with electro convulsive therapy as a treatment for severe depression. Additionally, and more recently, transcranial electromagnetic stimulation has also been gaining traction as a treatment for insomnia and other conditions [55,56]. The vagus nerve originates in the brain and vagal nerve stimulators electronically signal the vagus nerve (more specifically, they stimulate the afferent auricular branch of the vagus), which in turn stimulates the release of neurotransmitters in the brain, in order to generate a calming sensation. Stimulation of the vagal nerve also increases parasympathetic nervous system activity, which can potentially elicit a relaxation response. This can occur during the stimulation session, but also has longer lasting effects to decrease tension, if used daily. Surgically implantable vagal nerve stimulators are available and have been used to effectively treat seizures and depression. Wearable devices are now available that provide transcutaneous (tc) stimulation (and which do not require surgery). As of 2016, a device called *Nervana* offers an FDA-approved tc nerve stimulator, which combines music with vagal nerve stimulation in the ear canal, using ear buds.

8. Clinical Tips: Prescribing MB Skills Practice

One of the most important recommendations for prescribing the practice of MB skills to pediatric patients is to start small, such as a prescription for MB practice for only three to five minutes, once or twice a day. MB skills are best taught in an organized sequential manner, making certain that pediatric clients master each step along the way, as follows:

(1) Mind-Body Awareness
   a. Learn to discriminate (objectively) the mind-body differences between sympathetic nervous system arousal (stress) and parasympathetic nervous system dominant states (relaxation response).

(2) Mind-Body Self-Regulation
   a. Learn to modulate (first in a controlled environment) a given psychological or physiological function, in a therapeutic direction, consistently.

(3) Mind-Body Skill Transfer
   a. Apply this ability to self-regulate the mind and body in appropriate life situations, as needed, "in the moment".

(4) Mind-Body Reset
   a. Restructure (CNS) and rebalance (baseline ANS) with regular daily practice to a calmer, happier, emotionally resilient pattern long-term.

It is also necessary to prescribe daily practice in two different modes; consistent daily practices to reset the neurological baseline, along with recommending an "in-the-moment", brief application of techniques and technology, to manage acute situations in real life (e.g., feeling stressed, having a headache, trouble sleeping, getting angry). Have clients try and practice a variety of MB skills and gadgets so that they can figure out what works best for them. It is also ideal to have multiple options in one's "self-care toolkit" and to request that parents provide rewards for regular practice and effort shown. Clients should also focus on keeping a symptom diary, and describe practice frequency, length, and daily situations they find challenging, stating whether any MB skills that they had tried were helpful. A summary of potential MB resources to recommend to patients is listed in Table 2.

Table 2. List of MB resources.

Biofeedback	Other Technology-Assisted Relaxation Techniques	Mobile Apps
HRV Biofeedback www.heartmath.com	**AVE-Audio Entrainment** www.soundstrue.com www.centerpointe.com www.hemisynch.com	**Breathing** www.t2health.dcoe.mil www.breathing.zone www.bellybio.com
EDA Biofeedback www.thepip.com	**AVE-Audio Visual Entrainment** www.mindalive.com www.mindmachines.com www.deepakchopradreamweaver.com	**Me Moves** www.thinkingmoves.com
EMG Biofeedback www.lifematters.com	**CES** www.alpha-stim.com www.cesultra.com www.fisherwallace.com	**Healing Buddies Comfort Kit** www.healingbuddiescomfort.org

Table 2. *Cont.*

Biofeedback	Other Technology-Assisted Relaxation Techniques	Mobile Apps
TEMP Biofeedback www.mindfield.de	**tc-VNS** www.experiencenervana.com www.cerbomed.com	**Meditation** www.buddhify.com www.stopbreathethink.org www.stressedteens.com www.smilingmind.com.au
EEG Biofeedback www.choosemuse.com		**Yoga** www.adventuresofsuperstretch.com www.kidsyogaverse.com
MULTIMODAL BF www.wilddivine.com		

HRV: heart rate and variability; AVE: audio-visual entertainment; EDA: electrodermal activity; CES: cranial electrotherapeutic stimulation; EMG: electromyography; tc-VNS: transcutaneous vagal nerve stimulation; TEMP: temperature; EEG: electroencephalograph; BF: biofeedback.

9. Conclusions

The intention of this commentary was to provide an entertaining and informational perspective on the interface of technology, mind-body skills, and effective patient care for pediatric healthcare providers of all kinds. The reality is that computer games, interactive mobile apps, and other health-related gadgets are no longer just a trivial activity played by individuals for fun, but can now be utilized for various educational and therapeutic purposes. Consequently, the author intends to highlight the benefits of utilizing technology-assisted relaxation devices and strategies to enhance the practice of MB skills in children and youth in the service of healing and wellness promotion.

Well-designed computer games/apps have the potential to engage the player and are often designed to be intrinsically motivating, in order to encourage frequent use (the *Journey to Wild Divine* home biofeedback system serves as a good example of this) [57]. If technology-assisted relaxation devices and software provide positive reinforcement, mastery, and curiosity, kids and teens will be more willing to utilize them again, and therefore, therapeutic benefits can be gleaned from this approach. Although the use of technologies can be increasingly problematic in the life of children and teens, they can also be harnessed and adapted for therapeutic purposes. Technology-assisted relaxation can be quite useful (when carefully explained, prescribed, monitored, and utilized) as a culturally-syntonic vehicle to facilitate the regular practice of health-promoting MB therapies, such as breathwork, yoga, biofeedback-based relaxation, and mindfulness meditation. Therefore, healthcare providers should focus on understanding the latest technology available, and promoting self-regulation through MB skills training, which is known to provide benefits to humans of all ages.

In this age of rapid technological advancements, we could begin to imagine what the next frontier looks like: combining the best of the graphic design and multimedia arts, music, play, computerized hardware/software applications, and new miniaturized technologies for the creation of "therapeutic play" products, tools, and techniques for the next generation. Will the most effective therapists and pediatricians deliver their training on tablets and touch screen cellphones? Will clients check in regularly online via these devices? Will physiologic sensors be added into clothing or jewelry for additional information and options for more precise control of mind and body? As we continue to explore the interface of the arts, biomedical technologies, and healthcare endeavors in the service of healing, tremendous potential is available to develop new ways in which electronic media can enhance health and healing for kids and teenagers across a variety of settings, although vigilance is still needed to combat the potential downside to the overuse of technology [34].

Technology-assisted relaxation devices, in the form of computer games and electronic mobile apps, will certainly be part of the future of pediatric healthcare. Design features that optimize these healing technologies must take into account the specific client's play style, audio and visual preferences, developmental stage, and attention span. These products should support patients in a variety of ways, including promoting health literacy and improving self-regulatory abilities, both physically and psychologically. From a personalized healthcare perspective, computerized games utilized to promote health and wellness can provide a new source of information about patient preferences, health status, psychophysiological response patterns, and self-care abilities. Healthcare providers will hopefully find creative ways to utilize technology in care planning, as a way to enhance treatment adherence with recommendations to practice MB skills, and ultimately, to improve outcomes for the children, teenagers, and families we serve.

Author Contributions: Timothy Culbert is a developmental/behavioral pediatrician who is also board-certified in medical hypnosis, biofeedback, and holistic medicine. He has training in mindfulness meditation, functional medicine, nutrition, and clinical aromatherapy. Dr. Culbert is an author, lecturer, and product-developer in the area of natural therapies, self-regulation skills, and MB techniques for children, adults, and teens. Additionally, he has also written four books for children on holistic approaches for common problems, and co-edited the Oxford Series textbook "Integrative Pediatrics". He currently serves as Medical Director for Integrative Medicine at PrairieCare Medical Group in Minnesota.

References

1. AAP Section On Integrative Medicine. Mind-body therapies in children and youth. *Pediatrics* **2016**, *138*, e20161896.
2. Sibinga, E.M.S.; Kemper, K.J. Complementary, Holistic, and Integrative. Meditation Practices for Pediatric Health. *Pediatr. Rev.* **2010**, *31*, e91. [CrossRef] [PubMed]
3. Culbert, T.; Banez, G. Pediatric Applications. In *Biofeedback: A Practitioner's Guide*; Schwartz, M.S., Andrasik, F., Eds.; Guilford Publications: New York, NY, USA, 2015.
4. Culbert, T.; Friedrichsdorf, S.; Kuttner, L. Mind-body skills for children in pain. *Clin. Pain Manag. Pract. Appl. Proced.* **2007**, *138*, e20161896.
5. Greenland, S.K. *The Mindful Child: How to Help Your Kid Manage Stress and Become Happier, Kinder, and More Compassionate*; Simon and Schuster: New York, NY, USA, 2010.
6. Rosenkranz, M.A.; Davidson, R.; MacCoon, D.; Sheridan, J.; Kalin, N.; Lutz, A. A comparison of mindfulness-based stress reduction and an active control in modulation of neurogenic inflammation. *Brain Behav. Immun.* **2013**, *27*, 174–184. [CrossRef] [PubMed]
7. Gruzelier, J.H. A review of the impact of hypnosis, relaxation, guided imagery and individual differences on aspects of immunity and health. *Stress* **2002**, *5*, 147–163. [CrossRef] [PubMed]
8. Nassau, J.H.; Tien, K.; Fritz, G.K. Review of the literature: Integrating psychoneuroimmunology into pediatric chronic illness interventions. *J. Pediatr. Psychol.* **2008**, *33*, 195–207. [CrossRef] [PubMed]
9. Saltzman, A. *A Still Quiet Place: A Mindfulness Program for Teaching Children and Adolescents to Ease Stress and Difficult Emotions*; New Harbinger Publications: Oakland, CA, USA, 2014.
10. McCallum, S. Gamification and serious games for personalized health. *Stud. Health Technol. Inform.* **2012**, *177*, 85–96. [PubMed]
11. McQueen, A.; Cress, C.; Tothy, A. Using a tablet computer during pediatric procedures: A case series and review of the "apps". *Pediatr. Emerg. Care* **2012**, *28*, 712–714. [CrossRef] [PubMed]
12. Luxton, D.D.; McCann, R.; Bush, N.; Mishkind, M.; Reger, G. mHealth for mental health: Integrating smartphone technology in behavioral healthcare. *Prof. Psychol. Res. Pract.* **2011**, *42*, 505. [CrossRef]
13. Donker, T.; Petrie, K.; Proudfoot, J.; Clarke, J.; Birch, M.R.; Christensen, H. Smartphones for smarter delivery of mental health programs: A systematic review. *J. Med. Internet Res.* **2013**, *15*, e247. [CrossRef] [PubMed]
14. Kato, P.M. Video games in health care: Closing the gap. *Rev. Gen. Psychol.* **2010**, *14*, 113. [CrossRef]
15. Baranowski, T. Playing for real: Video games and stories for health-related behavior change. *Am. J. Prev. Med.* **2008**, *34*, 74–82. [CrossRef] [PubMed]
16. Handel, M.J. mHealth (mobile health)—Using apps for health and wellness. *EXPLORE J. Sci. Heal.* **2011**, *7*, 256–261. [CrossRef] [PubMed]
17. O'Keeffe, G.S.; Clarke-Pearson, K. The impact of social media on children, adolescents, and families. *Pediatrics* **2011**, *127*, 800–804. [CrossRef] [PubMed]

18. Radesky, J.S.; Schumacher, J.; Zuckerman, B. Mobile and interactive media use by young children: The good, the bad, and the unknown. *Pediatrics* **2015**, *135*, 1–3. [CrossRef] [PubMed]
19. Kabali, H.K.; Irigoyen, M.M.; Nunez-Davis, R.; Budacki, J.G.; Mohanty, S.H.: Leister, K.P.; Bonner, R.L. Exposure and use of mobile media devices by young children. *Pediatrics* **2015**, *136*, 1044–1050. [CrossRef] [PubMed]
20. Kemper, K.J.; Vohra, S.; Walls, R. The use of complementary and alternative medicine in pediatrics. *Pediatrics* **2008**, *122*, 1374–1386. [CrossRef] [PubMed]
21. Barnes, P.M.; Bloom, B.; Nahin, R.L. Complementary and alternative medicine use among adults and children: United States, 2007. *Natl. Health Stat. Rep.* **2008**, *12*, 1–23.
22. Harris, P.E.; Cooper, K.; Relton, C.; Thomas, K. Prevalence of complementary and alternative medicine (CAM) use by the general population: A systematic review and update. *Int. J. Clin. Pract.* **2012**, *66*, 924–939. [CrossRef] [PubMed]
23. Sussman, G.D.; Culbert, T. Pediatric self-regulation (Chapter 91). In *Developmental-Behavioral Pediatrics*, 4th ed.; Carey, W.B., Crocker, A.C., Coleman, W.L., Elias, E.R., Feldman, H.M., Eds.; Saunders Elsevier: Philadelphia, PA, USA, 2009; pp. 911–922.
24. El-Sheikh, M.; Erath, S.; Buckhalt, J.; Granger, D.; Mize, J. Cortisol and children's adjustment: The moderating role of sympathetic nervous system activity. *J. Abnorm. Child Psychol.* **2008**, *36*, 601–611. [CrossRef] [PubMed]
25. Bauer, A.M.; Quas, J.A.; Boyce, W.T. Associations between physiological reactivity and children's behavior: Advantages of a multisystem approach. *J. Dev. Behav. Pediatr.* **2002**, *23*, 102–113. [CrossRef] [PubMed]
26. Wyller, V.B.; Eriksen, H.R.; Malterud, K. Can sustained arousal explain the Chronic Fatigue Syndrome? *Behav. Brain Funct.* **2009**, *5*, 10. [CrossRef] [PubMed]
27. Shonkoff, J.P.; Garner, A.; Siegel, B.; Dobbins, M.; Earls, M.; McGuinn, L.; Pascoe, J.; Wood, D. The lifelong effects of early childhood adversity and toxic stress. *Pediatrics* **2012**, *129*, e232–e246. [CrossRef] [PubMed]
28. Mathews, H.L.; Janusek, L.W. Epigenetics and psychoneuroimmunology: Mechanisms and models. *Brain Behav. Immun.* **2011**, *25*, 25–39. [CrossRef] [PubMed]
29. Zannas, A.S.; West, A.E. Epigenetics and the regulation of stress vulnerability and resilience. *Neuroscience* **2014**, *264*, 157–170. [CrossRef] [PubMed]
30. Birdee, G.S.; Yeh, G.Y.; Wayne, P.M.; Phillips, R.S.; Davis, R.B.; Gardiner, P. Clinical applications of yoga for the pediatric population: A systematic review. *Acad. Pediatr.* **2009**, *9*, 212–220. [CrossRef] [PubMed]
31. Black, D.S.; Milam, J.; Sussman, S. Sitting-meditation interventions among youth: A review of treatment efficacy. *Pediatrics* **2009**, *124*, e532–e541. [CrossRef] [PubMed]
32. Rosen, L.; French, A.; Sullivan, G. Complementary, Holistic, and Integrative Medicine: Yoga. *Pediatr. Rev./Am. Acad. Pediatr.* **2015**, *36*, 468. [CrossRef] [PubMed]
33. Barnes, A.J. Childhood Stress and Resilience. In *Health Promotion for Children and Adolescents*; Springer: New York, NY, USA, 2016; pp. 85–98.
34. AAP Council on Communications and Media. Media and young minds. *Pediatrics* **2016**, *138*, e20162591.
35. Buchman, D.D.; Funk, J.B. Video and computer games in the 90s: Children's time commitment and game preference. *Child. Today* **1996**, *24*, 12. [PubMed]
36. Gentile, D.A.; Walsh, D.A. A normative study of family media habits. *J. Appl. Dev. Psychol.* **2002**, *23*, 157–178. [CrossRef]
37. Loftus, G.R.; Loftus, E.F. *Mind at Play; The Psychology of Video Games*; Basic Books, Inc.: New York, NY, USA, 1983.
38. National Center for Telehealth and Technology. Available online: www.t2health.dcoe.mil/apps/breathe2relax.com (accessed on 21 January 2017).
39. Stressed Teens. Available online: www.stressedteens.com (accessed on 21 January 2017).
40. Stop, Breathe and Think App. Available online: www.stopbreathethink.org (accessed on 21 January 2017).
41. Smiling Mind. Available online: www.smilingmind.com.au (accessed on 21 January 2017).
42. The Adventures of Super Stretch. Available online: www.adventuresofsuperstretch.com (accessed on 21 January 2017).
43. Let It Go Yoga. Available online: www.letitgoyoga.com/yoga-by-teens/ (accessed on 21 January 2017).
44. Kids Yogaverse. Available online: www.kidsyogaverse.com (accessed on 21 January 2017).
45. Me Moves. Available online: www.thinkingmoves.com (accessed on 21 January 2017).
46. Mindfield Biosystems. Available online: www.mindfield.de (accessed on 21 January 2017).

47. Life Matters. Available online: www.lifematters.com/biofeedback-machines.asp (accessed on 21 January 2017).
48. Kirsch, D.L.; Nichols, F. Cranial electrotherapy stimulation for treatment of anxiety, depression, and insomnia. *Psychiatr. Clin. N. Am.* **2013**, *36*, 169–176. [CrossRef] [PubMed]
49. Kirsch, D.L.; Smith, R.B. The use of cranial electrotherapy stimulation in the management of chronic pain: A review. *NeuroRehabilitation* **2000**, *14*, 85–94. [PubMed]
50. Gilula, M.F.; Kirsch, D.L. Cranial electrotherapy stimulation review: A safer alternative to psychopharmaceuticals in the treatment of depression. *J. Neurother.* **2005**, *9*, 7–26. [CrossRef]
51. Alpha-Stim. Available online: www.alpha-stim.com (accessed on 21 January 2017).
52. Siever, D. Applying audio-visual entrainment technology for attention and learning. *Biofeedback Mag.* **2008**, *31*, 1–15.
53. Huang, T.L.; Charyton, C. A comprehensive review of the psychological effects of brainwave entrainment. *Altern. Ther. Health Med.* **2008**, *14*, 38. [PubMed]
54. Boersma, F.J.; Gagnon, C. The use of repetitive audiovisual entrainment in the management of chronic pain. *Med. Hypnoanal. J.* **1992**, *7*, 80–97.
55. Clancy, J.A.; Mary, D.; White, K.; Greenwood, J.; Deuchars, S.; Deuchars, J. Non-invasive vagus nerve stimulation in healthy humans reduces sympathetic nerve activity. *Brain Stimul.* **2014**, *7*, 871–877. [CrossRef] [PubMed]
56. George, M.S.; Sackeim, H.; Rush, J.; Marangell, L.; Nahas, Z.; Husain, M.; Lisanby, S.; Burt, T.; Goldman, J.; Ballenger, J. Vagus nerve stimulation: A new tool for brain research and therapy. *Biol. Psychiatry* **2000**, *47*, 287–295. [CrossRef]
57. Wild Divine. Available online: www.wilddivine.com (accessed on 21 January 2017).

16

Family-Based Mindful Eating Intervention in Adolescents with Obesity

Seema Kumar [1,*], Ivana T. Croghan [2], Bridget K. Biggs [3], Katrina Croghan [4], Rose Prissel [5], Debbie Fuehrer [6], Bonnie Donelan-Dunlap [2] and Amit Sood [6]

1 Division of Pediatric Endocrinology, Department of Pediatric and Adolescent Medicine, Mayo Clinic, Rochester, MN 55905, USA
2 Primary Care Internal Medicine, Mayo Clinic, Rochester, MN 55905, USA; croghan.ivana@mayo.edu (I.T.C.); DonelanDunlap.bonnie@mayo.edu (B.D.-D.)
3 Department of Psychiatry and Psychology, Mayo Clinic, Rochester, MN 55905, USA; biggs.bridget@mayo.edu
4 Cancer Center, Mayo Clinic, Rochester, MN 55905, USA; croghan.katrina@mayo.edu
5 Endocrinology/Nutrition, Mayo Clinic, Rochester, MN 55905, USA; prissel.rose@mayo.edu
6 General Internal Medicine, Mayo Clinic, Rochester, MN 55905, USA; fuehrer.debbie@mayo.edu (D.F.); sood.amit@mayo.edu (A.S.)
* Correspondence: kumar.seema@mayo.edu

Abstract: Mindfulness has gained attention in the treatment of obesity. However, there is a paucity of data on family-based training in mindful eating in children. The objective of this pilot randomized clinical trial was to evaluate the feasibility and acceptability of a family-based mindful eating intervention (MEI) in adolescents with obesity, and to compare the efficacy of the MEI versus standard dietary counseling (SDC) for decreasing weight and improving cardiometabolic risk markers. Twenty-two adolescents (age 14.5–17.9 years) and parent pairs were randomized to the MEI or SDC. The MEI was administered in four 90-min sessions over 10 weeks and SDC was provided at baseline, 12 weeks, and 24 weeks. Despite the requirement of more frequent visits with the MEI, adolescents and parents attended 100% of the sessions and there were no dropouts in that group. High density lipoprotein (HDL) cholesterol increased in the SDC group, but not in the MEI group. Adolescents receiving the MEI demonstrated an increase in awareness at 24 weeks ($p = 0.01$) and a decrease in distraction during eating at 12 weeks ($p = 0.04$), when compared with the SDC group. The family-based MEI showed feasibility and acceptability in adolescents with obesity. Future studies with more intense therapy and larger sample sizes are warranted to examine the role of mindful eating in treating pediatric obesity.

Keywords: mindful eating; obesity; adolescents

---

1. Background

The problem of childhood obesity has reached epidemic proportions [1]. Currently, 18.5% of children in the United States have obesity and 6% have severe obesity [1]. Childhood obesity is associated with several adverse health consequences, including type 2 diabetes, dyslipidemia, and hypertension [2–4]. If established by adolescence, obesity, and its associated health problems, is likely to persist into adulthood [2]. While lifestyle modification is considered the cornerstone of pediatric obesity treatment, the efficacy of behavioral modification programs to address obesity through the promotion of healthier eating and an active lifestyle is modest and is limited by dropout rates of 27–73% [5–9]. Additionally, there is limited evidence for the long-term sustainability of weight loss in children with obesity [10–12]. Therefore, additional strategies are warranted to enhance the efficacy and sustainability of lifestyle modifications, including dietary habits, in the management of childhood obesity.

Mindfulness is defined as "the awareness that arises from paying attention on purpose, in the present moment and non-judgmentally" [13]. Eating behaviors play an important role in excess weight gain. Mindfulness has gained attention as an avenue for the treatment of obesity through modification of problematic eating behaviors, such as excess caloric intake in response to external cues (e.g., portion size) [14–17]. Studies investigating the effects of mindfulness on obesity-related eating behaviors have focused almost exclusively on adult samples, with only two including late-adolescent/young adult participants [15]. Several studies have demonstrated the benefits of mindfulness-based weight loss intervention for adults [18,19]. Mindfulness-based interventions have demonstrated effectiveness in improving binge eating, emotional eating, and external eating behaviors [15], as well as improving self-control [20]. Mindfulness techniques have been adapted for use with adolescents and children as young as preschool age, with at least 15 reported studies supporting their feasibility and acceptability when taught to children or to children and parents together [21,22]. The limited research suggests mindfulness can improve adolescents' self-regulation, particularly in response to stress [23]. However, there is a paucity of data on the effect of family-based mindful eating interventions (MEI) in the management of pediatric obesity or in young people's eating behaviors [24].

The objectives of this pilot randomized clinical trial were to (i) evaluate the feasibility and acceptability of a family-based MEI in adolescents with obesity and (ii) compare the efficacy of a family-based MEI versus standard dietary counseling (SDC) for decreasing weight and improving cardiometabolic risk markers in adolescents with obesity.

2. Subjects and Methods

2.1. Design Overview

This was a two-arm, parallel-group, pilot, randomized, blinded (outcome assessor and statistician), dietary counseling group controlled clinical trial in adolescents with obesity. The trial was registered on ClinicalTrials.gov (NCT01764113), and was approved by the Mayo Clinic Institutional Review Board (12-006349).

2.2. Setting and Participants

Adolescents between the ages of 14–17 years were considered eligible if their body mass index (BMI) was at or above the 95th percentile for age and gender. Age and gender-specific BMI percentiles and *z*-scores were calculated using the standards recommended by the Centers for Disease Control and Prevention [25].

Exclusion criteria included: (i) currently attending a supervised weight loss program; (ii) underlying genetic or endocrine cause for weight gain; (iii) type 1 or type 2 diabetes mellitus; (iv) ongoing treatment with receiving insulin, metformin, or oral hypoglycemic medications; (v) use of oral glucocorticoids in the previous two months; (vi) current cancer; (vii) established diagnosis of psychiatric illness in the previous six months; (viii) inability of the participant or parent to provide informed assent/consent or inability of the same parent to attend all of the intervention sessions and (ix) study visits along with their adolescent.

Participants were recruited from primary care practices (general pediatrics and family medicine) and pediatric specialties at the Mayo Clinic, Rochester, MN, USA.

2.3. Randomization and Interventions

Participants and one parent were randomized in a 1:1 ratio to the MEI group or SDC. Randomization was performed using a computer-generated randomization schedule. The same parent was required to attend the intervention sessions, as well as the study visits, in either group throughout the duration of the study.

Informed assent was obtained from the adolescents and informed consent was obtained from the parent who had enrolled in the study. Interventions for both the arms were group based (3–4 adolescent and parent pairs per group). The sessions in both the MEI and SDC treatment arms were conducted in an outpatient clinic setting on a weekday between 6 p.m. and 7:30 p.m. A healthy meal consisting of a sub sandwich with low fat meats and veggies with fruit, baked chips, and zero calorie lemonade was served before the meetings at 5:30 p.m.

The mindful eating program was administered over four 90-min sessions (baseline, 1 week, 6 weeks, and 10 weeks) by a team comprised of a physician and a trained mind-body therapist.

The adolescents and parents in the MEI arm attended concurrent sessions (one for adolescents and the other one for parents only) held in different rooms and met each other at the end of the session only. The program had two components: an approach toward mindfulness, and an application of the mindfulness principles to eating. The first session emphasized mindfulness and stress management strategies, including brief practices to improve attention and bring greater gratitude and compassion in life. In the next three sessions, participants learned mindful eating principles, including learning to be more cognizant of what one is eating, attuning with one's body to assess hunger and appropriate size of serving, cultivating gratitude for food and its preparers, relaxing for a moment prior to eating, paying purposeful attention to the color and aroma of food, eating slowly in small bites, enjoying each bite fully, and paying attention to the sensation of fullness from the stomach. Participants were also taught skills to avoid automatic eating, develop better self-control when offered appetitive calorie dense foods, and shopping with better awareness of the calorie density and nutritive value of foods. Each session offered a combination of a scientific perspective combined with stories and specific skills in mindfulness and mindful eating.

Adolescent/parent pairs in the SDC arm received three 90-min sessions of dietary counseling (parents and adolescents together) by a registered pediatric dietician at baseline, 12 weeks, and 24 weeks. The dietary counseling in the SDC group focused on portion control, decreasing intakes of calorie dense fast food/convenience store foods, and substituting with healthier foods consistent with routine care for youth with obesity. Throughout each session, the focus was on further educating teens and their caregiver through discussion and utilization of educational tools, such as using the provided meal to discuss portion control, satiety, energy density, and the nutrients provided in the food. In addition, using meaningful food labels, food models, and various plate, cup, and bowl sizes to engage thought provoking discussion were used along with the didactic means of educating teens and their care provider.

2.4. Outcomes and Follow Up

Participants were evaluated by study staff at baseline, 12 weeks, and 24 weeks. The primary outcomes measures were change in weight, BMI, and BMI *z*-score. The secondary outcomes measures were change in fasting glucose, insulin, lipids, high sensitivity C-reactive protein (hs-CRP), and domains in the mindful eating questionnaire (MEQ) and weight-efficacy lifestyle questionnaire (WEL).

Weight, height, and blood pressure were obtained at baseline, 12 weeks, and 24 weeks, and were collected by trained research assistants using standardized instruments. Blood glucose, insulin, total cholesterol, high density lipoprotein (HDL) cholesterol, triglycerides, and hs-CRP were obtained after a 10–12 h overnight fast at baseline and at 24 weeks. Plasma glucose was measured by hexokinase enzymatic assay, and serum insulin was measured using commercial electrochemiluminescence immunoassay kits. Total cholesterol, HDL cholesterol, and triglyceride levels were measured by an enzymatic calorimetric assay. Non-HDL cholesterol was calculated as total cholesterol minus HDL cholesterol. Low density lipoprotein (LDL) cholesterol was calculated using the equation: LDL = total cholesterol − HDL cholesterol − (triglycerides/5). Measurement of hs-CRP was performed using particle-enhanced immunonephelometry (Siemens Healthcare Diagnostics, Deerfield, IL, USA).

The MEQ [26] and WEL [27] were administered at baseline, 12, and 24 weeks. The MEQ is a 28-item scale designed to assess non-judgmental awareness of physical and emotional cues associated with eating. For each item, respondents rate the frequency of the listed behavior and items are scored 1–4, with 4 indicating higher mindfulness. Resulting scores include a summary score and five subscales: disinhibition, awareness, external cues, emotional response, and distraction. The WEL is a 20-item eating self-efficacy scale consisting of a total score and five situational factors: negative emotions, availability, social pressure, physical discomfort, and positive activities. For each item, respondents rate their level of confidence in their ability to resist eating in the given situation on a 10-point scale, from 0—"not confident", to 9—"very confident".

2.5. Sample Size Calculation and Statistical Analysis

A priori power analysis conducted using G*Power 3 [28] indicated that a sample size of 40 participants (20 for each arm) would be required to detect the medium to large effect sizes observed in similar previous research assuming 0.80 power with a two-tailed test and α set at 0.05. Since the trial was of a pilot nature and the primary aim was to examine the feasibility and acceptability of the MEI, recruitment was discontinued at the end of the trial despite a total enrollment of only 22 participants.

Continuous variables were summarized with mean $\pm$ standard deviation (SD), or median and interquartile range (IQR), as appropriate. Categorical variables were summarized as a frequency and percentage. Differences between time points were assessed within each study group with Wilcoxon signed-rank tests, and the paired differences were compared between study groups with Wilcoxon rank-sum tests. p-Values less than 0.05 were considered statistically significant. All analyses were performed using SAS version 9.3 (SAS Institute Inc., Cary, NC, USA) [29]. Subgroup analyses were not performed due to the small sample size.

3. Results

A total of 22 adolescents (age range 14.5–17.9 years) were enrolled in the study (Figure 1). Out of 45 adolescents that were called in and prescreened for the study, 31 passed the phone screen and 14 did not meet the study criteria (Figure 1). Twenty-nine adolescents consented to the study and two declined. Seven out of the 29 consented adolescents withdrew consent and; therefore, 22 adolescents were randomized to either of the study arms (11 in each group). The study was conducted between 7 December 2012 and 19 December 2013.The interventions were conducted at two different times of the year due to the convenience in the recruitment timing. The first group of 14 participants (8 males, 6 females) began intervention in winter (February 2013) and these were equally divided between the MEI and SDC (7 in each group). The remaining 8 patients (4 males, 4 females) began receiving the intervention in June 2013 and these were also equally split between the two intervention groups (4 in each group).

Anthropometric and laboratory characteristics of the participants are detailed in Table 1.

Age, gender, and race were not different between the two groups ($p > 0.05$). The median age (quartile, Q1, Q3) was 15.6 (15.2, 16.8) years in the SDC group and 17.1 (15.5, 17.4) years in the MEI group. There were 12 male and 10 female participants, with 7/11 (63.6%) participants in the SDC group (63.6%) and 5/11 (45.5%) participants in the MEI group were male. Nineteen out of 22 participants were white and three were non-white (one in the SDC group and two in the MEI group).

Baseline BMI was not significantly different between the two groups (median (Q1, Q3): 32.9 (30.9, 36.2) kg/m^2 and 34.9 (32, 36.6) kg/m^2 in the SDC and MEI group, respectively; $p > 0.05$). Baseline BMI z-score also was not different between the two groups (median (Q1, Q3): 2.4 (1.9, 3.2) and 2.5 (2.3, 3.0) in the SDC and MEI group, respectively; $p > 0.05$). There were no differences in the laboratory parameters between the two groups ($p > 0.05$, Table 1).

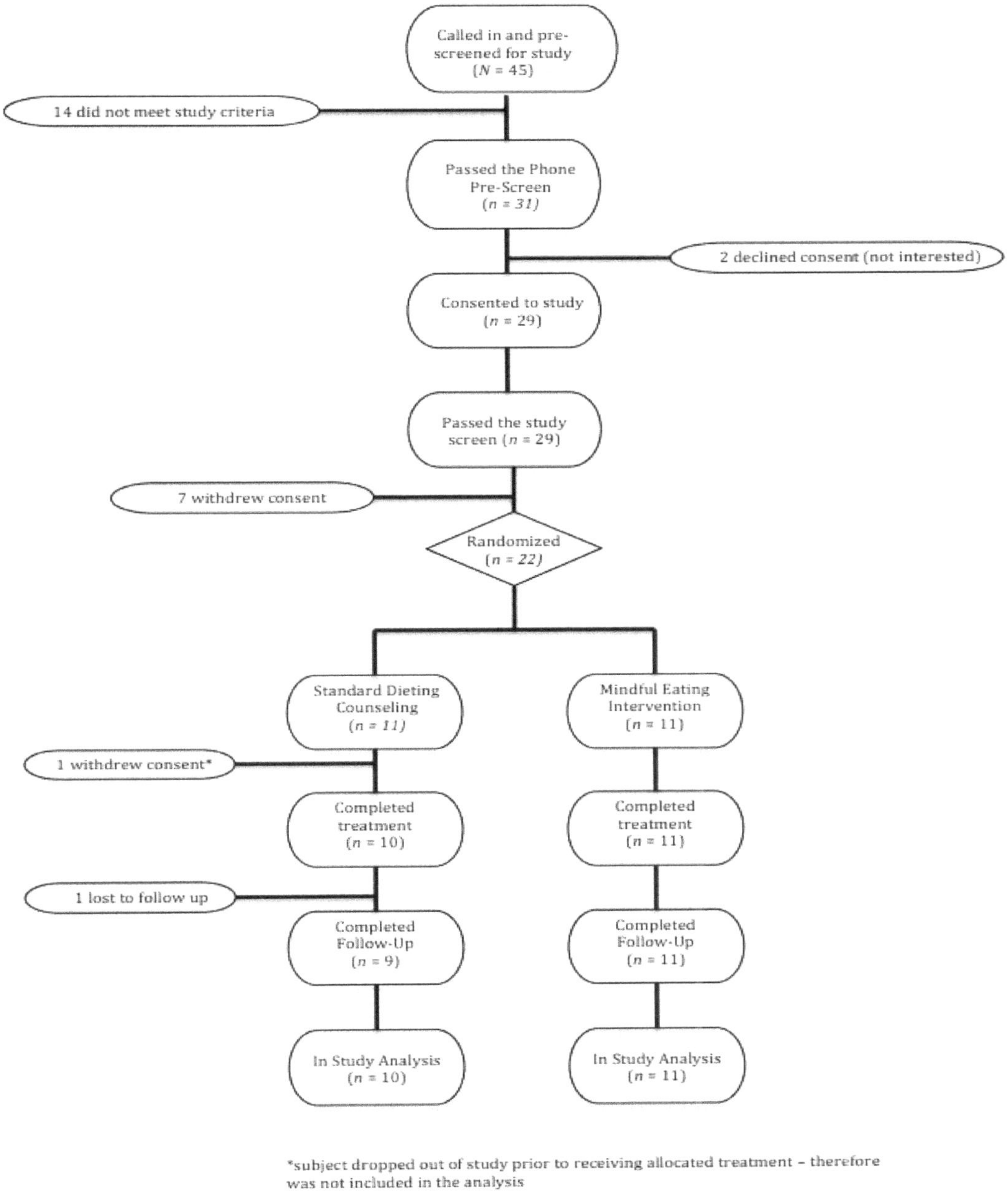

Figure 1. Study flow.

Table 1. Anthropometric and laboratory characteristics of study participants.

	Standard Dietary Counseling (n = 11)		Mindful Eating Intervention (n = 11)		Difference between the Two Arms
	Median	Q1, Q3	Median	Q1, Q3	p-Value
Age (years)	15.6	15.2, 16.8	17.1	15.5, 17.4	NS
Weight (kg)	103.7	87, 123	98.7	95.9, 106.4	NS
BMI (kg/m^2)	32.9	30.9, 36.2	34.9	32, 36.6	NS
BMI z-score	2.4	1.9, 3.2	2.5	2.3, 3.0	NS
Glucose (mg/dL)	88	81, 96	92	88, 99	NS
Insulin (mcIU/mL)	21.8	17.7, 24.5	29.3	15.6, 35.1	NS
Total cholesterol (mg/dL)	176	133, 183	144	124, 180	NS
HDL cholesterol (mg/dL)	41	33, 53	35	31, 48	NS
LDL cholesterol (mg/dL)	101	69, 106	81	77, 112	NS
Non-HDL cholesterol (mg/dL)	126	91, 146	108	93, 132	NS
Triglycerides (mg/dL)	174	81, 219	104	80, 134	NS
hs-CRP (mg/L)	1.7	0.5, 4.3	3.2	0.4, 5.7	NS

NS, $p > 0.05$. BMI, body mass index; HDL, high density lipoprotein; LDL, low density lipoprotein; hs-CRP, high sensitivity C-reactive protein; Q, quartile.

All 11 adolescent and parents in the MEI group attended all four intervention sessions, as well as the study visits, at 12 weeks and 24 weeks. Therefore, there were no drop outs in the MEI group. One participant in the SDC group dropped out after the first session and did not return for the 12-week or 24-week visit. Data from 10 participants in the SDC group and from 11 participants in the MEI group were included in the analysis.

Body mass index and BMI *z*-score in the MEI group were higher at 12 weeks and 24 weeks ($p < 0.05$) relative to baseline (Table 2). Body mass index and BMI *z*-scores in the SDC group were higher ($p < 0.05$) at 24 weeks compared to baseline (Table 2). However, there were no significant differences in the change in weight, BMI, and BMI *z*-score from baseline to 12-week or 24-week time points between the two groups ($p > 0.05$ for all, Table 2).

Table 2. Change in anthropometric and laboratory measures during follow up.

		Standard Dietary Counseling (n = 10)		Mindful Eating Intervention (n = 11)		Difference between the Two Groups
Parameter	**Time**	**Median**	**Q1, Q3**	**Median**	**Q1, Q3**	***p*-Value**
Weight (kg)	Week 12	−0.1	−1.4, 1.2	2.3	−0.7, 3.2	NS
	Week 24	2.5	1.5, 3.3	4.0	−0.2, 5.2	NS
BMI (kg/m^2)	Week 12	−0.3	−0.9, −0.1	0.6	−0.2, 1.2	NS
	Week 24	1	0.4, 1.1	0.9	0.2, 2.3	NS
BMI *z*-score	Week 12	−0.1	−0.2, 0	0.1	0, 0.2	NS
	Week 24	0.2	0.1, 0.2	0.2	0, 0.4	NS
Glucose (mg/dL)	Week 24	2	−3, 6	−4	−8, 6	NS
Insulin (mcIU/mL)	Week 24	3.5	1.4, 6.6	0.3	−4.5, 4.8	NS
Total cholesterol (mg/dL)	Week 24	14	4, 24	3	−11, 28	NS
LDL cholesterol (mg/dL)	Week 24	1	−7, 12	8	−11, 20	NS
HDL cholesterol (mg/dL)	Week 24	7	2, 10	−1	−2, 3	0.0245
Triglycerides (mg/dL)	Week 24	9	2, 27	7	−8, 24	NS
hs-CRP (mg/L)	Week 24	0.3	0.2, 0.4	0.2	−1.4, 1.2	NS

NS, $p > 0.05$.

There was a statistically significant difference in the δ HDL cholesterol between the SDC and MEI groups, with HDL cholesterol increasing in the SDC group (median (Q1, Q3): 7 (2, 10) mg/dL), but not in the MEI group ((−1 (−2, 3) mg/dL); $p = 0.0245$). There was no difference in changes in other laboratory measures between the two groups.

No adverse side effects were reported by study participants in either of the groups.

Adolescents in the MEI group demonstrated an increase in awareness at 24 weeks and a decrease in distraction during eating at 12 weeks relative to the SDC group ($p = 0.01$ and $p = 0.04$, respectively, Table 3).

Table 3. Changes in mindful eating questionnaire (MEQ) and weight-efficiency lifestyle questionnaire (WEL) domains.

	Standard Dietary Counseling (SDC) (n = 10)			Mindless Eating Intervention (MEI) (n = 11)		
	Baseline [a]	**Week 12** [a]	**Week 24** [a]	**Baseline** [a]	**Week 12** [a]	**Week 24** [a]
Mindful eating questionnaire						
Awareness	2.5 (0.6)	2.5 (0.7)	2.4 (0.7)	2.1 (0.5)	2.4 (0.4)	2.5 (0.5) *
Disinhibition	2.7 (0.7)	2.7 (0.6)	2.6 (0.8)	3.0 (0.4)	2.9 (0.3)	2.9 (0.4)
Distraction	3.7 (0.3)	3.6 (0.3)	3.7 (0.5)	3.8 (0.2)	3.4 (0.4) **	3.6 (0.4)
Emotional	2.6 (0.3)	3.1 (0.4)	2.9 (0.3)	2.9 (0.4)	2.8 (0.5)	2.9 (0.3)
Weight efficacy lifestyle questionnaire						
Total score	6.2 (2.0)	6.5 (1.9)	6.5 (2.0)	7.0 (1.2)	6.5 (1.2)	7.0 (1.1)
Negative emotions	6.5 (2.5)	6.4 (2.8)	6.9 (2.4)	6.8 (2.2)	6.7 (1.7)	7.0 (1.6)
Availability	5.2 (2.2)	5.7 (2.3)	5.6 (2.2)	5.9 (1.5)	5.4 (1.9)	6.1 (1.4)
Social pressure	5.8 (2.7)	6.3 (2.4)	5.7 (2.0)	7.0 (1.2)	6.2 (1.7)	6.8 (1.5)
Physical discomfort	6.9 (1.8)	7.3 (1.6)	7.4 (1.9)	7.7 (1.2)	7.3 (1.3)	7.7 (1.4)
Positive activities	6.7 (1.8)	7.0 (1.7)	6.8 (2.1)	7.4 (1.1)	7.0 (0.8)	(0.9)

[a] Data are presented as mean ± SD (standard deviation); difference between MEI and SDC groups with regards to change from baseline: * MEQ awareness (week 24-baseline difference), $p = 0.01$; ** MEQ distraction (week 12-baseline difference), $p = 0.04$.

4. Discussion

We demonstrate the feasibility and acceptability of a family-based mindful eating intervention in adolescents with obesity. To our knowledge, this is the first randomized clinical trial to test the feasibility, acceptability, and short term weight loss efficacy of a family-based mindful eating intervention in adolescents with obesity.

Despite the need for four 90-min sessions for adolescents and their parents over a period of 10 weeks, we noted 100% attendance in the four training sessions by adolescents and their parents. In addition, all participants in the MEI group returned for assessments at 12 weeks and 24 weeks. This level of attendance in the intervention sessions and retention over the 24-week period is remarkable given reported dropout rates in behavioral treatments for pediatric obesity [9], and the scant data on the feasibility and acceptability of a mindful eating-based intervention in children and adolescents with obesity [30]. In contrast to our findings, Daly and colleagues reported only 57% retention in a randomized feasibility study aimed at weight loss in adolescent Latino females [30]. The mindful eating intervention in that study was administered to adolescents recruited in a public high school in southwestern United States and was not delivered to parents. The differences in retention rates may be related to differences in the ethnicity and gender distribution of participants as the majority of our study participants were white, and males comprised more than half of our study population. Additionally, there were several differences in the specifics of the mindful eating intervention, such as the frequency of the intervention sessions (90-min session every week for six weeks in the study by Daly versus four 90-min sessions over a period of 10 weeks in our study), time of the day (afterschool setting versus evening time in our study), and setting (classroom versus outpatient clinic in our study). The mindful eating intervention in our study, on the other hand, was conducted in the late evening with an evening meal provided to all participants and their parents. Finally, involvement of the family, as was required in our study, could have also contributed to a greater retention. Our finding of a higher retention in the MEI group is all the more remarkable in view of the longer follow up period in our study (24 weeks versus 10 weeks in the study by Daly and colleagues [30]).

The MEI was not efficacious in decreasing BMI or BMI *z*-score at 12 weeks or 24 weeks in our study. Participants in both groups had an increase in BMI and BMI *z*-scores at 24 weeks. These findings are not surprising given the modest efficacy of behavior modifications on severity of adiposity [31]. Similar to our study, overweight/obese adolescent females in another study by Shomaker and colleagues also exhibited an increase in BMI despite receiving mindfulness-based group intervention [32]. In contrast, a 1.4 kg/m^2 decrease in BMI was noted at 10 weeks in Latino adolescent females receiving MEI, but no subsequent BMI measurements were available at 24 weeks in their study [30]. The greater frequency of MEI in the study in Latino adolescent females (six weekly 90-min sessions) compared to our study (four 90-min sessions over a period of 10 weeks) may partly account for differences in the effects on BMI. Mindful eating-based interventions have been shown to result in weight loss among children with Prader-Willi syndrome [33–35]. Several studies in adults have also demonstrated modest benefits in adults [18,19,36], with a mean weight loss of 4 kg and a mean decrease in BMI of 1.3 kg/m^2 in one study [19]. The lack of improvement in weight or BMI in the participants in our MEI or SDS groups may be due to the low intensity of the intervention, with only 6 h of contact over a period of six months, despite the most recent The United States Preventive Task Force guidelines recommending >26 h "over a period of 2–12 months" [37]. It remains unknown if an addition of a greater number of hours of mindfulness-based intervention would lead to an improvement in outcomes of adolescents with obesity.

We noted improvements in awareness and in reduced distraction during eating among the adolescents receiving the mindful eating intervention. No differences in mindfulness awareness were noted in adolescent Latino females receiving a mindful eating intervention [30]. Unfortunately, changes in these domains did not result in an improved weight status during the study period. The inclusion of dietary assessments in future studies would further the understanding of whether changes in these mindful eating domains translate into changes in dietary quality or caloric intake that could, over time, lead to changes in weight status.

The strengths of our study include the randomized clinical trial design with the presence of a control group receiving standard dietary counseling on a low fat, portion controlled dietary plan. We had excellent retention with follow up on all but one out of the 22 participants at six months from the time of enrollment.

The most significant limitation of our study is its pilot nature and small sample size. The study was underpowered to determine the efficacy of the MEI on weight and cardiometabolic risk factors in adolescents with obesity. Another limitation was the low intensity of the intervention, with the total number of hours of contact of 6 h being significantly below the >26 h "over a period of 2–12 months" recently recommended by national experts [37]. The duration of follow up was short and, therefore, outcomes beyond six months could not be assessed. Other important limitations were the lack of information regarding pubertal staging and body composition, and lack of data on disordered eating patterns, such as binge eating and emotional eating, as well as on quality/quantity of dietary intake and physical activity. Finally, the study findings cannot be generalized due to a lack of ethnic and racial diversity among the participants.

5. Conclusions

A family-based mindful eating intervention was found to be feasible and acceptable in adolescents with obesity. No beneficial changes in weight, BMI, or any of the cardiometabolic risk factors were observed. Further studies with a greater intensity of interventions and larger sample size are warranted to examine the role of mindful eating interventions in the treatment of childhood obesity.

Author Contributions: Conceptualization, S.K. and A.S.; Methodology, S.K., A.S., I.T.C., B.K.B., R.P. and A.S.; Validation, S.K., I.T.C. and A.S.; Formal Analysis, S.K., A.S. and I.T.C.; Investigation, S.K., K.C., and A.S.; Resources, I.T.C., A.S. and S.K.; Writing-Original Draft Preparation, S.K.; Writing-Review & Editing, S.K., I.T.C., B.K.B., A.S., K.C., D.F., B.D.-D. and R.P.; Supervision, I.T.C. and A.S.; Project Administration, I.T.C., K.C., R.P., D.F., B.D.-D.; Funding Acquisition, S.K. and A.S.

References

1. Skinner, A.C.; Ravanbakht, S.N.; Skelton, J.A.; Perrin, E.M.; Armstrong, S.C. Prevalence of obesity and severe obesity in us children, 1999–2016. *Pediatrics* **2018**. [CrossRef] [PubMed]
2. Kelly, A.S.; Barlow, S.E.; Rao, G.; Inge, T.H.; Hayman, L.L.; Steinberger, J.; Urbina, E.M.; Ewing, L.J.; Daniels, S.R. Severe obesity in children and adolescents: Identification, associated health risks, and treatment approaches: A scientific statement from the american heart association. *Circulation* **2013**, *128*, 1689–1712. [CrossRef] [PubMed]
3. Weiss, R.; Dziura, J.; Burgert, T.S.; Tamborlane, W.V.; Taksali, S.E.; Yeckel, C.W.; Allen, K.; Lopes, M.; Savoye, M.; Morrison, J.; et al. Obesity and the metabolic syndrome in children and adolescents. *N. Engl. J. Med.* **2004**, *350*, 2362–2374. [CrossRef] [PubMed]
4. Skinner, A.C.; Perrin, E.M.; Moss, L.A.; Skelton, J.A. Cardiometabolic risks and severity of obesity in children and young adults. *N. Engl. J. Med.* **2015**, *373*, 1307–1317. [CrossRef] [PubMed]
5. Barlow, S.E. Expert committee recommendations regarding the prevention, assessment, and treatment of child and adolescent overweight and obesity: Summary report. *Pediatrics* **2007**, *120*, S164–S192. [CrossRef] [PubMed]
6. Epstein, L.H.; Valoski, A.M.; Vara, L.S.; McCurley, J.; Wisniewski, L.; Kalarchian, M.A.; Klein, K.R.; Shrager, L.R. Effects of decreasing sedentary behavior and increasing activity on weight change in obese children. *Health Psychol.* **1995**, *14*, 109–115. [CrossRef] [PubMed]

7. Whitlock, E.P.; O'Connor, E.A.; Williams, S.B.; Beil, T.L.; Lutz, K.W. Effectiveness of weight management interventions in children: A targeted systematic review for the uspstf. *Pediatrics* **2010**, *125*, e396–e418. [CrossRef] [PubMed]
8. Ho, M.; Garnett, S.P.; Baur, L.; Burrows, T.; Stewart, L.; Neve, M.; Collins, C. Effectiveness of lifestyle interventions in child obesity: Systematic review with meta-analysis. *Pediatrics* **2012**, *130*, e1647–e1671. [CrossRef] [PubMed]
9. Skelton, J.A.; Beech, B.M. Attrition in paediatric weight management: A review of the literature and new directions. *Obes. Rev.* **2011**, *12*, e273–e281. [CrossRef] [PubMed]
10. Butryn, M.L.; Wadden, T.A.; Rukstalis, M.R.; Bishop-Gilyard, C.; Xanthopoulos, M.S.; Louden, D.; Berkowitz, R.I. Maintenance of weight loss in adolescents: Current status and future directions. *J. Obes.* **2010**, *2010*, 789280. [CrossRef] [PubMed]
11. Nguyen, B.; Shrewsbury, V.A.; O'Connor, J.; Steinbeck, K.S.; Lee, A.; Hill, A.J.; Shah, S.; Kohn, M.R.; Torvaldsen, S.; Baur, L.A. Twelve-month outcomes of the loozit randomized controlled trial: A community-based healthy lifestyle program for overweight and obese adolescents. *Arch. Pediatr. Adolesc. Med.* **2012**, *166*, 170–177. [CrossRef] [PubMed]
12. Mameli, C.; Krakauer, J.C.; Krakauer, N.Y.; Bosetti, A.; Ferrari, C.M.; Schneider, L.; Borsani, B.; Arrigoni, S.; Pendezza, E.; Zuccotti, G.V. Effects of a multidisciplinary weight loss intervention in overweight and obese children and adolescents: 11 years of experience. *PLoS ONE* **2017**, *12*, e0181095. [CrossRef] [PubMed]
13. Paulson, S.; Davidson, R.; Jha, A.; Kabat-Zinn, J. Becoming conscious: The science of mindfulness. *Ann. N. Y. Acad. Sci.* **2013**, *1303*, 87–104. [CrossRef] [PubMed]
14. Godsey, J. The role of mindfulness-based interventions in the treatment of obesity and eating disorders: An integrative review. *Complement. Ther. Med.* **2013**, *21*, 430–439. [CrossRef] [PubMed]
15. O'Reilly, G.A.; Cook, L.; Spruijt-Metz, D.; Black, D.S. Mindfulness-based interventions for obesity-related eating behaviours: A literature review. *Obes. Rev.* **2014**, *15*, 453–461. [CrossRef] [PubMed]
16. Sojcher, R.; Gould Fogerite, S.; Perlman, A. Evidence and potential mechanisms for mindfulness practices and energy psychology for obesity and binge-eating disorder. *Explore* **2012**, *8*, 271–276. [CrossRef] [PubMed]
17. Dunn, C.; Haubenreiser, M.; Johnson, M.; Nordby, K.; Aggarwal, S.; Myer, S.; Thomas, C. Mindfulness approaches and weight loss, weight maintenance, and weight regain. *Curr. Obes. Rep.* **2018**, *7*, 37–49. [CrossRef] [PubMed]
18. Tapper, K.; Shaw, C.; Ilsley, J.; Hill, A.J.; Bond, F.W.; Moore, L. Exploratory randomised controlled trial of a mindfulness-based weight loss intervention for women. *Appetite* **2009**, *52*, 396–404. [CrossRef] [PubMed]
19. Dalen, J.; Smith, B.W.; Shelley, B.M.; Sloan, A.L.; Leahigh, L.; Begay, D. Pilot study: Mindful eating and living (meal): Weight, eating behavior, and psychological outcomes associated with a mindfulness-based intervention for people with obesity. *Complement. Ther. Med.* **2010**, *18*, 260–264. [CrossRef] [PubMed]
20. Hendrickson, K.L.; Rasmussen, E.B. Effects of mindful eating training on delay and probability discounting for food and money in obese and healthy-weight individuals. *Behav. Res. Ther.* **2013**, *51*, 399–409. [CrossRef] [PubMed]
21. Black, D.S.; Fernando, R. Mindfulness training and classroom behavior among lower-income and ethnic minority elementary school children. *J. Child Fam. Stud.* **2014**, *23*, 1242–1246. [CrossRef] [PubMed]
22. Black, D.S.; Milam, J.; Sussman, S. Sitting-meditation interventions among youth: A review of treatment efficacy. *Pediatrics* **2009**, *124*, e532–e541. [CrossRef] [PubMed]
23. Adams, C.E.; McVay, M.A.; Kinsaul, J.; Benitez, L.; Vinci, C.; Stewart, D.W.; Copeland, A.L. Unique relationships between facets of mindfulness and eating pathology among female smokers. *Eat* **2012**, *13*, 390–393. [CrossRef] [PubMed]
24. Dalen, J.; Brody, J.L.; Staples, J.K.; Sedillo, D. A conceptual framework for the expansion of behavioral interventions for youth obesity: A family-based mindful eating approach. *Child. Obes.* **2015**, *11*, 577–584. [CrossRef] [PubMed]
25. Kuczmarski, R.J.; Ogden, C.L.; Guo, S.S.; Grummer-Strawn, L.M.; Flegal, K.M.; Mei, Z.; Wei, R.; Curtin, L.R.; Roche, A.F.; Johnson, C.L. 2000 CDC growth charts for the united states: Methods and development. *Vital Health Stat.* **2002**, *11*, 1–190.
26. Framson, C.; Kristal, A.R.; Schenk, J.M.; Littman, A.J.; Zeliadt, S.; Benitez, D. Development and validation of the mindful eating questionnaire. *J. Am. Diet. Assoc.* **2009**, *109*, 1439–1444. [CrossRef] [PubMed]

27. Clark, M.M.; Abrams, D.B.; Niaura, R.S.; Eaton, C.A.; Rossi, J.S. Self-efficacy in weight management. *J. Consult. Clin. Psychol.* **1991**, *59*, 739–744. [CrossRef] [PubMed]
28. Faul, F.; Erdfelder, E.; Lang, A.-G.; Buchner, A. G*Power 3: A flexible statistical power analysis program for the social, behavioral, and biomedical sciences. *Behav. Res. Methods* **2007**, *39*, 175–191. [CrossRef] [PubMed]
29. SAS Institute Inc. *Sas/Stat User's Guide—Version 9.4*; SAS Institute: Cary, NC, USA, 2017.
30. Daly, P.; Pace, T.; Berg, J.; Menon, U.; Szalacha, L.A. A mindful eating intervention: A theory-guided randomized anti-obesity feasibility study with adolescent latino females. *Complement. Ther. Med.* **2016**, *28*, 22–28. [CrossRef] [PubMed]
31. McGovern, L.; Johnson, J.N.; Paulo, R.; Hettinger, A.; Singhal, V.; Kamath, C.; Erwin, P.J.; Montori, V.M. Clinical review: Treatment of pediatric obesity: A systematic review and meta-analysis of randomized trials. *J. Clin. Endocrinol. Metab.* **2008**, *93*, 4600–4605. [CrossRef] [PubMed]
32. Shomaker, L.B.; Bruggink, S.; Pivarunas, B.; Skoranski, A.; Foss, J.; Chaffin, E.; Dalager, S.; Annameier, S.; Quaglia, J.; Brown, K.W.; et al. Pilot randomized controlled trial of a mindfulness-based group intervention in adolescent girls at risk for type 2 diabetes with depressive symptoms. *Complement. Ther. Med.* **2017**, *32*, 66–74. [CrossRef] [PubMed]
33. Singh, N.N.; Lancioni, G.E.; Singh, A.N.; Winton, A.S.; Singh, A.D.; Singh, J. A mindfulness-based health wellness program for individuals with Prader-Willi syndrome. *J. Ment. Health Res. Intellect. Disabil.* **2011**, *4*, 90–106. [CrossRef]
34. Singh, N.N.; Lancioni, G.E.; Singh, A.N.; Winton, A.S.; Singh, J.; McAleavey, K.M.; Adkins, A.D. A mindfulness-based health wellness program for an adolescent with Prader-Willi syndrome. *Behav. Modif.* **2008**, *32*, 167–181. [CrossRef] [PubMed]
35. Singh, N.N.; Lancioni, G.E.; Singh, A.N.; Winton, A.S.; Singh, J.; McAleavey, K.M.; Adkins, A.D.; Joy, S.D. A mindfulness-based health wellness program for managing morbid obesity. *Clin. Case Stud.* **2008**, *7*, 327–339. [CrossRef]
36. Lillis, J.; Hayes, S.C.; Bunting, K.; Masuda, A. Teaching acceptance and mindfulness to improve the lives of the obese: A preliminary test of a theoretical model. *Ann. Behav. Med.* **2009**, *37*, 58–69. [CrossRef] [PubMed]
37. Force, U.S.P.S.T.; Grossman, D.C.; Bibbins-Domingo, K.; Curry, S.J.; Barry, M.J.; Davidson, K.W.; Doubeni, C.A.; Epling, J.W., Jr.; Kemper, A.R.; Krist, A.H.; et al. Screening for obesity in children and adolescents: US preventive services task force recommendation statement. *JAMA* **2017**, *317*, 2417–2426.

Permissions

All chapters in this book were first published by MDPI; hereby published with permission under the Creative Commons Attribution License or equivalent. Every chapter published in this book has been scrutinized by our experts. Their significance has been extensively debated. The topics covered herein carry significant findings which will fuel the growth of the discipline. They may even be implemented as practical applications or may be referred to as a beginning point for another development.

The contributors of this book come from diverse backgrounds, making this book a truly international effort. This book will bring forth new frontiers with its revolutionizing research information and detailed analysis of the nascent developments around the world.

We would like to thank all the contributing authors for lending their expertise to make the book truly unique. They have played a crucial role in the development of this book. Without their invaluable contributions this book wouldn't have been possible. They have made vital efforts to compile up to date information on the varied aspects of this subject to make this book a valuable addition to the collection of many professionals and students.

This book was conceptualized with the vision of imparting up-to-date information and advanced data in this field. To ensure the same, a matchless editorial board was set up. Every individual on the board went through rigorous rounds of assessment to prove their worth. After which they invested a large part of their time researching and compiling the most relevant data for our readers.

The editorial board has been involved in producing this book since its inception. They have spent rigorous hours researching and exploring the diverse topics which have resulted in the successful publishing of this book. They have passed on their knowledge of decades through this book. To expedite this challenging task, the publisher supported the team at every step. A small team of assistant editors was also appointed to further simplify the editing procedure and attain best results for the readers.

Apart from the editorial board, the designing team has also invested a significant amount of their time in understanding the subject and creating the most relevant covers. They scrutinized every image to scout for the most suitable representation of the subject and create an appropriate cover for the book.

The publishing team has been an ardent support to the editorial, designing and production team. Their endless efforts to recruit the best for this project, has resulted in the accomplishment of this book. They are a veteran in the field of academics and their pool of knowledge is as vast as their experience in printing. Their expertise and guidance has proved useful at every step. Their uncompromising quality standards have made this book an exceptional effort. Their encouragement from time to time has been an inspiration for everyone.

The publisher and the editorial board hope that this book will prove to be a valuable piece of knowledge for researchers, students, practitioners and scholars across the globe.

List of Contributors

Terry Polevoy
33-285 Sandowne Dr., Waterloo, ON N2K 2C1, Canada

Adrienne L. Adler-Neal, Abigail Cline and Travis Frantz
Center for Dermatology Research, Department of Dermatology, Wake Forest School of Medicine, Winston-Salem, NC 27101, USA

Lindsay Strowd and Sarah Taylor
Department of Dermatology, Wake Forest School of Medicine, Winston-Salem, NC 27101, USA

Steven R. Feldman
Center for Dermatology Research, Department of Dermatology, Wake Forest School of Medicine, Winston-Salem, NC 27101, USA
Department of Pathology, Wake Forest School of Medicine, Winston-Salem, NC 27101, USA
Department of Public Health Sciences, Wake Forest School of Medicine, Winston-Salem, NC 27101, USA

Dario Esposito and Arianna Belli
Child Neurology and Psychiatry Unit, Department of Human Neurosciences, Sapienza University of Rome, 00185 Rome, Italy

Raffaele Ferri
Sleep Research Centre, Oasi Research Institute–IRCCS, 94018 Troina, Italy

Oliviero Bruni
Department of Developmental and Social Psychology, Sapienza University of Rome, 00185 Rome, Italy

Andrea Stevenson Won
Department of Communication, Cornell University, 417 Mann Library Building, Ithaca, NY 14853, USA

Jakki Bailey, Jeremy Bailenson and Christine Tataru
Department of Anesthesiology and Perioperative Medicine, Stanford University, 300 Pasteur Dr. H3580A, Stanford, CA 94305, USA

Isabel A. Yoon
Department of Anesthesiology and Perioperative Medicine, Stanford University, 300 Pasteur Dr. H3580A, Stanford, CA 94305, USA
Department of Anesthesia, Stanford University School of Medicine, Stanford, CA 94305, USA

Hilary McClafferty, Audrey J. Brooks, Mei-Kuang Chen and Victoria Maizes
Department of Medicine, Arizona Center for Integrative Medicine, University of Arizona, Tucson, AZ 85724, USA

Michelle Brenner
Department of Pediatrics, Eastern Virginia Medical School/Children's Hospital of the King's Daughters, Norfolk, VA 23507, USA

Melanie Brown
Department of Pediatrics, University of Chicago Comer Children's Hospital, Chicago, IL 60637, USA

Anna Esparham and Joy Weydert
Department of Pediatrics, University of Kansas School of Medicine, Kansas City, KS 66160, USA

Dana Gerstbacher, Ann Ming Yeh and John Mark
Department of Pediatrics, Stanford University School of Medicine, Palo Alto, CA 94304, USA

Anne Herbert
Gottlieb Memorial Hospital, Loyola University Health System, 701 North Ave, Melrose Park, IL 60160, USA

Anna Esparham
Division of Integrative Medicine, University of Kansas Medical Center, 3901 Rainbow Blvd, Mailstop 1017, Kansas City, KS 66160, USA

Megan E. Voss and Mary Jo Kreitzer
Center for Spirituality and Healing, University of Minnesota, Minneapolis, MN 55455, USA

Lynn C. Waelde
Pacific Graduate School of Psychology, Palo Alto University, Palo Alto, CA 94304, USA
Department of Psychiatry and Behavioral Sciences, Stanford University School of Medicine, Stanford, CA 94305, USA

Brenda Golianu
Department of Anesthesia, Perioperative and Pain Medicine, Stanford University, Palo Alto, CA 94304, USA
Department of Anesthesiology and Perioperative Medicine, Stanford University, 300 Pasteur Dr. H3580A, Stanford, CA 94305, USA

Amanda B. Feinstein, Rashmi Bhandari and Anya Griffin
Department of Anesthesia, Stanford University School of Medicine, Stanford, CA 94305, USA

Missy Hall and Susanne M. Bifano
Child Life Department, NewYork-Presbyterian Morgan Stanley Children's Hospital Columbia University Medical Center, 3959 Broadway, New York, NY 10032, USA

Leigh Leibel
Division of Hematology/Oncology, Columbia University Medical Center, 161 Ft. Washington Ave, Suite 922, New York, NY 10032-3789, USA

Linda S. Golding
Pastoral Care, NewYork-Presbyterian Milstein Columbia University Medical Center, 622 W. 168th St., New York, NY 10032-3789, USA

Shiu-Lin Tsai
Division of Pediatric Emergency Medicine, Department of Emergency Medicine, Columbia University College of Physicians and Surgeons, 3959 Broadway, CHN-W116, NY 10032, New York

Anju Sawni
Department of Pediatrics, Hurley Children's Hospital/ Hurley Medical Center, Michigan State University College of Human Medicine, Flint, MI 48503, USA

Cora Collette Breuner
Department of Pediatrics, Adolescent Medicine Division and Department of Orthopedics and Sports Medicine, Seattle Children's Hospital, University of Washington, Seattle, WA 98105, USA

Genevieve D'Souza, Christina Almgren, Alexandra C. Ross and Amanda Marshall
Department of Anesthesia, Perioperative and Pain Medicine, Stanford University, Palo Alto, CA 94304, USA

Anava A. Wren
Department of Pediatrics, Division of Pediatric Gastroenterology, Hepatology and Nutrition, Stanford University, Palo Alto, CA 94304, USA

Claudia Calvano and Petra Warschburger
Counseling Psychology, University of Potsdam, Potsdam 14469, Germany

Martina Groß
Deutsche Morbus Crohn/Colitis ulcerosa Vereinigung (DCCV e.V.), Berlin 10179, Germany

Nicholas Chadi
Department of Pediatrics, Boston Children's Hospital, Harvard Medical School, 300 Longwood Avenue, Boston, MA 02115, USA

Elli Weisbaum
Institute of Medical Sciences, University of Toronto, 1 King's College Circle, Room 2374, Toronto, ON M5S 1A8, Canada

Catherine Malboeuf-Hurtubise
Department of Psychology, Bishop's University, 2600 College Street, Sherbrooke, QC J1M 1Z7, Canada

Sara Ahola Kohut
Department of Psychiatry, Hospital for Sick Children, University of Toronto, 555 University Avenue, Toronto, ON M5G 1X8, Canada

Christine Viner
Department of Pediatrics, Downstate Medical Center, State University of New York, 450 Clarkson Ave Brooklyn, NY 11203, USA

Miriam Kaufman
Division of Adolescent Medicine, Department of Pediatrics, Hospital for Sick Children, University of Toronto, 555 University Avenue, Toronto, ON M5G 1X8, Canada

Jake Locke
Department of Child and Adolescent Psychiatry, British Columbia Children's Hospital University of British Columbia, Vancouver, BCV6H 3N1, Canada

Dzung X. Vo
Division of Adolescent Health and Medicine, Department of Pediatrics, BC Children's Hospital, University of British Columbia, 4480 Oak St, Vancouver, BC V6H 3N1, Canada

Pamela Kaiser and Rebecca L. Kajander
National Pediatric Hypnosis Training Institute (NPHTI), 29 Western Terrace, Minneapolis, MN 55426, USA

Daniel P. Kohen
National Pediatric Hypnosis Training Institute (NPHTI), 29 Western Terrace, Minneapolis, MN 55426, USA
Partners-in-Healing, 10505 Wayzata Blvd #200, Minnetonka, MN 55305, USA
Department of Pediatrics, University of Minnesota, 717 Delaware St SE #353, Minneapolis, MN 55414, USA

Melanie L. Brown
Department of Pediatrics, University of Minnesota, 717 Delaware St SE #353, Minneapolis, MN 55414, USA
Children's Hospitals and Clinics of Minnesota, 2525 Chicago Ave, Minneapolis, MN 55404, USA

Andrew J. Barnes
National Pediatric Hypnosis Training Institute (NPHTI), 29 Western Terrace, Minneapolis, MN 55426, USA
Department of Pediatrics, University of Minnesota, 717 Delaware St SE #353, Minneapolis, MN 55414, USA

Timothy Culbert
PrairieCare Medical Group, Chaska, MN 55419, USA

Seema Kumar
Division of Pediatric Endocrinology, Department of Pediatric and Adolescent Medicine, Mayo Clinic, Rochester, MN 55905, USA

Ivana T. Croghan and Bonnie Donelan-Dunlap
Primary Care Internal Medicine, Mayo Clinic, Rochester, MN 55905, USA

Bridget K. Biggs
Department of Psychiatry and Psychology, Mayo Clinic, Rochester, MN 55905, USA

Katrina Croghan
Cancer Center, Mayo Clinic, Rochester, MN 55905, USA

Rose Prissel
Endocrinology/Nutrition, Mayo Clinic, Rochester, MN 55905, USA

Debbie Fuehrer and Amit Sood
General Internal Medicine, Mayo Clinic, Rochester, MN 55905, USA

Index